Psychosocial Nursing Assessment and Intervention

A DAVID T. MILLER BOOK

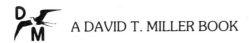

J.B. Lippincott Company   Philadelphia

London   Mexico City   New York   St. Louis   São Paulo   Sydney

Patricia D. Barry

R.N., M.S.N., C.S.

Psychiatric Liaison Clinical Specialist in Nursing
St. Francis Hospital and Medical Center
Hartford, Connecticut

Lecturer, University of Hartford Department of
Adult Education
Hartford, Connecticut

Nursing consultant in private practice

Foreword by
Barbara J. Lowery, R.N., Ed.D.

Psychosocial Nursing Assessment and Intervention

Sponsoring Editor: David T. Miller
Manuscript Editor: Elizabeth P. Lowe
Indexer: Donald Smith
Art Director: Tracy Baldwin
Production Supervisor: N. Carolyn Kerr
Production Assistant: S. M. Gassaway
Compositor: McFarland Graphics & Design, Inc.
Printer/Binder: The Murray Printing Company

*To my family and to
all nurses and their patients*

6   5   4   3

Library of Congress Cataloging in Publication Data

Barry, Patricia D.
    Psychosocial nursing assessment and intervention.

    Bibliography: p.
    Includes index.
        1. Sick—Psychology.   2. Sick—Family relationships.
3. Nursing—Psychological aspects.   I. Title. [DNLM:
1. Nursing process.   2. Nurse-patient relations.
3. Adaptation, Psychological—Nursing texts.   4. Attitude
to health.   5. Sick role. WY 100 B281p]
R726.5.B36   1984   616'.001'9   83-13586
ISBN 0-397-54392-1

The author and publisher have exerted every effort to
ensure that drug selection and dosage set forth in this text
are in accord with current recommendations and practice
at the time of publication. However, in view of ongoing
research, changes in government regulations, and the
constant flow of information relating to drug therapy and
drug reactions, the reader is urged to check the package
insert for each drug for any change in indications and
dosage and for added warnings and precautions. This is
particularly important when the recommended agent is a
new or infrequently employed drug.

Foreword

At the heart of nursing is its caring for people who hurt. Nurses have always known intuitively that people who develop physical illness suffer from more than the physical symptoms themselves. The adolescent who is badly burned worries about scars and limited range of motion, but the severe worries are that others will reject him, especially peers and loved ones. The father who has suffered a coronary clearly fears another, and death itself. But these fears are multiplied by concerns about who will take care of his family and how they will manage if he cannot work at his former pace. Interestingly, children suffering from leukemia, with all its insults to body integrity, often worry deeply about whether their parents can remain strong and hopeful as the children approach death. The sick child may be the strongest support the parents have throughout the ordeal.

Nurses know the many ways in which physical illness impacts on life. Unlike physicians, they cannot enter the patient's life for a few minutes each day and then withdraw. Regardless of the heartache involved, the nurse must have the knowledge, the skill, and often the courage to be with patients and their families for long hours each day throughout the illness. *Psychosocial Nursing Assessment and Intervention* calls our attention to the rich potential that emanates from such relationships.

Although they are acutely aware of the difficulties patients encounter, nurses often feel unprepared to respond to these problems. Occasionally nurses will say that they are too busy keeping patients alive to worry about their mental health or their family's mental health. But most realize that the alternatives are not intervention vs. no intervention but rather planned vs. unplanned intervention. Each interchange with the patient or family can impact on their response to the illness. That impact can be either positive or negative depending upon the knowledge and skill of the nurse. Given the number of interchanges involved, nurses are in a better position to provide psychosocial help than any other health-care givers.

Fortunately, nurses need no longer trust only their intuitions in dealing with the emotional problems that impact on the lives of patients and their families. There are basic principles of psychosocial assessment and intervention that they can use to foster positive adjustment.

Until now, however, the literature in nursing has not focused on these concerns. Admittedly, there are references to the broader application of mental-health principles in most basic psychiatric nursing texts. Moreover, most texts in other specialities offer some comment on the psychological concerns related to patient problems. *Psychosocial Nursing Assessment and Intervention* brings together admirably content that nurses would formerly have had to glean from a variety of sources. In addition, it synthesizes current literature from nursing, psychiatry, systems theory, and family theory and applies them to a number of different clinical contexts. Such a book has clearly been needed to serve as an adjunct text in basic medical-surgical or psychiatric nursing courses. It should also be made available as a standard resource wherever nurses are caring for patients, regardless of the clinical focus. The book is about principles and as such can be adapted to people in trouble whether they are children, adults, or the aging. In each chapter, Patricia Barry draws heavily on her mental-health background to describe nursing intervention with physically ill patients and their families. Her experience as a psychiatric liaison nurse is clearly evidenced in the clinical vignettes and her thoughtful description of the theory and practice associated with them. Because it truly integrates mental-health principles with care of the physically ill, her book sets a precedent that others are sure to follow.

The insights provided serve several purposes: 1) they offer guidelines for assessing the patient's and family's response to the illness; 2) they suggest interventions that can be fairly readily applied by most nurses; and 3) perhaps most importantly, they provide the nurse with a barometer by which he or she can judge the need for outside consultation. Fortunately, most hospitals are beginning to recognize the need for psychiatric nursing specialists to serve as consultants for both patients and staff. Mrs. Barry's book offers a clear guide about when to call for help, certainly an important first step in the utilization of these nurses.

Psychosocial Nursing Assessment and Intervention is well written, well organized, and best of all, interesting. I therefore do not hesitate to recommend it to my nursing colleagues, trusting that they will find it as valuable as I have.

Barbara J. Lowery, R.N., Ed.D.
Associate Professor of Nursing
School of Nursing
University of Pennsylvania
Philadelphia, Pennsylvania

Preface

Physical illness has been a part of human experience since time began, as has the emotional pain that accompanies it. During the rehabilitation process, the patient and his family resume their normal life styles. If adaptation to the changes brought about by the illness does not occur, the outcome can be a decreased quality of life for the individual and his family.

Increasingly, there is attention to the psychosocial aspects of illness in the curricula of the various health-care disciplines. A large body of literature has been developed on intrapsychic, family systems, and social system functioning within the fields of psychiatry and psychology. It has not been well integrated, however, in the care of the patient and members of his family who are responding to the stress of physical illness. Through research on individual and family responses to changed health status, we are becoming aware that maladaptation to physical illness leads to long-term disruption of the lives of all concerned.

In *Psychosocial Nursing Assessment and Intervention* I have used general psychiatric concepts to develop a psychosocial assessment and intervention model that can be used by nurses in the general hospital and out-patient settings. This book differs from traditional psychiatric nursing textbooks because it describes assessment and intervention techniques related to the intrapsychic and social functioning of *normal* people who are responding to the stress of physical illness.

During the past decade we have seen the advent of the integrated curriculum in nursing schools, emphasis on the nursing process in both the educational and clinical settings, primary nursing, nursing diagnoses with a strong psychosocial orientation, and a definition of nursing by the American Nurses Association that describes nursing as the diagnosis and treatment of the *human response to illness. These changes have increased the need for a psychosocial theoretical base that nurses can use to provide total care of the physically ill patient and his family.*

The material in this book has been prepared for students in basic and graduate programs in nursing. Special attention has also been given to the needs of staff nurses and directors of care who are trying to meet the needs of patients who are maladapting to physical illness.

The book includes many clinical examples of medical–surgical patients who are demonstrating specific types of responses to the stress of illness. The initial chapters in the book present general information on current psychiatric concepts and the theoretical frameworks of major theorists in the field of human psychological development.

The remainder of the book covers new areas of content not usually addressed in nursing textbooks, including the following chapter topics:

1. The identification of adaptive and maladaptive uses of defense mechanisms (Chapter 4)
2. The recognition of particular personality styles in general hospital patients and an explanation of the underlying dynamics, as well as recommended nursing approaches that can reduce the patient's level of anxiety (Chapter 5)
3. An analysis of the major causes of maladaptation by patients with physical illness (Chapter 6)
4. A review of general and family systems dynamics that can promote or undermine an individual and his family's adaptation (Chapters 7 and 8)
5. Theories pertaining to psychosocial responses to stress, including the following:
   a. A clarification of the coping process
   b. The psychosocial mediation of stressful events
   c. The psychobiology of stress mediation
   d. The effect of stress on the development of physical illness (Chapter 9)
6. Extensive information on organic brain syndrome and its many etiologies (Chapter 11)
7. An indepth discussion of counseling techniques for nurses (Chapter 12)
8. A tool for psychosocial assessment and a conceptual model for evaluation of psychosocial maladaptation (Chapters 13 and 14)
9. Crisis intervention with the patient or family member who is at risk or is maladapting to physical illness (Chapter 15)
10. Recommended nursing interventions with patients who are presenting challenges to nurses because of maladaptation, for example the patient with excessive depression, anxiety, anger, sexual acting-out, noncompliance, and so on (Chapter 16)
11. Assessment and intervention approaches to patients with specific conditions, such as infertility, birth anomalies, hysterectomy and menopause, and disfiguring conditions such as amputation, ostomies, and burns (Chapter 17)
12. Recommendations for promoting adaptation in all patients with chronic illness. In addition, there are subsections on coronary artery disease (medically and surgically treated), cancer, chronic obstructive pulmonary disease (COPD), stroke, and spinal cord injuries (Chapter 18)
13. Assessment and intervention recommendations about working with the dying patient and the family with an extensive review of the normal grief process and maladapative grief (Chapter 19)
14. Recommendations to promote the nurse's own self-understanding and acceptance in the nursing care of the dying patient (Chapter 20)
15. Ways to promote the nurse's well-being and ability to work in a stressful health-care environment (Chapter 21)

Patricia D. Barry, R.N., M.S.N., C.S.

Acknowledgments

Psychosocial Nursing Assessment and Intervention is the result of my long-held hope of being able to contribute to an improved quality of life for individuals who are coping with physical illness and their families. Dianne Schilke Davis, Donna Diers, Barbara Gallo, and Dorothy Sexton played supportive roles as I began to think about undertaking this project.

When the manuscript was developing, I asked five readers to critique the content. Their encouraging comments helped to keep me on target. They are Mona Branchini, a baccalaureate nursing student; Holly Burnes, a psychiatric liaison clinical nurse-specialist; Jackie Dowling, a graduate student in pediatric oncology; Mary Nemeth, a nurse in an out-patient setting; and Dr. Robert Woodhouse, a psychiatrist in private practice. I am deeply indebted to them for their commitment, perceptivity, and support during the many months of the manuscript preparation.

In addition, several other persons read chapters that were related to their areas of clinical expertise. They are Dianne Davis, Chapter 9; Pat Duclos, Chapters 1, 12, and 13; Trish Helm and Mary Scully, Chapters 7 and 8; Marilyn Prouty, Chapter 21; Drs. Peter DeBell and Jonathan Pincus, Chapter 11; and Dr. Austin McCawley, Chapters 5 and 11. Their assistance in clarifying these chapters was helpful.

I am grateful also for the assistance of Mona Branchini in compiling the glossary. The library staff at St. Francis Hospital and Medical Center were exemplary in their conscientious assistance. Pam Jaiko and Caroline Wilcox were always available, it seemed, when an elusive subject needed to be obtained. I must say a word of thanks also for the availability of the splendid medical library at the University of Connecticut Medical School in Farmington, whose facilities have been a pleasure for me to use over the years.

My conversations and correspondence with David Miller, Vice President and Editor, Nursing Department, J.B. Lippincott Company, helped to provide extra structure and substance, as well as ongoing momentum for the developing manuscript. His quick thinking and positive manner were never-failing.

I have deep admiration and gratitude to Pat Gatzen who so professionally deciphered my original handwritten drafts and returned them to me in beautiful form. Her positive encouragement about the content during the year and a half we worked together was heartwarming.

Finally, I must thank the nurses I have worked with over the years whose eagerness to know more about the psychosocial aspects of physical illness gave me the impetus to write this book. I hope they will find it meaningful.

The clinical examples in this book are all based on actual cases. However, names, ages, sex, and other distinguishing characteristics have been changed in order to protect the privacy of the patients and their families.

Part One
**A Theoretical Base for Psychosocial
Nursing Assessment** 1

1 **Characteristics of Psychosocial
Nursing Assessment** 3
Liaison Psychiatry 3
Intuitive Characteristics of Nurses 4
The Importance of Speaking a Professional
Language 5
The Differences in the Medical vs. the
Nursing View of the Patient 6
The Nurse as Patient Advocate 7
What is Adaptation? 7
Psychosocial Assessment Factors 10
Conclusion 13

2 **The Building Blocks of Personality** 15
Drive Theory 15
Affect 16
Object Relations 17
The Id, the Ego, and the Superego 17
The Conscious, the Preconscious, and the
Unconscious 19
Bonding 19
Inborn Personality Characteristics 21
Conclusion 22

3 **Major Theories of Personality
Development** 23
Mahler: The First Two Years of Life 23
Piaget: The Cognitive Stages of
Development 25
Skinner: Operant Conditioning 26
Freud: Psychosexual Stages of
Development 28
Erikson: Psychosocial Stages of
Development 30
Maslow: Hierarchy of Human Needs 31
Conclusion 32

4 **The Use of Defense Mechanisms in
Physical Illness** 33
The Importance of Recognizing Patients'
Use of Defense Mechanisms 34
Is There a Difference Between Coping and
Defense Mechanisms? 35
Development of Defense Mechanisms 35
Levels of Defense Mechanisms 36
Narcissistic Defense Mechanisms 37

Contents

Immature Defense Mechanisms   38
Neurotic Defense Mechanisms   41
Mature Defense Mechanisms   44
*Conversion: An Unclassified Defense
    Mechanism   45*
Conclusion   47

**5   Personality Styles Seen in General
      Hospital Patients**   49
State vs. Trait Characteristics   50
Major Personality Styles   50
The Dependent, Demanding Patient   50
The Controlled, Orderly Patient   51
The Dramatizing, Emotionally Involved,
    Captivating Patient   52
The Suspicious, Complaining Patient   53
The Long-Suffering, Self-Sacrificing
    Patient   54
The Patient With Superiority Feelings   55
The Uninvolved, Aloof Patient   55
The Antisocial Patient   56
The Inadequate Patient   57
Conclusion   58

**6   Major Psychosocial Issues of Patients
      With Physical Illness**   59
Major Developmental Issues   60
Trust   60
Self-esteem   61
Control   66
Loss   68
Guilt   70
Intimacy   72
Conclusion   73

**7   General Systems Theory in Clinical
      Practice**   75
What Is a System?   75
Types of Systems   76
General Systems Theory   77
Conclusion   80

8   The Family as a System   81
Family Systems Terminology   82
Differentiation of Self   82
What is the Self?   83
The Levels of Self-Differentiation   83
*Other Concepts of Family Systems
    Theory   85*
Conclusion   93

**9   Stress: Its Implications in Physical
      Illness**   95
Part One:
Specific Subsystem Responses to
Stress   96
Physiological Stress   96
*Psychological Stress and the Coping
    Process   96*
Social Stress   99
Part Two:
Psychosocial Mediation of Stressful
Events   99
Adaptation to a Major Life Event   99
Types of Responses to Stress   101
Part Three:
Biopsychosocial Mediation of Stressful
Events   102
*The Psychobiology of Stress Mediation: The
    Mind-Body Bridge   102*
*Historical Development of a Systems
    Approach to Stress   103*
*Effect of Stress on the Development of
    Physical Illness   104*
*A Comprehensive Model for Evaluating
    Stress   105*
Conclusion   105

10   The Mental Status Examination   107
*The Difference Between the Symptoms of
    Functional and Organic Psychiatric
    Disorders   108*
*The Importance of Mental Status
    Observation   108*
*The Categories of Mental Status
    Evaluation   110*
Conclusion   116

11   Organic Brain Syndrome   119
*Importance of Nurses as Observers of Early
    Symptoms of Acute Organic Brain
    Syndrome   119*
*The Difference Between the Etiologies of
    Functional Psychiatric Disorder and
    Organic Brain Syndrome   120*
Types of Organic Brain Syndrome   120
Causes of Organic Brain Syndrome   122

*Categories of Organic Brain
  Syndrome   123*
*Prevalent Types of Organic Brain
  Syndrome   133*
Conclusion   138

**12   Counseling Techniques for
       Nurses**   *139*
*Which Patients Are Appropriate for Nursing
  Intervention?   140*
Empathy vs. Sympathy   140
*The Difference Between Informal and
  Formal Counseling Relationships   141*
The Patient's Readiness for Help   141
*Important Personal Qualities of a
  Counselor   141*
*A Counseling Deterrent: "Professional
  Distancing"   142*
*The Nurse's Attitude Toward
  Counseling   142*
The Meaning of Support   142
The Importance of Assessment   143
Content and Process   144
*Specific Characteristics of the
  Relationship   144*
*Underlying Dynamics of the
  Relationship   144*
Different Types of Relationships   146
*Attending Behaviors in the Nurse
  Counselor   147*
Leading Skills   148
*Other Characteristics of the
  Relationship   150*
Support Groups   151
Conclusion   154

Part Two
**Application of Psychosocial Nursing
Theory to the Nursing Process**   *155*
The Nursing Process   155

**13   Psychosocial Nursing Assessment and
       Diagnosis**   *157*
*Justification for Importance of Psychosocial
  Nursing Assessment   158*
*The Psychosocial Nursing Assessment
  Interview   158*
*Psychosocial Nursing Assessment
  Process   159*

*Rationale for Psychosocial Assessment
  Categories   159*
*Nursing Diagnosis of Psychosocial
  Maladaptation   170*
*Documentation of the Psychosocial Nursing
  Process   172*
Conclusion   172

**14   A Model for Psychosocial Nursing
       Process**   *175*
*Is It Realistic to Teach a Patient New
  Coping Skills?   176*
*Psychosocial Intervention With General
  Hospital Patients   176*
The Nurse as a Change Agent   177
*A Model for Promotion of Psychosocial
  Adaptation   177*
*Conceptual Approach to Psychosocial
  Nursing Intervention   178*
Conclusion   180

**15   Crisis Intervention With the
       Maladapting Patient**   *183*
Coping Ability in a Crisis   184
Critical Time for Crisis Resolution   186
Nursing Process in Crisis Intervention   187
*When Nursing Crisis Intervention Is Not
  Enough   190*
Potential for Crisis   191
Conclusion   196

**16   Nursing Intervention With the
       Emotionally Complex Patient**   *197*
The Anxious Patient   198
The Depressed Patient   201
The Suicidal Patient   203
The Unmotivated Patient   205
The Alcoholic Patient   206
*The Patient With Sexual Dysfunction as the
  Result of Physical Illness   208*
*The Demanding or Noncompliant
  Patient   211*
The Medication-Dependent Patient   214
The Organic Brain Syndrome Patient   215
Sensory Disturbances   217
Conclusion   218

17 Psychosocial Aspects of Specific Physical Conditions 219

Infertility 219
Exceptional Child or Child With Congenital Anomalies 221
Hysterectomy and Menopause 223
Disfiguring Conditions 228
Isolation for Communicable Diseases and Immunosuppressive Conditions 235
Conclusion 237

18 The Coping Challenge of Chronic Illness 239

Major Effects of Chronic Illness on Psychosocial Stress of Patients, Families, and Nurses 239
The Patient With Cancer 241
The Patient With Coronary Artery Disease 244
The Stroke Patient (Cerebral Vascular Accident) 247
The Patient With Chronic Obstructive Pulmonary Disease 249
The Patient With a Spinal Cord Injury 250
Conclusion 252

19 The Dying Patient and the Family 255

What Does Death Mean to a Dying Person? 256
Fears of the Dying 256
The Process of Resolution of Loss 257
The Effect of the Social Environment on the Grieving Person 260
The Normal Emotional Response to Loss 260

Anniversary Reaction 262
Maladaptive Grieving Process 263
The Consequences of Unresolved Grief for Family Members 263
Nursing Diagnosis of Maladaptive Coping in Family Members 264
Conclusion 265

20 The Nurse and the Dying Patient 267

Specific Issues of Caring for Dying Patients 267
Reasonable Limits of the Nurse's Emotional Involvement With the Dying Patient 276
Conclusion 278

Part Three
Adaptation to Nursing 279

21 Stress in Nursing Practice 281

Stress: What's It All About? 281
Can We Change the Way We Respond to Stress? 281
Basic Principles of Stress That Relate to Nursing 282
Professional Stress in Nursing 287
Changing the Climate in Hospitals 289
Conclusion 292

Appendix 293

Glossary 325

Bibliography 335

Index 347

The first part of this book includes theoretical perspectives that can form the base on which you develop the nursing process of assessment and diagnosis, planning the intervention, intervening, and evaluating the intervention. This section will include material perhaps already familiar to you from introductory courses in psychology as well as many new concepts that have not been generally available to nurses. These concepts are integrated with recent theory that has been developed to provide you with a deeper understanding of the psychosocial responses of human beings to the stress of illness.

This section is designed to present the normal to abnormal range of psychosocial reactions you will observe in patients and family members who are responding to physical illness. Theories about the cause, effect, and signs of psychosocial maladaptation are emphasized.

Part One

A Theoretical Base for Psychosocial Nursing Assessment

Psychological functioning is abstract; it covers a vast array of processes that are essential for normal human development. These functions operate in human beings at all times. They are so essential that, without them, adult human beings would still be lying in cribs. It is psychological functioning that determines motivation, motor ability, intellectual development, perception, speech, decision-making ability, and many other characteristics that are the basis of full human functioning (Small, 1979). (A fuller explanation of these functions is included in Chap. 2.) Depending on a person's physical and mental health, these functions will work to promote well-being. If the person is under physical or emotional stress or has a longstanding psychological problem, then one or more of these functions may not work properly and may cause distress for the patient as well as for those around him.

All patients in a hospital setting experience increased physical stress. All, except those who are unconscious (and this can be debated), are under increased mental stress because of concern about their physical well-being. Finally, all patients enter the hospital with unique personalities. With the stress of illness, certain unhealthy personality characteristics that were acquired during the patient's development may surface. They can undermine his ability to adapt to the hospital environment and to the changes brought about by his illness. Psychosocial maladaptation can occur and become permanent.

In this book, psychosocial maladaptation to physical illness is differentiated from psychiatric illness. Psychosocial maladaptation will be addressed here as an outcome of illness that causes temporary or permanent changes in a person's normal personality functioning, his relationships with others, and his normal roles within his family and social groups. Although he and his family may experience chronic emotional stress and a decrease in the quality of normal social functioning, these changes are not severe enough to be classified as functional psychiatric illness. It is important to point out, however, that if psychosocial maladaptation is marked—if, for example, a person has a severe depressive reaction to a change in health status—functional psychiatric illness can result.

Liaison Psychiatry

Awareness of the strong effects of stress on all persons with physical illness is increasingly being

1

Characteristics of Psychosocial Nursing Assessment

recognized by nurses and by patients themselves. A new clinical science has emerged that concentrates on understanding the emotional dynamics of the person with physical illness. It is called *liaison psychiatry* (Hackett, 1978; Robinson, 1974). The word *liaison*, which is taken directly from the French, is the key to understanding the main function of liaison psychiatry. Liaison is defined as intercommunication for the purpose of mutual understanding. In the hospital a clinician trained in this theory works with the patient and all caregivers. He or she explains the behavior of the patient and, if necessary, the family to the caregivers in order to ease the adaptation process for everyone. In turn, the patient and family may need assistance in understanding the hospital care system. Liaison psychiatry borrows heavily from the theory of general psychiatry and combines it with theory gained in observing the stages or processes that normal persons experience in their emotional and physical adaptation to major surgery, chronic illness, or anticipated death.

The Response of the Family to Illness

This theory also pertains to the reactions of families when they have an ill member. The importance of examining the responses of family members can be understood if you recall, for example, the reaction of your mother when you were a child and had a bad bruise. Most likely you received love and understanding and felt better as a result. You can probably still remember the effect her concern had on you. If you did not receive love, you can remember that effect also.

When a person becomes ill, the response of the patient and *each* of the family members will be different. The response of one will affect the responses of the others. If a child is ill, for example, the mother will respond to her child based on what the child's illness means to her and the way that the child responds to the illness. The father, in turn, will respond based on his perceptions of the child's illness and his own normal personality and coping style. Remember, too, the child's illness introduces a whole new dynamic in the mother-father relationship, and this new stress can affect the parents' ability to support the child and each other. To complicate the picture further, the emotional responses of these three family members are never static. New dynamics enter and can cause daily changes in the way family members react to one another and to illness.

Does this all sound very complex? When we begin to examine these aspects of a patient's care, they may initially seem so. Without a theoretical approach that separates and looks at the components involved in the psychosocial functioning of patients, these ideas can seem very confusing. Lacking the ability to perform *reliable* psychosocial assessment, we may seriously undermine the rehabilitative potential of many patients.

Monitoring the Psychosocial Response of the Patient to Illness

It may surprise you to realize that nurses may be in the best position of any member of the caregiving team to monitor and evaluate the patient's and family's psychosocial response to illness. They spend more time with the patient than any other member of the health care team. Accordingly, they have the best opportunity to observe the patient's response to his illness. They also can see the patient interact with his family, friends, and other members of the health care team. If psychosocial problems develop, they are most frequently observed by the nurse (Robinson, 1974; Schwab, 1968).

Nurses are usually viewed by patients as nurturing, supportive people. Patients frequently are able to talk about their feelings with their nurses *if* their nurses are aware of these feelings and are able to accept them. When nurses are aware of emotional disruption in their patients, they have the opportunity to alert the patients' physicians to the problem.

Intuitive Characteristics of Nurses

Women make up 97% of the total membership of nursing (Greenleaf, 1978). The personality characteristics normally applied to women are also used to describe the characteristics of nurses. One of these characteristics is *intuition*. Intuition is the ability to gain knowledge without using conscious reasoning. The intuitive ability of women has been recognized for a long time by other women but has not generally been validated. The reason for this may be that observations based on intuition usually lack a series of logical, deductive steps. Accordingly, persons who arrive at intuitive judgments may not be able to explain or articulate their reasoning. Women may understand, intuitively, the statements of other women. Frequently no rationale is necessary for them to agree on the same conclusion.

To illustrate this point, think about the way in which nurses communicate with one another about patient care or related issues in nursing reports at changes of shifts. Their communication frequently consists of a few spoken words and hand and facial gestures. Look around at the other nurses present and see the nods of understanding. If a male physician were present and were asked after the report to describe the conditions of patients based on what he learned in the report, he would have a difficult time doing so. He has been socialized in a different way. His scientific training has not prepared him to be receptive to an intuitive type of communication. He does not know how to speak this type of nursing language. Male nurses who enter the profession gradually become socialized into a type of communication that relies heavily on nonverbal and intuitive exchange of information.

A woman psychoanalyst, Jean Baker Miller (1975), has written about the development of women's intuition, which she calls "mysterious gifts that are in fact skills, developed through long practice, in reading many small signals, both verbal and nonverbal."

It is important to recognize and to value this intuitive ability. As a nurse, you will frequently observe signs in patients that are clues that the patient is not coping well with his illness. It could be the way a patient sighs, stares blankly out the window, lacks motivation to eat, or interacts with his family in a strained way.

The Importance of Speaking a Professional Language

In relaying your concerns, which are good nursing observations, it is essential that you speak a language that physicians can understand.

Nurses develop a combination of nonverbal and verbal communication skills as part of their professional language. This language works when they communicate with each other. It does *not* serve nurses or their patients well when they communicate their observations to physicians or other members of the health care team in this manner. The physician may disregard the nurse's

concerns if he or she presents them in this way. For example:

Dr. Atwood, I'm worried about Mrs. Flaherty.

Remember that the nonpsychiatric physician is trained to be aware of bodily processes, not emotional ones. On hearing the nurse's concern, he will mentally expect to hear a physical symptom as the clue to Mrs. Flaherty's problem.

Yes, Miss Weber, what seems to be the problem?

Dr. Atwood, she doesn't look right. She seems sort of out of it, like she's given up trying. Do you know what I mean? She's been different the last few days.

The physician is now left to decide what this statement means. If he asked the nurse to explain further, she might persist and say, "I don't know, she just isn't the same as she was at first." Because of the nurse's use of slang and lack of description of behavioral signs, the physician may not take her observation seriously.

Instead, consider the following comments by the nurse:

Dr. Atwood, I'm concerned about Mrs. Flaherty. She appears depressed. When she was admitted she was pleasant and friendly. She had many visitors and talked with other patients. She has been here for 5 days now. She is not eating well. It is hard to rouse her in the morning. She stays in her room and says that she wants to be alone. She stares out of the window much of the day, and several of us have seen her crying. She refuses to talk to us about her concerns. She has a hard time falling asleep at night, although we give her medication. She awakens two or three times a night. Her husband told us that she is not acting like her usual self.

Although the nurse in the first example was using all the behavioral clues described in the second example as part of her nursing assessment process, she did not realize the importance of articulating them in a professional language to the physician. It is surprising how often this happens in hospitals. It may be one of the reasons why the nursing profession does not receive more respect from the medical profession.

It is essential that you discipline yourself to speak in complete sentences, avoid using slang, and state *all* the behavioral clues you have observed rather than using one or two general adjectives to explain why you think a patient is experiencing psychological distress. When we sound as if we know what we're talking about, people *will* listen to us.

The use of categories and defining characteristics from the St. Louis classification nursing diagnosis conference groups is recommended to describe the psychosocial maladaptation clues you see (see Chap. 13: Psychosocial Nursing Assessment and Diagnosis). Nurses who use these terms when describing their observations have informally reported that physicians understand and respect their opinions; they are usually open to nursing recommendations for medical assistance to reverse the maladaptation process. The same is true for nursing recommendations given to other hospital caregivers, such as social workers and physical therapists.

The Differences in the Medical vs. the Nursing View of the Patient

Nurses in hospitals occasionally become angry that physicians are not more aware of emotional distress in their patients. Frequently, nurses complain that doctors are insensitive to their patients' emotional needs; they seem unaware of the effect that a catastrophic or chronic illness can have on a person and the members of his family.

The following explanation may help you to understand some of the reasons why this is so. Physicians have been charged with the responsibility of keeping people alive. As a result, they closely monitor all physiological responses of the patient and work to bring these responses within normal limits.

At times, in order to save the patient's life, efforts to cure the patient physically cause the patient psychological distress. For example, if a patient has cancer of the head or neck, surgery may cure the cancer but the psychosocial consequences of that surgery may cause the patient to wish he were dead. The same may be true for a severely burned patient facing a long hospitalization and permanent disfiguration or a leukemic adolescent forced to live in a germ-free hospital environment.

Because physicians are caring people, it can be distressing for them to be aware of the emotional hardships that their "cures" may impose on patients. If physicians were fully aware of the emotional hardships that they impose on some of their patients in order to keep them alive, they probably could not continue being physicians. Instead, a form of denial occurs. The mechanism of denial is an unconscious protection that the mind develops so that physicians can continue their work. It pushes from their minds the awareness of the sometimes awful consequences of their treatment. This is not necessarily bad. If it did not happen, a physician could spend an evening in tears as, for example, he remembered the look in the eyes of the young woman on whom he had performed a bilateral mastectomy the day before. We nurses may feel badly about the young woman described above, but at least we know we didn't cause her pain. Instead, we can care for her physically and support her emotionally.

Obviously, physicians have varying degrees of denial about their patients' emotional problems, but it is important to remember that, within reasonable limits, this is a healthy defense for physicians. When nurses are aware of this, they can then recognize their own importance to both the physician and the patient in monitoring the patient's response to illness. Another important point to remember is that the physician may spend only a few minutes a day with the patient, compared to the several hours a day that a nurse spends with the patient. An additional reason why the physician may not observe developing problems is because of the patient's attitude toward his physician. In the United States, physicians still are one of the most admired professional groups. The doctor is a very important authority figure for all persons. Most patients are very eager to please their physicians and try to be on their best behavior when talking with them.

When a person is hospitalized, he usually feels very dependent on his doctor; indeed, his *life* is in the physician's hands. The patient reasons that if he displeases his physician, the physician may lose interest or even retaliate and not give him the best care possible. Even worse, he or she may abandon the patient by turning him over to another physician. It therefore becomes vital to the patient to withhold all unessential, unpleasant information. If the patient is feeling worried, depressed, or angry or is having trouble talking with his family about his illness, he will usually not tell his physician. Patients usually do not have the same unconscious fear about being abandoned by nurses and find it easier to confide their fears to them. Another factor in the patient's choice to confide in the nurse is that he or she is available for longer periods and more consistently than the physician.

A clinically observant and objective nurse who knows how to assess a patient's adaptation to physical illness can promote the patient's ability to regain his previous level of psychic and physical functioning. Remember that living with the results of disfiguring surgery or chronic illness can seriously impair, *sometimes permanently,* a person's ability to enjoy life. It can also detrimentally affect the lives of family members for months and years.

When we care for patients in an acute care setting, it is possible for them to be unaware of the long-term (postdischarge) consequences of illness. The effects of illness can have an impact on *all* aspects of a patient's functioning: physiological; intrapsychic; interpersonal, including intrafamilial and the general social environment; and economic well-being.

The Nurse as Patient Advocate

Because of the reasons explained above, the nurse may also be in the best position to be the patient's advocate. Patient advocacy is a catchword of the consumer protection era of the 1970s. Hospitals are now required to employ persons as patient advocates in order to safeguard patients' rights and well-being and speak out on their behalf. The advocacy role, however, continues to be unofficially carried out by nurses on behalf of their patients.

Nurses are able to monitor the response of the health care system to patients' needs. They are also able to monitor patients' responses to the health care system's interventions. Accordingly, the nurse should be able to identify those patients who are at risk for maladaptation and mobilize the health care system's resources to assist such patients in the adaptation process. If nurses do not identify those patients who are at risk for long-term psychosocial maladaptation, then who else will?

What Is Adaptation?

Adaptation is the process of adjusting to change. The term *adaptation* implies that a person has accommodated and adjusted to a changed set of internal or external conditions in his life. Whenever change occurs, however, the adjustments may not be positive ones. For example, a newly diagnosed young woman with diabetes may become sullen and withdrawn. This response to change, if it becomes permanent, is maladaptive.

For ease of explanation, *adaptation* will be used here to describe positive adjustment to change; that is, after the event is over, the person's quality of life returns to normal or improves. *Maladaptation,* on the other hand, is the development after a major change of long-term or permanent negative characteristics that have a harmful effect on the patient's physical, emotional, or social spheres.

The most important factor in successful adaptation is the ability of the person to cope. Coping is a combination of conscious and unconscious mental maneuvers that are used to maintain emotional stability (Weisman, 1978). (These will be explained in more detail in Chaps. 4 and 9.) Some people are emotionally stronger than others. The difference between those who are identified as emotionally strong and those who are called emotionally weak is actually the difference in the way that they cope with new situations.

For example, a newly admitted patient who will undergo open-heart surgery is faced with a very stressful situation. His ability to cope with the surgery and convalescence will be largely determined by his previous experiences and the way he normally copes with stress. In the past, if he has folded easily under pressure, he will be more at risk for maladaptation than someone who has coped well with a variety of difficult situations during previous years.

Roy (1976) has identified four modes of adaptation that challenge the human being: physiological, self-concept, role function, and interdependence. If failure to adapt occurs in any or all of these modes, then the person is not functioning at his former level. His functioning can be compared to a four-cylinder car that is trying to operate on three cylinders. The entire engine is working harder than normal, yet its ability and power are lessened.

In order to simplify the forms of adaptation, consider that there are only *two* areas in which a person must adjust if he is to maintain his normal level of functioning: the physiological, which includes his physical response to change, and the psychosocial, which is the way his psyche reacts and the way in which he interacts with other people and the environment. Actually, these two aspects of psychosocial functioning are interrelated.

The Physiological Mode of Adaptation

The physiological mode of adaptation may initially sound as if it were separate from the emotional domain of the patient. It is not. The emotions and physical processes of the body interact and are inseparable (Engel, 1962).

This essential fact is frequently overlooked by the sciences of medicine and nursing. As a result, the patient's disease process is often evaluated with only physical examination data. In some instances, psychological factors can be the presenting symptoms of an undiagnosed physical problem, as in the case of thyroid disease, for example (Martin, 1979). The psychosocial realm is usually considered by clinicians only when the patient maladapts psychologically *after* illness occurs. In a large majority of cases, this approach is like putting the cart before the horse. *Instead, it may be the patient's physiological response to emotional stress that actually causes a physical disease process to occur* (Holmes and Rahe, 1967). Unless a diagnostician includes an evaluation of the current intrapsychic and social stressors in the patient's life, diagnosis of the actual root cause of the physical problem may be overlooked. The implications of stress and its role in the development of physical illness will be discussed in detail in Chapter 9.

The physiological mode is regulated partially by the *autonomic nervous system* (Snyder, 1980). The autonomic nervous system controls involuntary bodily functions, which include the following major organs: the eyes, salivary glands, blood vessels, lungs, heart, gastrointestinal tract, liver, gall bladder, pancreas, adrenal glands, sweat glands, kidneys, bladder, and internal and external genitalia. The autonomic nervous system is subdivided into the sympathetic and parasympathetic divisions. Both divisions fall under the influence of the hypothalamus gland. The pituitary gland, which is called the master gland of the body, is actually controlled by the hypothalamus. The hypothalamus is a tiny anatomical structure located deep within the limbic system. The limbic system is the seat of emotions in human beings (Arthur, 1979). It is possible that the hypothalamus is the "missing link" between the emotional and physical domains in the human being.

To help understand the significance of the effect of emotions on the body, think for a moment of your body's response when you almost have a serious accident; your heart beats rapidly, blood pressure rises, pupils dilate, mouth feels dry, gastrointestinal activity slows down, and bronchial tubes dilate to allow more oxygen to enter the lungs. It is the emotion of fear that causes the sympathetic nervous system to activate the various physiological responses in the body. Once the fear has subsided, the parasympathetic system takes over again and all organ systems return to their normal level of functioning.

Research into the relationship between stress and disease development is ongoing. Many surprising results are being found that prove the existence of a far greater association between the physiological and the psychological subsystems of human beings than had previously been known (Hurst and colleagues, 1979).

The Concept of Unitary Man: A Holistic Approach to Physical Illness

Nursing, in its approach to physical illness, has integrated the physiological and behavioral responses to illness. The concept of *unitary man* was proposed by Rogers in 1970. Rogers states that the human being is an open system consisting of many elements or subsystems. (In case the term system is unfamiliar to some readers, Chap. 7, General Systems Theory in Clinical Practice, will help to explain the concept of a system.) Essentially, systems theory teaches that all the subsystems of a human being—gastrointestinal, cardiovascular, genitourinary, and so on—are constantly interacting with his or her intrapsychic subsystem, social system, and the environment or ecological system. This is an ongoing, dynamic process.

Rogers' concept of unitary man has been synthesized here to form the basis for holistic nursing assessment and nursing diagnosis (see the chart on p. 9).

The holistic health care movement began to grow in the early 1970s. The term *holistic health care* involves the concept of many different aspects of wellness: "the integration of mind and body, the importance of the family and other social support systems, and a conception of health as more than the absence of disease" (Gillette, 1980). Its philosophy is to promote the concept of healing body, mind, and spirit rather than healing the body alone. Care of the total person is emphasized. A preventive approach to optimal health is administered by holistically oriented physicians, nurse specialists, clergy, and counselors (Gillette, 1980; Van Vorst and Root, 1980). This approach to health care has been strongly advocated by the

Characteristics of Unitary Man: Framework for Classification of Nursing Diagnosis (1980)

Factor I: Interaction

Exchanging—interchange of matter and energy between man and environment
    Assessment factors: eating, drinking, eliminating, breathing, giving-receiving, approval, advice

Communicating—interchange of information between man and environment
    Assessment factors: verbal, nonverbal

Relating—connecting with other persons or objects
    Assessment factors: spacing, touching, eye contact, belonging, referencing

Factor II: Action

Valuing—the assigning of worth
    Assessment factors: philosophical beliefs regarding health, spirituality, human interaction
    Empirical indicators: locus of control; health goals and priorities; meaning of life and immortality; religious practices and beliefs

Choosing—the selection of one or more alternatives
    Assessment factors: judgment-decision capacity regarding alternatives, consequences, commitments
    Empirical indicators: health choices and practices; perceived alternatives; perceived consequences; congruence of choice and value/belief patterns

Moving—activity within the environment
    Assessment factors: mobility rhythm/patterns (spatial, temporal, frequency of exercise and activity)
    Empirical indicators: locomotion characteristics (type, frequency, balance, equilibrium); control of intentional movement; joint flexibility; goal-directed movement (ADL, self-care practices); activity tolerance

Factor III: Awareness

Waking refers to levels of arousal
    Assessment factors: position and movement, verbal expression
    Empirical indicators: REM time, alterations in moving, alterations in speech

Feeling refers to quality of sensation and mood
    Assessment factors: position and movement, verbal expression
    Empirical indicators: alterations in intake; alteration in movement (such as smiling, wringing of hands), alteration in mood (such as repetitive speech, laughing, crying)

Knowing refers to meaning associated with a world view
    Assessment factors: position and movement, verbal expression
    Empirical indicators: wrinkled brow, puzzled look, participation in planned regime, frequent questioning about phenomenon, personal verification ("I don't know what's happening" or "I do know"), reports time, place, and person, for example, reports limited information, reports inaccurate information

(Roy C: Historical perspective of the theoretical framework for the classification of nursing diagnosis [1980]. In Kim M, Moritz D [eds]: Classification of Nursing Diagnosis: Proceedings of the Third and Fourth National Conferences, pp. 244–245. New York, McGraw-Hill, 1982)

nursing profession, since it embodies most of the ideals of nursing (Zbilut, 1980). Roy (1982) states that "nurses were probably among the first health care professionals to look at the patient holistically" (p. 241).

A Case Example

The process of adaptation involves the interaction of both the patient's mind and body. In order to understand this process more fully, a clinical example is presented and discussed below. Some terms used in the case example may be unfamiliar to you; they will be explained in the following chapters.

> Tom, a 17-year-old high school junior, is a first-string football player and was recently named to his state's all-star football team. He has above-average intelligence. He comes from a lower-middle-class family in which there are five children. He is the oldest child. His life aspirations include attending college on a football scholarship and becoming a civil engineer. One week ago he experienced some disturbing symptoms in his left leg. After being examined by his physician, he was admitted to the hospital, where a malignant tumor of the tibia was diagnosed. In order to save his life, his leg was amputated.

His life may indeed by saved by the surgery. The surgical wound should heal rapidly because of his age. If, however, he reacts to this surgery with prolonged anger, resentment, or depression, it is possible that his physiological well-being could be affected. Can you remember the effects strong anger have on you? When a person is very angry, his body responds the same way it does to extreme fear. Think of the detrimental effect these strong emotions could have on the vital signs of blood pressure, pulse, and respiration if they persisted for a long time. In Tom's case, his physiological integrity could be seriously undermined. It has also been discovered that prolonged sadness about the loss of something valuable can depress the immunological system of the body (Bartrop and colleagues, 1977); the body's resistance to infection can thus be lowered.

Because of the various mind-body interactions in this case, the young man could be more prone to postoperative complications if he experiences strong and prolonged negative emotion of *any* type. Awareness of the impact of the emotions on the autonomic nervous system is critical in evaluating the patient's adaptation in the physiological mode. Perhaps this case example can teach us just how difficult it is to separate the psychosocial and physiological realms.

Psychosocial Adaptation to the Stress of Physical Illness

The psychosocial adaptation process is the more complex and less understood of the two modes of adaptation. The intrapsychic aspect of this mode is abstract and can only be observed behaviorally. It is a process that is different in every human being. No two human beings *ever* respond emotionally in the same way to the same event. This is in contrast to physiological adaptation, which is objectively observable and more predictable.

The complexities of personality development and the resulting intrapsychic dynamics in the human mind result in an infinite number of possible responses. This differs from a purely physical response, such as the body's reaction to an inflamed appendix. The physiological response consists of the classic symptoms of appendicitis; increased white blood cell count, abdominal tenderness, and so on. The body reacts the *same* way in the majority of persons.

Psychosocial adaptation to the stress of illness imposes many new stressors on the patient. He has usually never experienced these stressors before; accordingly, he does not have a repertoire of coping mechanisms to relieve them. His family, which usually is a major support, is subjected to many new stressors and may temporarily be unable to meet the increased emotional needs of its loved one.

The process of promoting psychosocial adaptation to illness involves awareness of several factors in the patient's psychosocial functioning before and during illness. The following categories have been devised in order to provide structure as you work with the patient in order for him to return to his presickness level of psychosocial, as well as physical, functioning.

The substance of the remaining chapters will include the specific information to help you assess these factors.

Psychosocial Assessment Factors

Psychosocial adaptation after a major illness depends on the following factors:

1. *Social history.* This includes information about a patient's life style and availability of persons who can support him emotionally during a difficult event.
2. *Level of stress during the year before admission.* This factor assesses the patient's current life situation, which includes the major stressors he has experienced during the past year.
3. *Normal coping pattern.* People respond to difficult times in certain ways. When asked, most patients can describe what they normally

do to cope when they have a serious problem or are experiencing high levels of stress.

4. *Neurovegetative changes.* These are signs of differences in a person's normal psychophysiological functions. They include changes in sleep patterns, appetite, bowel functioning, energy levels, and sexual functioning.

5. *Patient's understanding of illness.* Does the patient fully understand what is now happening and will continue to happen to him as a result of his illness? How threatening is *this* illness to *this* patient? Think, for a moment, of Tom, described in the case example. How long has he had to prepare psychologically for the effects his illness will have on his future?

6. *Mental status.* Is there any evidence of emotional, intellectual, or perceptual dysfunctioning at *this* time?

7. *Personality style.* This is the way a person normally interacts socially with others. Sometimes someone's personality style causes problems in his ability to adapt to hospitalization and caregivers and to his illness.

8. *Major issues of illness.* Illness can cause many types of psychosocial stress for the patient and his family. These include disruptions in his ability to trust, maintain self-esteem, retain a sense of control, tolerate a major loss, avoid feelings of guilt, and maintain intimacy in his close relationships.

The effects of these factors in Tom's psychosocial adaptation are discussed below:

1. *Social history.* Tom describes his family as normal. He and his parents and siblings get along well. His next-younger brother is a year younger. They have a close relationship. Tom's best friend has been his classmate since kindergarten. He has a girl friend he has been going out with for 2 years.

2. *Level of stress during year before admission.* Tom's last year in school has been "a good one." His family has experienced no major losses through death or separation from loved ones.

3. *Normal coping style.* In questioning Tom about how he normally handles pressure, he reports that he has always "blown off steam" by playing sports. After a fight with his parents, for example, he normally has gone to the high school to run at the track or has played an extra hard game of tennis. This information should raise a warning flag. Tom's usual way of coping with pressure has been lost to him. It would be better for him if he normally becomes

angry and shouts, does transcendental meditation, or uses any other form of conscious coping strategy that would not necessitate using his legs. When rehabilitated, he should be able to play sports again. Meanwhile, during the immediate postoperative period and the sometimes frustrating and discouraging rehabilitative process, his capacity for psychological adaptation will be inhibited until, and if, he develops a new way to cope consciously with the stress of illness.

4. *Neurovegetative changes.* Tom reports that since he noticed the bump on his leg, he has had trouble falling asleep at night. His appetite has decreased as well.

5. *Patient's understanding of illness.* Tom is aware of the possibility of cancer and the amputation that is made necessary by such a diagnosis. In Tom's case, this is considered a catastrophic illness. It is threatening in many ways. Most important, he knows he may die if the disease is not arrested. Second, he had intended to finance his college education with an athletic scholarship. Because his family is poor, they cannot afford to send him to the college he had hoped to attend. His dream of attending a good college has suddenly been threatened. A third concern is that he might not be able to pursue his career choice, civil engineering, which requires physical agility. The degree of threat of this illness is high. Warning flag number two should go up. As soon as Tom's medical condition was suspected, he was admitted to the hospital, subjected to many diagnostic procedures, and operated on. Only 1 week elapsed between the time he suspected a problem and the time a mid-thigh amputation was performed. This is a rapid series of events for a young man to integrate in such a short time. Warning flag number three is raised.

6. *Mental status.* Tom seems anxious at this time, but not beyond what would be considered normal for his situation. There is no evidence of intellectual or perceptual difficulty.

7. *Personality style.* Tom is a very pleasant young man with no unusual personality traits or characteristics.

8. *Major issues of illness.* The threat of amputation, cancer, and possibly death has the potential to undermine all Tom's major psychosocial issues: trust, self-esteem, control, loss, guilt, and intimacy. Many more warning flags are raised. Tom is at risk for psychosocial maladaptation.

Psychosocial Assessment as the Basis of the Nursing Process

Using the eight psychosocial assessment factors, nurses should be able to predict with a good level of accuracy whether a patient will be able to adapt to a sudden change in health status. If one or more of the indicators points out a potential problem, then the nurse can observe the patient's responses closely. He or she can immediately begin to provide stronger supportive care, especially in those areas of psychosocial functioning in which warning indicators are initially observed.

The nurse is not able to *make* the person cope. Rather, when the nurse provides external emotional support, it facilitates the patient's own internal coping ability to return to *normal*. Remember that the stress of illness usually causes the normal coping ability to regress in all patients (Hackett, 1978). It is impossible to expect patients to cope better than they did when they were well. That would be like hoping that a boat half filled with water and riding low will suddenly become buoyant.

In Tom's case, several areas where potential problems can occur have been identified. What supportive interventions can we use after surgery to promote psychosocial adaption? Before surgery, Tom used physical running activity as an outlet. He will not be able to work off stress in this way, at least in the immediate future. The nurse should point out the loss of this normal outlet to the physician and emphasize the reasons for providing a substitute outlet.

The nurse can ask the physician to order physical therapy as soon as possible so that Tom can exercise *all* parts of his body. The nurse should call the physical therapy department to explain the reasons for total body exercise. At times, nurses assume that other departments will carry out the requests they receive from nursing staff. It is possible that, without understanding the rationale for total body exercise, the physical therapy department would use a normal amputee exercise program. Nursing is often the liaison between the various caregivers. This is an important role to promote proper integration of all patient services.

The inclusion of such activity in Tom's care plan is important for three reasons: (1) it provides an outlet for the anger and anxiety he is experiencing; if anger is not released, it can turn inward and lead to depression (Jacobson, 1971), (2) it gives Tom hope because he is starting the rehabilitative process with no delay, and (3) it is a positive form of diversion for a young man who has always been very active.

The second warning indicator in Tom's case is the degree of threat of the illness to him. The greatest threat of this illness is that Tom may die if the disease is not arrested. Because of the swiftness of surgery and the small tumor discovered, Tom's prognosis is good. He will receive a course of chemotherapy as a precautionary measure.

Tom will benefit from being able to talk to his nurse and physician about his concerns. He should be encouraged to express these concerns, no matter how insignificant they seem to him. The health care team should answer Tom's questions honestly and give him a chance to express his thoughts and feelings about their answers. In addition, every day his nurse should find some time to sit with him and ask him how he feels about what is happening to him. In this way, his level of coping can continually be assessed.

It can be expected that Tom will wonder if he will be able to use his body as he once did. He also will wonder if people will accept him if he has only one leg. With many physical conditions, patients report that one of the most helpful aids in developing a positive outlook is to meet someone who has experienced a similar illness. This concept is used by many organizations: the Reach to Recovery program sponsored by the American Cancer Society, in which women who have had mastectomies visit recent mastectomy patients in the hospital, or the Mended Hearts Club, in which persons who have undergone cardiac surgery visit patients scheduled for surgery.

When patients meet someone who has successfully mastered the challenges of a particular condition, it gives them hope. The patient is able to voice his concerns and ask questions of his visitor. This approach would be an excellent one for a young man in Tom's circumstances. With justification by his nurse, the physical therapy department can help to arrange such a meeting.

Tom's concern about people's acceptance of him can be partially resolved by the positive reactions of his family and his friends of both sexes. Three other ways in which he can test the acceptance of others will need facilitation by the nursing staff. He can be placed in a room with another young person as soon as possible. Nursing can, on occasion, relax the normally rigid rules about the number of visitors allowed for each patient; a supportive group of young friends can be a great morale booster to a young man who doubts his own worth after disfiguring surgery. Another consideration is the possibility of a day pass on a weekend before discharge. Being with his family and having them do special things for him is also reassuring. During the period of rehabilitation, Tom's family and friends will benefit from support by nurses as well.

The major psychosocial issues of illness are trust, self-esteem, control, loss, guilt, and intimacy. Although never formally addressed between most nurses and their patients, these issues are constantly present. If the patient has a consistent relationship with a nurse, the dynamics of many of these issues will be present. Can he trust his caregivers and himself? Will he have any value after the surgery? What if he can't control his sadness or his anger? Will his life ever be normal again after all the losses the amputation will cause? Was there anything he could have done to prevent the cancer? Will anyone *really* love him with only one leg?

A sensitive nurse can listen for clues that one or more of these issues may be troubling a patient. A caring nurse who pulls up a chair next to the bed can allow the patient to examine some of these issues and begin to resolve them before they become more deeply troubling to him after discharge.

Immediately after a sudden illness, the adaptive mode of the psyche usually assists the patient by not being aware of the long-term implications of an illness. The immediate concerns of staying alive and avoiding rejection are all that the ego can tolerate, and it will defend itself by using unconscious defense mechanisms. (The use of defense mechanisms by patients will be explained in Chap. 4.) If, toward the end of his hospitalization, Tom begins to question his future functioning, his questions should be answered honestly. This approach is preferable to the hollow reassurances that he will recognize as untruths. The avoidance of the truth by hospital personnel only causes more feelings of anger and alienation for intelligent patients who are seeking the truth about their conditions and, in Tom's case, for adolescent patients who are struggling to be in charge of their own lives.

Essential Nursing Role in Psychosocial Assessment

In defending the need for nurses to develop more knowledge about the emotional functioning of patients, Rawnsley (1980) has pointed out that the difference between medicine and nursing is "nursing's primary concern for the person who is experiencing physiological or emotional disruption to well-being, as opposed to medicine's interest in the clinical problem that he happens to be manifesting" (p. 244). In a similar statement, Fields (1980) has written:

> Many nursing leaders stress the difference between nursing and medicine. Biomedical research is concerned with the causes of disease and its treatment, they say, while nursing care aims to help patients cope with illness, learn to care for themselves, and get better more quickly [p. 6].

Note that Fields has described that it is our job to help patients cope. If the nurse is not able to assess the patient's ability to cope and to design interventions when maladaptation occurs, then he or she will not be able to carry out the second and third functions described by Fields: teaching patients to cope for themselves and helping them to get better more quickly. The nurse's efforts will be thwarted because of the patient's maladaptation. The use of nursing diagnosis in the nursing process involves the need for an astute psychosocial assessment based on sound theory. This is necessitated by the fact that the majority of the nursing diagnosis categories developed by the St. Louis Conferences on Nursing Diagnosis are psychosocial. Once a psychosocial nursing diagnosis is established, there is a need for good counseling techniques and knowledge of intervention theory relating to psychosocial maladaptation in physical illness.

Knowledge of psychosocial assessment theory is mandatory if we are to support our patients' adaptation. Knowledge of theory is the first essential, since we must know *what we* are looking for. The second part, equally essential, is to know *how* to intervene when a problem is spotted. The following chapters will present clinical psychosocial assessment information and intervention models that have been developed in the clinical setting.

Conclusion

Medicine has traditionally not been active in developing psychosocial support techniques for the physically ill patient. Accordingly, the door to giving patient care in this area is open wide to the nursing profession. Every day, patients face the crisis of physical illness, which has the potential to overwhelm them. If these crises are not averted or worked through, maladaptation can cause a chronic or permanent deterioration in the quality of life for patients *and* their families. The psychosocial care of patients offers great opportunities for creativity, ingenuity, and deep personal reward to all nurses.

The human mind is one of the most complex systems in existence. Many psychoanalysts, psychiatrists, and psychologists have developed theories about how the psyche develops in humans. Some of these theories may be familiar to you. Those presented in this chapter have been chosen because they are essential in understanding patients' reactions to illness, performing psychosocial assessment, and developing interventions when maladaptation is anticipated.

The *personality* is the combination of unique characteristics and behaviors acquired by a person during his developmental process. It begins to develop at birth and is shaped by the interactions between his inherited disposition, the responses of other persons in his environment, and significant external events. Every person has a different personality, and it will determine how others react to him during his lifetime.

Drive Theory

Before attempting to absorb the teachings of the various theorists about personality development, it is important to understand one of the basic concepts of the force that causes the newborn to become aware of his environment and gradually interact with it in his own unique way. This force, which occurs naturally in all humans, has usually been called *instinct*. Most psychologists today use the word *drive* instead of instinct. It is generally believed that there are two main drives in every person: the drive to feel pleasure and the aggressive drive (Blanck and Blanck, 1979).

These two drives are present from the moment of birth. They can be seen in the infant as he frantically searches for his mother's nipple. If you stimulate a newborn's lips with your finger, his head will turn in the direction he believes the breast or bottle is located, his mouth will grope excitedly, and he will make grunting sounds until he finds the nipple. Once he finds the nipple, his body will suddenly relax; total tranquility will ensue, and the infant will demonstrate a remarkable peace. This is an example of the drive for pleasure; this is also called *libidinal drive* or *libido*. The baby seeks the nipple because, once obtained, it feels so good. His body is at rest.

The libidinal drive is the infant's major motivating force during his first years of life. Thereafter, the aggressive drive becomes equal to the libidinal drive, and the two operate together for the remainder of a person's life. The *libidinal drive* has been described as the force that connects and

2

The Building Blocks of Personality

seeks to establish unity. The *aggressive drive,* on the other hand, is the force that serves to undo connections in order to promote growth (Blanck and Blanck, 1979).

These drives operate in all human beings. They are essential to full human development. Without them, the human being lacks the motivation to attain his needs. In some people, one or both of the drives may become dysfunctional if severe frustration occurs over a prolonged period. For example, the main drive of the infant during the first year is to feel pleasure through his mouth and to receive gratification. One of the ways he does this is by being loved by his mother and developing a sense of security in her. If the baby cries and his mother fails to respond for a long period and continually fails him in this regard, he will experience frustration in his search for the pleasure of her love. It has been found that babies can become seriously depressed if their need for love is constantly frustrated (Spitz, 1965). This was learned by studying babies in orphanages. Because their need for love was rarely, if ever, fulfilled, they seemed to give up. They did not cry for attention any longer. Eventually, some of them became ill and died.

Another example of frustration of drive is a toddler who wants to be free to explore. His aggressive drive is experienced as an internal need to satisfy his curiosity and also his newfound ability to walk. If his caregiver does not allow some flexibility to this active youngster, and if, at the age of 2 years, he is still kept in a playpen most of the day with a very limited number of toys, the frustration of his aggressive drive may result in an intellectually and physically inhibited child. It is the aggressive and libidinal drives that spur the child toward full emotional, intellectual, and physical development.

In order to understand the importance of drive in the human being, read these important words of Spitz (1965):

> We speak often enough of the aggressive drive, it is rarely spelled out that the aggressive drive is not limited to hostility. Indeed, by far the largest and most important part of the aggressive drive serves as the motor of every movement, of all activity, big and small, and ultimately of life itself [p. 106].

In working with physically ill patients in the clinical setting, many clinicians find the statement that the aggressive drive is ultimately *the motor of life itself* to be remarkably true. It is as if it were a life force. There are physically ill persons about whom physicians say, "I don't understand why he is going downhill so quickly." Actually, these human beings demonstrate a total lack of the aggressive drive. They have given up, even before their bodies are ready to die. Other patients who are critically ill remain alive, sometimes to the wonderment of their caregivers. They cling tenaciously to life. In each case the aggressive drive, sparked by various motivations, keeps them alive. An example is the cancer patient who maintains that she will attend her son's wedding 2 weeks hence. After attending the wedding she may then slip into a coma and die by morning.

Affect

Affect is the overall feeling state observed in patients. Affect is the feeling side of a thought or idea or the emotional reaction to a person or object (Kaplan and Sadock, 1981). Affect can also be the visible sign of a drive. For example, some of the affects seen as a result of the aggressive drive are anger, rage, and hate. The term *affect* is sometimes interchanged with the term *mood.* Actually, mood should be used to describe the internal feelings experienced by a person. Affect is used when referring both to mood and to the external signs of a person's feelings (Hinsie and Campbell, 1977).

During your nursing career, you will be asked to describe your patients' affect frequently both in nursing reports and in describing the patient to physicians and other caregivers. The ability to detect accurately the affect observed in patients will help you to give sensitive and understanding care. Indeed, you may be the only person in the hospital who really understands how the patient is feeling and allows him to talk about it. The following list contains many common emotions:

Emotional States

Aloofness	Disgust
Anger	Disillusionment
Anxiety	Elation
Bitterness	Enthusiasm
Boredom	Envy
Compassion	Faith
Complacency	Fear
Curiosity	Fretfulness
Cynicism	Fury
Depression	Gloating
Despair	Grief

Emotional States (continued)

Guilt	Relief
Gullibility	Resignation
Hate	Reverence
Homesickness	Sadism
Hope	Sarcasm
Jealousy	Shame
Joy	Shyness
Love	Smugness
Masochism	Trust
Mysticism	Wistfulness
Peace	Wonder
Petulance	

Object Relations

Another concept that is crucial in understanding patients' and families' responses to illness is object relations theory. *Object relations* are internal images of self and others and the emotional energy invested in them. Psychoanalytic theorists believe that an object can only be another person or the self.

As you learned earlier, all human beings have two main drives: the drive to seek pleasure and the aggressive drive. In order to obtain pleasure or fulfill the aggressive drive, it is necessary that the energy of these drives be invested in something. Think, for example, of the emotional reaction of a mother who never finished high school as she watches her daughter receive her college degree; years of hope and love were invested in her daughter's development and also in her own dream that someday her daughter would attend college. How would you feel if this were your child?

The son whose mother is dying of chronic obstructive pulmonary disease is losing one of the most important objects in his life. Another type of object relations that affects nurses is their attachment to the patients they care for. The nurse experiences loss when his or her favorite patient either goes home or dies.

Although object relations theory may be a new idea to you, you will discover, upon proceeding through this book, why it applies to every patient you will ever care for. Although it is a simple concept, it is of great importance to people struggling with the effects of illness.

The Id, the Ego, and the Superego

In order to understand how the personality develops, it is essential to understand the abstract structures of the psyche. These structures were first described by Sigmund Freud. Freud was a theorist who explored his own thoughts and feelings and delved deep within himself in his analysis of his past experiences and their association to present experiences. During this process, his *structural theory* evolved. He proposed that there are three main structures or parts of the psyche: the *id,* the *ego,* and the *superego.*

The Id

The psyche of a newborn infant is composed almost entirely of id. The id contains the basic drives of a person: the pleasure seeking or sexual drive and the aggressive drive. Freud taught that these drives are primarily biological in origin. The id is totally unconscious; a person is never fully aware of its functioning. When a person feels compelled to do something and does not quite understand why, the motivation is usually id-related. As the child matures to adulthood, the illogical drives of the id are usually held in check by the ego and superego. Observe a 2-month-old baby who has just lost his bottle, and you will see unchannelled id being unleashed on the world. In an adult schizophrenic who is displaying psychotic behavior, you will also see many id derivatives (DiCaprio, 1974; Kaplan and Sadock, 1981; Hinsie and Campbell, 1977; Carson, 1979).

The Ego

The ego is the regulator of the personality. It watches over the instinctual energy of the id and channels it into acceptable ways of satisfying the person's drives. Unlike the id, the ego is in touch with the world. It has conscious and unconscious components (Kaplan and Sadock, 1981).

The most important job of the ego is to adapt to reality. It is like a buffer between the drives of the id and the external judgmental environment. It consists of a large number of functions that are essential for normal human development. As you read the following list, stop and think of the complexity of functions that the ego performs automatically (Small, 1979).

Ego Functions

1. *Consciousness*
2. *Mastery of motor skills*
3. *Mobility.* The ability to move around the environment.
4. *Perception.* The ability to scrutinize the environment. This is done by the various senses of vision, hearing, smell, touch, and taste, all of which are controlled by the ego.
5. *Judgment.* The ability to interpret these observations.
6. *Sense of reality.* The ability to separate one's self from other people and the environment. This includes a realistic view of one's self and encompasses such concepts as self-esteem and body image.
7. *Regulation and control of emotions and impulses.* All of a person's feelings are channeled and controlled by the ego.
8. *Object relations.* Described previously. The ego controls the intensity of feelings we have about objects. It is possible for there to be too much or too little feeling about objects, depending on the undercontrol or overcontrol of the ego.
9. *Memory.* This includes long-term and recent memory. Long-term memory is the ability to file away mentally the different steps in a nursing procedure, the normal laboratory values of human blood, and what your kindergarten teacher looked like, for instance. Recent memory examples are remembering what happened this morning or a laboratory value read to you over the telephone. Whenever there is an organic impairment of the physiological functions of the brain, such as the effects of old age or a toxic reaction to an illness, the recent memory will fail before the long-term memory.
10. *Thinking.* The ability to know and learn is included in this category. Reasoning and problem solving and all cognitive processes are controlled by this function of the ego.
11. *Defense mechanisms.* These include the maneuvers that the mind uses to defend itself against threatening reality. All of us have defense mechanisms that we use unconsciously. They are our greatest ally in coping with the stress of life. The defense mechanisms will be described in Chapter 4.

The ego exists at birth but constitutes a very small part of the infant's psyche (Blanck and Blanck, 1979). The above list shows that the maintenance of consciousness and the senses are actually the only ego functions present in the newborn. The remainder of the baby's psyche is controlled by the id. The rest of the ego functions are acquired little by little as the infant becomes a toddler, a child, and finally an adult. In a retarded adult, or one who is emotionally ill, the ego functions are less developed than they would be in an adult whose development has proceeded normally. The ego develops in human beings as a result of the interaction between the child and his caregivers. The result of the interaction between mother and child during the early years of a child's life molds his personality for *the rest of his life* (Bowlby, 1973; Thomas and Chess, 1980). The care given by the father, other family members, or surrogate mothers in a child-care setting may have an effect on the infant and the child, but not as influential an effect as the mother-child relationship, which is a special bond.

The Superego

The superego is the third structure in the psyche. It is not present at birth (Fenichel, 1945). The superego begins to develop as a result of the child's interacting with his mother and father and the environment at large (Fenichel, 1945). One of the main needs of the infant and child is to obtain love and approval. Anything that displeases mother, father, and other authority figures causes a loss of love. The mother becomes an external conscience for the 10-month-old infant or the 2-year-old child. The lay term for the superego is the *conscience.*

During early childhood, the superego develops rapidly. It occurs with the help of the ego. The ego allows the development of a set of moral judgments that will ensure the infant, and later the child, the love of mother, father, and all the other important persons in his life (DiCaprio, 1974; Carson, 1979). Actually, what the child does unconsciously is to internalize the teachings and opinions of these people (Fenichel, 1945). For example, have you ever seen a toddler behave in a certain way with one person and quite differently with another? A stern and disapproving grandmother instills a certain sense of dread in the toddler, so that he thinks twice before he picks up her ashtray and bangs it on the table. If his mother is a relaxed, casual person, he will operate under fewer prohibitions in his own home.

The superego has two main roles. The first is to caution the person; it has a threatening quality that says, "You *shouldn't* do that!" The second function establishes goals for the person, saying, "You *should* do that." The most rapid development of the superego occurs during the Oedipal stage (ages 4 to 6 years), the time when the youngster is attracted to the parent of the opposite sex and fears the punishment that he or she may receive from the parent of the same sex (Fenichel, 1945).

The development of the superego is nearly over by the age of 6 years. It is very strict and unyielding. It is subject to modification during the early and middle school years as the child is exposed to an ever-widening social group.

Through the adolescent years it is necessary for some modification of the harsh superego to occur. If this does not happen, the result will be an adult who is not able to fully participate in life (Carson, 1979). In order for this process to occur, the adolescent will rebel to some degree. The rebellion, which is outwardly directed at the parents, is actually raging to a larger degree in the superego. It is healthy for the adolescent to be given a reasonable degree of freedom so that he can mediate these internal prohibitions in a manner that will result in his becoming a well-adjusted young adult. If there is too much parental or environmental disapproval, the adolescent will never be able to allow these modifications in his conscience. He will become an adult whose participation in life will be rigid and inhibited. Accordingly, if few restrictions are placed on him in adolescence, his superego may be modified in too radical a direction and he may lack the discipline to become a responsible adult (Carson, 1979).

The superego works unconsciously. The effect that we feel when we go against it actually comes from the ego. These feelings include guilt, remorse, and anxiety (DiCaprio, 1974).

The Conscious, the Preconscious, and the Unconscious

The terms *conscious* and *unconscious* have already been used here. These concepts were also described by Freud (1924a). He became aware of them because in his own analysis and his work with patients he discovered that there are certain psychological processes of which a person is not aware. Stop and think of the times when you do something and then say to yourself, "*Why* did I do that?"

The Conscious

The *conscious* involves the awareness of what is happening at *a specific moment*. This awareness includes what a person is thinking and feeling, that is, his internal environment. The remainder of his awareness is of the external environment, that is, where he is, whom he is with, and so on.

The Preconscious

The *preconscious* consists of memories that a person is not constantly thinking about but that can easily be recalled. This includes remembering the time and date of a dental appointment next week or a relative's telephone number.

The Unconscious

The *unconscious* is a psychologic process that a person is not aware of and cannot control. It has been compared to a rosebud or an onion. It consists of layer upon layer of repressed memories and experiences surrounding the core of the id drives. The id itself is also part of the unconscious (DiCaprio, 1974; Kaplan and Sadock, 1981; Freud, 1933; Hinsie and Campbell, 1977; Thomas, 1973; Carson, 1979).

Bonding

Bonding is a concept that has gained in importance in the fields of obstetrics and neonatology (the care of the newborn infant, a subspecialty of pediatrics). The nursing profession has advocated the importance of the bonding process to the mother-father-child *triad*. A triad is a close relationship between three persons (Bowen and Miller, 1980; Clark and Affonso, 1976; Cropley and colleagues, 1976). It is possible that one of the reasons for the widespread acceptance of this concept by nurses is that many female obstetricians, nurses, midwives, obstetrics nursing educators, and obstetrics staff nurses have personally experienced the mother-infant bonding process or were blocked by hospital policies that frustrated their desire to be with their new infants during the first 24 hours of life.

Bonding is an attachment process that occurs very early in the infant's life. The most significant bond is formed between mother and child. Bonding is a two-way attachment. It is an attachment of the helpless infant to his mother in a manner that

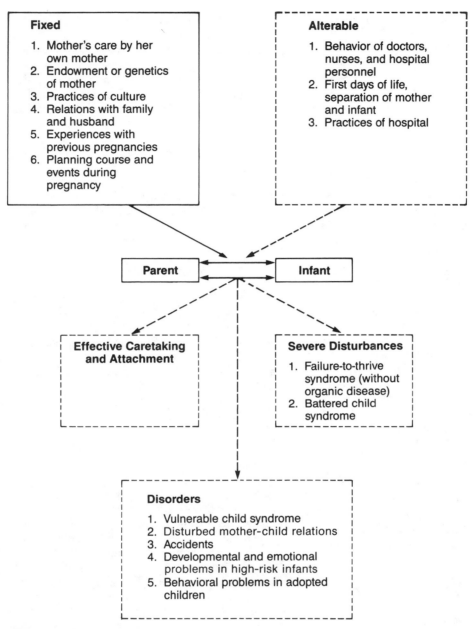

Fixed

1. Mother's care by her own mother
2. Endowment or genetics of mother
3. Practices of culture
4. Relations with family and husband
5. Experiences with previous pregnancies
6. Planning course and events during pregnancy

Alterable

1. Behavior of doctors, nurses, and hospital personnel
2. First days of life, separation of mother and infant
3. Practices of hospital

Parent ⟷ Infant

Effective Caretaking and Attachment

Severe Disturbances

1. Failure-to-thrive syndrome (without organic disease)
2. Battered child syndrome

Disorders

1. Vulnerable child syndrome
2. Disturbed mother-child relations
3. Accidents
4. Developmental and emotional problems in high-risk infants
5. Behavioral problems in adopted children

Figure 2-1.
Influences on maternal-infant bonding. Hypothesized diagram of the major influences on maternal behavior and the resulting disturbances. *Solid lines* represent unchangeable determinants; *dotted lines* represent alterable determinants. (Klaus M, Kennell J: Maternal-Infant Bonding, 1st ed, p. 13. St. Louis, CV Mosby, 1976)

meets the needs of his psychological dependency. It also involves the bonding of the mother to her baby: love for him and desire to meet his needs (Klaus and Kennell, 1976).

In a critical review of studies of parent-infant bonding, Siegel concluded that close contact between parents and infants during the postpartum period resulted in short and intermediate effects within families. Siegel also emphasizes that there are many other variables that promote positive parent-child interactions and favorable family dynamics. They include "family planning, comprehensive prenatal care, and particularly, family supports to reduce socio-environmental and psychological stresses (1982, p. 61).

Klaus and Kennell originally identified the maternal-infant bonding process immediately following birth as essential to the child's future capacity to form attachments in all relationships during his lifetime (1976). They modified their original position in a subsequent edition of their book. In it, they state that because of the adaptability of the human there are many other routes to positive relationships if the initial bonding opportunity between mother and newborn is thwarted (1982).

Many hospitals continue to use policies that deprive the infant and mother of closeness to one another during the first few days of life. This can be especially detrimental to the bonding process, according to Klaus and Kennell, who have described it as "a sensitive period in the first minutes and hours of life during which it is necessary that the mother and father have close contact with their neonate for later development to be optimal" (p. 14).

At special risk because of deprivation of contact with the mother are infants who are cared for in premature and intensive care nurseries. Without frequent exposure to their babies, the mothers of infants who have spent a prolonged time in such nurseries are found to lack the normal "instincts" of mothers (Clark and Affonso, 1976; Cropley and colleagues, 1976). Similarly, their babies frequently experience difficulties that reflect the "failure to thrive" phenomenon. In response to these findings, some hospitals have relaxed visiting hours in the intensive care and regular nurseries. Parents are encouraged to spend as much time as they want with their child.

Figure 2-1 presents a hypothetical diagram of the environmental influences on the mother and her baby and the problems that can result.

In order to understand your patients and their current level of personality functioning, it is important to realize that they are *who* they are as the result of a long continuum of development. Their psychic development actually begins when they are still fetuses and there is an awareness, id-dominated as it is, of the warm, dark, protective environment they are living in. Could a person ask for more comfort and security?

Various psychologists and obstetricians consider the process of birth to be a psychological insult to the child. They believe that the awareness of this experience actually remains stored in the psyche of all humans (Janov, 1971). It is one of the reasons why proponents of natural childbirth and "quiet births" beg for understanding of their beliefs (LeBoyer, 1975; Karmel, 1959).

Inborn Personality Characteristics

Formal psychiatric theorists rarely discuss the personality of the newborn. It is as if all children were born with a "blank screen" of personality characteristics and personality were then acquired as a result of inborn biochemical drives and the impact of caregivers as they gradually mold and shape an infant's behavior.

Berry Brazelton (1973), a pediatrician, has demonstrated in his research that newborns enter the world with as many as 26 different behavioral characteristics and 20 reflexes that can each be observed and rated (*Babies*, 1983). In other words, every baby is different. A baby is not born with a neutral personality. The formal theory proposed by Brazelton can be verified by observant mothers everywhere. Astute mothers have always been able to identify the differences evident in their offspring when compared to the child's earlier or later siblings. A mother with two, six, or ten children can report definite inborn traits, such as irritability, placidity, and alertness. Surprisingly, the observations of these mothers remain true as the child matures.

Some of Brazelton's specific observations about newborns include the following:

General State Observations

Alertness

General tone

Cuddliness

Motor maturity

Tremulousness

Activity

Irritability

Amount of startle reflex during examination

Lability of skin color

Lability of states

Self-quieting activity

Hand-to-mouth facility

Smiles

Response to light

General State Observations (continued)

Response to rattle

Response to bell

Response to pinprick

Orientation to various auditory and visual stimuli

Defensive movements

Consolability with intervention

Peak of excitement

Rapidity of buildup of excitement

Pull to sit

Conclusion

This chapter has presented information about the foundations of personality. At times, psychology textbooks skip over some of this information in their haste to present more complex concepts. Being aware of these dynamics in patients can help you to be more fully aware of their psychosocial responses to illness. Another important reason why this chapter is included is to increase your awareness of these dynamics, which are always operating in you. By being open to these dynamics in yourself, your capacity to engage in therapeutic relationships with your patients can be enhanced.

This chapter presents a general overview of the personality theories that have been developed by various social scientists. These theories are important for nurses to understand as they assess and approach the emotional, cognitive, and perceptual aspects of their patients' psyches. The *psyche* includes the mind and all its functions. For clarification, the emotional side of the psyche is affect. Affect is what a person feels. The cognitive side of the psyche is the intellect; it controls thinking, understanding, problem solving, and other cognition functions. Perception is the way that the mind interprets all external stimuli received through the various senses. Chapter 10, The Mental Status Examination, will explain these functions in more detail.

Some of the theories deal with specific periods of a person's life, and others concern themselves with the developmental continuum of an entire lifetime. All these theories have been developed from the specific viewpoint of the various theorists. Think about each theory, and compare it with your own experience or with observations of children, siblings, parents and grandparents, and adult patients of varying ages. By doing this, each theory will be more meaningful.

Instead of viewing patients from several separate personality viewpoints, try to integrate these theories into one overall way of viewing the patient. Trying to place all psychosocial observations of patients into separate distinct categories is not possible. This may be more easily understood by considering the physical body systems. It is impossible to consider each as totally separate from the others. For example, the kidneys in the urinary system depend on the circulatory system, the metabolic system, and the immunosuppressive system in order to function.

3

Major Theories of Personality Development

Mahler: The First Two Years of Life

Margaret Mahler (1974) is a psychoanalyst who, during her training years in the late 1920s, worked in a well-baby clinic in Austria. In watching the infants and their interactions with their mothers, she gradually began to observe certain psychological patterns of the infants. These patterns depended on the infants' ages and the quality of interaction between mother and child. Her research findings have provided important clues to the causes of emotional dysfunctioning. She believed that the most severe emotional afflictions develop during the first 2 years of life when there are severe problems in the mother–child dyad. (A *dyad* is any two-person relationship.) She has described the following substages.

The Autistic Phase (0 to 3 to 4 weeks)

The child is generally unaware of the environment in the autistic phase. He is unaware of any difference between his internal and external world. His psyche is governed by physiological needs, and his drives are in complete control. A form of psychopathology that results from inability to progress beyond this stage is severe autistic schizophrenia. The person is living in his own world; he never is able to communicate with others.

Symbiotic Phase (1 to 4 months)

In the symbiotic phase, the child becomes aware of his mother, and the bond between the mother and child is created. The infant is not able to differentiate between his mother and himself. During this stage, the infant invests emotional energy in his mother. He is very passive. He interacts with his mother and other persons and objects that are brought to him. He lacks mobility and is unable to explore anything beyond his immediate reach. If the interaction between mother and baby is positive, he has a sense of "confident expectation." When he cries, someone responds.

If interaction between the infant and his mother or consistent caregiver during this phase is markedly inadequate, then other forms of schizophrenia may result.

Separation–Individuation Phase

The separation-individuation phase includes four important subphases.

Differentiation subphase (5 to 10 months)
The child's ability to move away from his mother begins in the differentiation subphase. He may squirm and slide off her lap. He begins to crawl back to her quickly. The child needs to be able to see his mother or caretaker to continue feeling secure. If he should stray too far from mother, his security depends on her consistency in picking him up and returning him to her side.

Putting a child in a playpen in a room away from the mother for several hours when the child is awake causes him to feel insecure. However, he must be able to be away from her some of the time in order to develop an awareness of his own separateness and sense of self. Frequent frustration in his attempts to be near her will distort this process. It is during this subphase that the child's intense fear of strangers occurs, about 7 or 8 months of age. This further demonstrates his great need for security at this stage.

It is essential during this stage that the child have a minimal number of caregivers and that he can depend on them for his security. Ideally, the primary caregiver should be the mother, so that the child's sense of trust in the environment can develop fully. The quality of caregiving is also essential. The caregiver should be capable of transmitting love to the infant. If the child constantly lacks a feeling of trust in the environment because of undependable care (when he cries, no one comes), then the result can be tragic. It was found that orphaned infants in foundling homes who were 6 to 8 months of age died when they did not receive adequate care. Their deaths were attributed to their sense of being abandoned. This was described as severe depression (Spitz, 1965).

It is during these important months that a child begins to establish trust in his mother. If trust does not develop because of chronically inadequate care, this can form the basis of loss of trust in all persons as the child matures into adulthood. Remember that the words "inadequate care" refer to a major failure on the part of the predominant caregiver to meet the infant's emotional needs. Whenever the following situations occur chronically, for several months, the outcome may be severe: a child who cries for several hours with no one responding, whether or not someone is at home; a child who must spend several hours in a soiled diaper; a child who must cry for food for long periods; abusive verbal and physical treatment by a caregiver.

Mahler also emphasizes that it is healthy for the infant to experience a mild level of frustration in his need of his mother. If, for example, the child is with the mother during every waking and sleeping hour with *no* separation from her, he would *never* be able to begin the process of differentiation. It is also important to the mother's sense of self that she be able to maintain her own identity and have diversions away from the child.

Practicing subphase (10 to 18 months)
The practicing subphase is a developmentally active period. The infant's main drive in the first year of life is libidinal: looking for love and seeking

his mother. As he approaches his second year, he becomes more active. His aggressive drive eventually becomes dominant. The child takes pleasure in moving away from his mother. "At the same time, however, mother continues to be needed as 'home base' for what Furer named 'emotional refueling'" (Mahler, 1974, p. 97).

It is during this stage that the child's *self-esteem* is developed. The essential step that must occur at this point is for the mother to allow the infant to become more independent. If he is not allowed a moderate level of freedom, he will not be able to develop a sense of satisfaction with himself. Observe the face of a young toddler as he "escapes" from his mother. Have you ever seen such joy? His love of self will never be greater than it is at this time. Narcissism is considered a very healthy trait in a child of this age. He also becomes more interested in the environment at large. His ego is developing rapidly. Many of the ego functions listed earlier come into being at this time. Toward the end of this stage, at 16 to 18 months, he becomes more aware of his separateness from his mother. At times, he even seems pensive as this awareness sinks in.

Rapprochement subphase (18 to 22 months)

Rapprochement is a French word that means bringing near or drawing close. During this stage, the youngster learns that he can go away from his mother and come back. He becomes secure that he will still be loved and accepted even when he is separate from her or consciously opposes her wishes (Mahler, 1974).

Have you ever seen an angry, screaming toddler lying in the middle of the supermarket aisle kicking his feet in the air? This age is a period of intense ambivalence for the child (and very difficult for mothers also). As in all the phases, the mother's interaction with her child will determine the outcome. She should give neither too much nor too little love and approval. If the mother *always* allows the toddler to have his own way in order to avoid tantrums, the child will not be able to develop his own sense of restraint (the beginning of the super-ego). Consistent overprotectiveness by the mother can affect the youngster. If he is not allowed to express himself and his independence during this stage, he can become fearful of himself and the world. The tendency toward depression in adulthood is the outcome of incomplete mastery of this stage (Jacobson, 1971; Blanck and Blanck, 1979).

Object constancy subphase (22 to 28 months)

The object constancy subphase is the last stage that Mahler describes. During this stage, the toddler fully accepts his own separateness from his mother. He develops a stable image of himself and his mother. With her continued availability and support, his psychological growth proceeds. He develops the ability to cope with the frustrations he encounters, is able to test the reality of his world, and is eager to learn about his environment.

• • •

Another important form of pathology that can develop as a result of the child's inability to gratify his needs during the Mahler-described phases is a tendency toward addiction in later life. Drug and alcohol abuse may, in part, be due to inadequate care during the first 2 years of life (Frosch, 1970; Wiedner and Kaplan, 1969).

Piaget: The Cognitive Stages of Development

Jean Piaget was a Swiss psychologist who studied the intellectual stages of development of children. During a period spanning several decades in the mid-1900s, he studied this process by clinical interviewing, observing, and experimenting. He believed that there are four stages in the intellectual development of the child (Speeth and Tosti, 1973; Piaget and Inhelder, 1969).

Sensorimotor Stage (0 to 18 months)

During the sensorimotor stage the infant gradually learns through his senses. He pays attention to the things he sees and hears. He touches objects and explores the environment around him. He is able at times to predict the result of his actions. Testing his predictions can also become a game for him. This type of thinking also marks the beginning of simple problem solving and is the basis of all forms of higher intellectual development. If, for example, he throws his cereal bowl on the floor, he is quite certain what his mother's response will be.

Preoperational Thought Stage (1½ or 2 to 7 or 8 years)

The preoperational thought stage is characterized by rigid thinking. This is demonstrated by an inflexibility in the way the child views the environment at large. Once he has a thought or idea, it rarely changes during this stage. It is also normal for the child to be self-centered in his interactions. He is quite unable to comprehend the ideas of others if they differ from his own. This is called *ego-centricity.*

Another important aspect of this phase is that the child develops object permanence. *Object permanence* is the awareness in the child that, although people and objects may move in and out of his perceptual range, their absence no longer signifies lack of existence. During the sensorimotor stage, when an object disappeared, it signified total loss of the object. The child also begins to use elementary symbols in his thinking and communication. A *symbol* is a single idea or object that represents another more complex thought or thing; there is a common association between them (Kaplan and Sadock, 1981).

Stage of Concrete Operations (8 to 11 years)

During the stage of concrete operations, the child develops the concepts of moral judgment, numbers, and spatial relationships. The child is not yet capable of abstract reasoning. He understands things as he sees them and as they seem to be.

He would not, for example, be able to explain the abstract reasoning of the proverb, "You can lead a horse to water, but you can't make him drink." The abstract meaning of this proverb can be interpreted as follows: you can teach someone something but you can't *make* him learn. (Think of an adolescent diabetic patient in this case; you can't *make* him adhere to his diet and follow all medical instructions.) The child would explain the meaning of the proverb in a concrete and literal way, perhaps saying that you can put the horse's mouth *in* the bucket but you can't make him drink or that if the horse isn't thirsty, he may not drink any water.

Stage of Formal Thought (12 years to adulthood)

During the stage of formal thought, the young person is able to use sequential steps in his thinking to solve problems and form conclusions by deductive reasoning. He is able to think in an abstract manner, and he is able to form and test hypotheses.

• • •

Piaget's theories are important to nurses for many reasons. All nurses work in a pediatric setting at some time during their professional education. When patient teaching is necessary, it is important to understand the intellectual stage of cognitive development in which the child is functioning. If a nurse is preparing to teach a 9-year-old patient with diabetes about his illness, it is essential to avoid abstract concepts and those concepts that involve a level of reasoning that the child cannot perform.

These concepts are also essential in caring for adult patients, even though most adults have already progressed through these stages. An important point to remember in caring for patients is that illness and hospitalization are very threatening to them. A coping device that the ego uses in very threatening circumstances is regression. *Regression* is the return to an earlier level of functioning as a way of handling stress. It is an unconscious mechanism (Carson, 1979). Lewis and Levy (1982) have written, "Clearly, the most prominent psychological feature of the medically ill is regression" (p. 132).

When this occurs, a patient's level of comprehension is affected. He may regress to the stage of concrete operations or even to the preoperational stage of inflexible thinking. At times, we may think that an intelligent person is being resistant to our teaching. Instead, because of the tendency to regress, it is quite possible that the person is not capable of understanding what he is hearing. Remember, too, that some patients never develop beyond the stage of concrete operations or, possibly, a lesser stage of intellectual development. When a person's intellectual quotient (IQ) appears to be below normal, your teaching approach will be more successful if you use very basic, concrete explanations that will be more readily understood.

Skinner: Operant Conditioning

B. F. Skinner is a psychologist who founded the field of behavioral psychology. He was born in 1904 in Pennsylvania and holds a PhD in psychology from Harvard, where he continues to teach and carry out his studies. Skinner believes that desired behavior is obtained by giving rewards when the person does what is expected of him. He believes that personality develops because of the interaction of two variables: the intrapsychic makeup of the person (described above as id, ego, and so on) and the social environment (DiCaprio, 1974). The term *operant conditioning* derives its meaning from the fact that a person operates in his environment. Operant responses are voluntary, as opposed to involuntary or reflex behavior (Kaplan and Sadock, 1981).

Skinner discovered that a person's behavior is molded by the way that the social environment reacts to his behavior. He learns which of his behaviors are "good" and which are "bad."

If a woman complains to her family that she does not feel well, one of the ways family members can respond is to become more attentive, relieve her of tasks, and give her emotional support. This extra attention usually helps to decrease her level of tension. A week later she may have a similar problem, and her family may respond in the same manner. If this pattern continues, and the mother finds her needs met consistently, it is possible for her future behavior to be positively reinforced and a chronic sick role to occur. *Positive reinforcement* is similar to a reward. It increases the possibility that a person will continue his original behavior because the environment responds positively (Speeth and Tosti, 1973).

People can reshape the behavior of a person who originally was positively reinforced by ignoring further similar behaviors. Eventually the person will stop the behavior because of a lack of response and reinforcement from the environment. This is called *extinction* (Speeth and Tosti, 1973). In the example above, if the family tires of the extra demands of the mother, they may ignore her attention-seeking behavior, and she may respond by eventually returning to her normal way of interacting with her family.

Negative reinforcement is another important concept to understand when working with patients. *Negative reinforcement* is the rewarding of a stoppage of an undesirable event or behavior. Frequently this concept is confused with punishment. Perhaps the following examples can clarify the two (Speeth and Tosti, 1973).

Case Example

John has angina pectoris. Whenever he overexerts himself, he experiences sharp chest pain (aversive stimulus). When he takes a nitroglycerine tablet, the pain disappears (behavioral response causes removal of the aversive stimulus, and the person feels better).

Each time that a nitroglycerine tablet relieves John's chest pain, his medication-taking behavior is reinforced. Because it stops an aversive stimulus, it is called negative reinforcement. An *aversive* stimulus is any event that results in an unpleasant feeling in a person. The aversive stimulus always *precedes* the behavior. This is in contrast to punishment. With *punishment,* the aversive stimulus always follows the behavior. Because of punishment, the person may choose to eliminate the behavior that results in an aversive stimulus.

Case Example

Cathy injured her knee in a soccer accident. The physician told her not to play soccer for 4 weeks in order to allow the knee to heal properly. Because of an important game, she decided to play 1 week too soon (behavior). She pulled some muscles in the affected knee during the game (aversive stimulus). When she revisited the physician, she assured him that she would follow his directions carefully in order to prevent further injury. Four weeks later she resumed her soccer playing. (The punishment of reinjuring her knee brought about the desired behavior.)

The term *reinforcement* used in reference to teaching new information means that once something is learned, it will be remembered better if it is presented again. It has been found that if the material is presented in yet another form, it may be better understood and retained for a longer period. This is an important concept for nurses, who routinely do preventive health teaching in the inpatient and outpatient settings.

Because of the complexity of these terms, they will be presented again using an alcoholic (or drug addict) as an example.

Alcoholics or drug addicts frequently describe themselves as feeling "empty" inside. This unpleasant feeling prompts them to want a drink or a "fix." After they have it, they feel a reduction of tension. The alcohol or drug is a positive reinforcer. *Positive reinforcement* results in either a feeling of pleasure or a decrease in tension. This feeling is the final step of the positive reinforcement process. Without this internal feeling, no reinforcement can occur. If the original empty feeling of the addicted person was not replaced by the positive feeling, it is possible that he would not continue his habit.

Alcoholics and drug addicts thus do not respond well when we simply teach them about the harmful outcome of their substance addiction. Teaching reaches only the intellectual cognitive sphere. For the drug or alcohol addict, it is the affect-feeling sphere that needs relief. Such a person's feelings dominate and flood his intellect.

His tension or negative feeling must *first* be relieved or substituted with other feelings, such as accomplishment, before he can begin to break his habit.

An example of negative reinforcement of the alcoholic patient is the chronic family disapproval he experiences because of his drinking. In this example, the family's disapproval is the aversive stimulus. When the patient maintains sobriety, his family's disapproval is replaced by love and understanding. Their approval is a reinforcer that does away with the original negative behavior. It is important to remember that in negative reinforcement, the aversive stimulus (in this case, the disapproval of the family) *precedes* the behavioral response (sobriety), and then the negative behavior (excessive alcohol intake) is removed.

With punishment, the aversive stimulus *follows* the negative behavior. An example of punishment with the alcoholic patient is the way that he feels *after* he drinks too much. His negative behavior is his drinking. The aversive stimulus or punishment can be both the disapproval he senses from others *and* a miserable hangover. An example of punishment used with alcohol patients is the use of disulfiram (Antabuse). Disulfiram is a potent drug given to some alcoholics. If the person consumes even a small amount of alcohol, his body will react violently. He will experience acute respiratory distress, violent nausea and vomiting, chest pain, and many other negative physiological effects.

Understanding and applying these concepts can make the difference in the way that patients respond to nurses' teaching. Think of patients with the following conditions: cardiac disease, chronic respiratory and gastrointestinal disease, diabetes mellitus and other glandular conditions, and substance addictions (food, alcohol, drugs). In order to relieve these conditions, patients must undergo major modifications in their life styles. Nurses must be aware of the accompanying unpleasant feelings that these new regimens produce in patients. It is wise to develop a care plan that attends to the increased emotional needs that accompany the losses caused by the patient's treatment regimen. Patients like their regular habits. It is a loss to them if they must be given up. The clinical approach called behavior modification is based on the theories of Skinner.

Behavior modification is the restructuring of a patient's undesirable behavior by the use of conditioning techniques designed to bring about the desired behavior. These conditioning techniques are designed to obtain a specific outcome. The caregiver and patient together develop a plan that is agreeable to both in order to obtain a specific goal or outcome.

Freud: Psychosexual Stages of Development

Sigmund Freud developed a theory about the development of personality that is based on the concept of *libido*. Libido, the energy existing in a person, is the basis of his pursuit of pleasurable feelings. Freud taught that this energy was derived from the human being's physiological makeup.

Libido, according to Freud, is the impulse or drive to promote object relations with other persons. It involves avoidance of conflict in order to ensure pleasurable feelings (Blanck and Blanck, 1979). Early drive for pleasure in children is called *infantile sexuality* (Fenichel, 1945). The characteristics of infantile sexuality differ from those of adult sexuality, but they are experienced in the same positive manner. In addition, the ability to obtain pleasure sexually as an adult depends on earlier experiences of positive body sensations.

Freud taught that various parts of the body become the primary zones of gratification during early development, and he described the following stages of development.

Oral Stage (0 to 12 months)

During the oral stage, the infant's needs, perceptions, and modes of expression are centered in the mouth, lips, and tongue. The infant's expression of drives is as follows:

Libidinal: need to eat, be satiated, and sleep

Aggressive: biting, chewing, and spitting; rage while crying

Anal Stage (1 to 3 years)

During the anal stage of development, the toddler achieves neuromuscular control of the anal and urethral sphincters. His expression of drives is as follows:

Libidinal: pleasure in expelling and retaining feces; to a lesser degree, pleasure in releasing urinary sphincter

Aggressive: withholding feces from authority figures; ambivalence of the "terrible twos."

Phallic Stage (3 to 6 years)

During the phallic stage, the genital organs become sources of pleasure and are of prime interest. Children become aware of anatomical and social differences between men and women. Fantasies involving the parent of the opposite sex become predominant. This is called the *Oedipus complex.* Young boys love their mothers and ambivalently view their fathers as rivals and as models. Because of the sexual aspect of his love for mother, the young boy fears that his father, who is much bigger and stronger, may remove his penis. This fear is called *castration anxiety.* A similar process occurs in a young girl's reaction to her father. It is called the *Electra complex.* Because girls do not have a penis, they develop *penis envy.* Freud believed that the result of penis envy was that women undervalue the feminine role and overvalue the masculine role.

According to Freud, the seeds of neurosis are rooted in the phallic stage. Because many of the thoughts and feelings of this stage are disapproved of by parents, the child represses them. They are repressed whether or not the conflicts are resolved. The results of this repression are personality traits that the child carries into adulthood. The child's expression of drives is as follows:

Libidinal: Self-preoccupation (egocentricity); masturbation and fantasies common; enjoys social interaction with others

Aggressive: asserting own needs and rights

Latency Stage (6 to 12 years)

During the latency stage, the child's personality traits, developed during earlier stages, become more firmly established. No important dynamic changes occur during this stage. Freud considered this to be a neutral time that was not libidinally oriented like the first three stages. The child's expression of drives is as follows:

Libidinal: no dominant traits

Aggressive: energy invested in peer relationships (tendency toward cliques—exclusion of others), school work, and sports

Genital Stage (12 to 20 years)

During the genital stage, work on the permanent personality structure is completed. The intensification of both libidinal and aggressive drives frequently causes some aspects of the personality to regress to a previous level. Unresolved conflicts from the earlier level are reopened. The Oedipal and Electra complexes become dominant in many adolescents. This may be the cause of much of the emotional turmoil that adolescents and their parents experience. Conflicts with the parent of the same sex are common.

Some of the frequently observed adolescent traits are egocentricity, ambivalence, rebelliousness, heightened sense of guilt, and increase in religious feelings or rejection of religious beliefs, (DiCaprio, 1974; Kaplan and Sadock, 1981; Elkind, 1967; Stuart and Sundeen, 1979; Topalis and Aguilera, 1978). The changes in religious interests that occur actually may have two different dynamics. In the case of the youngster who develops more of an interest in religion than he previously had, it may be partially due to his need to ward off unaccustomed and unwelcome sexual feelings. Increased belief in God and adherence to religious teachings can help the adolescent to work through the accompanying guilt of this period in a more comfortable manner.

On the other hand, a child who has always attended religious services with his parents may suddenly, in his teens, decide that he no longer wants to go with them. This change may be due to the child's need to form his own identify, one separate from his parents and family. This does not mean that he actually wants to separate physically from his family. Instead, he wants to be accepted as a unique person within the family structure rather than as a member who follows the family indiscriminately with no thoughts or opinions of his own. His expression of drives is as follows:

Libidinal: initially same-sex friendships with large peer groups, developing into heterosexual relationships

Aggressive: ambivalence, conflict with authority figures, active sports involvement, emotional separation from parents (attains a sense of individuality)

Freud viewed the end of the genital stage as the final step in the development of personality. If the conflict of this and earlier stages are resolved, the outcome of the genital stage is *the ability to love and the ability to work* (DiCaprio, 1976; Erikson, 1963; Kaplan and Sadock, 1981; Freud, 1933, 1959; Hinsie and Campbell, 1977; Usdin and Lewis, 1979).

● ● ●

Freud believed in the need for all human beings to experience pleasure through the release of their instincts or drives. The main drive in a young baby is to have something in his mouth. There are no bounds in the child as he attempts to put *anything* in his mouth. Think about the tranquility of the infant once he begins nursing. If he loses the nipple, what is his reaction? It is total, overwhelming rage.

Essentially, these same forces operate in every human being during all the psychosexual stages, except that the primary zones of gratification are different. The drives are less obvious because they slowly come under the control of the ego and its defenses. At the same time, the child is gradually socialized by the authority persons in his environment, and he wants their approval. He develops self-restraint (superego). Freud believed that the amount of restraint and discipline imposed on the child determines, to a great extent, the successful resolution of each state. Too little restraint can be as detrimental as too much.

If too little or too much restraint is imposed on the developing child during the various stages, *fixations* can occur. A fixation is the incomplete working through of one of the earlier stages of psychosexual development. Results of incomplete maturing during the oral phase are, for example, persons who chain smoke or overeat compulsively. They are still seeking the oral pleasure of infancy. These fixations eventually become a part of a person's adult personality traits. *Personality traits* are ingrained behavior patterns that characterize the way an individual interacts with another (Kaplan and Sadock, 1981).

Erikson: Psychosocial Stages of Development

Erik Erikson was born in 1902 in Germany. His father abandoned his mother before he was born, and he was raised by his mother and stepfather. For many years he was unaware that his stepfather was not his real father. It is interesting that his main interests, as he developed his theories, dealt with identity and the confusion and crises that occur as man seeks to understand himself (Kaplan and Sadock, 1981).

He described the psychosocial development of the human being on a continuum from birth to death. He believed that there are four major phases in life: childhood, adolescence, adulthood, and old age. He further subdivided these phases into eight psychosocial stages with specific developmental tasks.

A *developmental task* is a challenge that a person's ego must work at and resolve during sequential stages of growth. Three steps mark each stage of development: the *immature phase*, when the ego first becomes aware of the challenge; the *critical phase*, when the ego works at the challenge; and the *resolution phase*, which occurs if the challenge is met and the outcome successful. The other possible outcome of the critical phase is failure to resolve the challenge of the crisis. Erikson believed that if the crisis is not worked through in the critical stage, the opportunity to resolve it will recur later.

The stages and the developmental challenges that are involved are described below. The desired personality trait is contrasted to the trait that develops if the critical phase of that stage is not resolved (DiCaprio, 1976; Erikson, 1963).

Early infancy (birth to 1 year)

Trust vs. mistrust
   Trust: result of receiving affection and feeling valued
   Mistrust: result of deprivation, abuse, isolation, lack of love, too early or too harsh weaning

Basic qualities acquired: drive and hope

Later infancy (1 to 3 years)

Autonomy vs. shame and doubt
   Autonomy: beginning of differentiation from parents; still dependent
   Shame and doubt: inhibition of self; poor self-confidence; afraid to develop new skills

Basic qualities acquired: self-control and will power

Compare these first two stages of Erikson's to Margaret Mahler's separation-individuation theory. Their theories were developed separately but contain very similar viewpoints.

Early childhood (4 to 5 years)

Initiative vs. guilt
   Initiative: begins to imitate and model self after authority figures; imagination flourishes; testing behavior
   Guilt: conscience is developing in too harsh a manner; lacking in spontaneity; evasive

Basic qualities acquired: direction and purpose

Middle childhood (6 to 11 years)

Industry vs. inferiority
   Industry: better able to set realistic goals for self; sense of accomplishment about efforts; motivated to adhere to social rules
   Inferiority: feelings of inadequacy; dooms self

before any new project is begun; does not assert self

Basic qualities acquired: method and competence

Puberty and adolescence (12 to 20 years)

Ego identity vs. role confusion
Ego identity: positive self-image and sense of identity (who am I?); idealistic; sexual preference for opposite sex; open to mentor relationships
Role confusion: self-conscious; poor value judgment; bisexual confusion; work role confusion

Basic qualities acquired: devotion and fidelity

This is the point at which Freud stops describing personality development. Erikson believed that a human being's personality continues to develop after adolescence is completed. He teaches that human beings continue to go through stages of conflict and crisis resolution during the remainder of life.

Early adulthood (20 to 40 years)

Intimacy vs. isolation
Intimacy: ability to commit self to others in meaningful relationships (Developmental challenge of trust may be reawakened.)
Isolation: aloof; overuse of avoidance or withdrawal in relationships; demeaning manner with others; promiscuous (This trait is actually a denial of one's own basic need of a lasting loving relationship.)

Basic qualities acquired: affiliation and love

Middle adulthood (40 to 60 years)

Generativity vs. stagnation
Generativity: productive; creative; establishing and guiding the next generation: children, younger co-workers, students
Stagnation: self-love excludes others' needs; nonproductive and noncontributing; chronic sickliness; hypochondriasis

Basic qualities acquired: productivity and ability to care for and about others

Late adulthood (60 years and older)

Ego integrity vs. despair
Ego integrity: satisfaction with self and the way that life has been lived; able to let go of past; complacent about future events; Sense of peace

Despair: fear of death; longing for past; wish to relive life and do things differently; regrets; feelings of disgust (may mask despair)

Basic qualities acquired: renunciation (letting go) and wisdom

Maslow: Hierarchy of Human Needs

Abraham Maslow was born in 1908 in New York City and died in 1970. His undergraduate and graduate degrees in psychology were obtained at the University of Wisconsin. He was chairman of the department of psychology at Brandeis University. Maslow was one of the founders of *humanistic psychology*. He believed that personality develops because of a person's need for satisfaction, happiness, and growth. This is contrasted to the theories of the other main schools of psychology: behavioral, in which the human being is motivated by the avoidance of punishment; and psychoanalysis, in which the human being develops because of the need to decrease or relieve the tension of drives (DiCaprio, 1974).

Maslow believed that there are five levels of needs in human beings. He called his theory the *hierarchy of human needs*. The main view of his theory is that the first level of needs must be met before one can strive for the next level of needs, the second level must be met before one can strive for the third, and so on. The needs are organized according to their potency and primacy (Kaplan and Sadock, 1981). Compare these needs with the theories of Freud, Erikson, and Skinner. Are there similarities? Differences? Think about them in relation to the adult with a major illness. In the last analysis, think of them in relation to yourself.

Physiological Needs

The needs for food, shelter, sleep, sexual gratification, physiological equilibrium, and lack of pain are physiological needs. They are essential to all human beings. If these needs are not met, death will result.

Safety Needs

All human beings need safety from harm and a predictable social and physical environment. Safety needs are required by all persons from birth through old age. Even the infant needs security. If the needs are partially unfulfilled, then, depending on the severity, serious emotional damage can occur because of the chronic effect of fear.

Love and Belonging Needs

All people need family, friends, social aceptance, and enduring intimacy. This need awakens in the older infant as he develops an awareness of the social environment and the people who care for him. He needs his family members. As he matures, he thrives on his interaction with them and with other people. This need level is essential for full social development but is not achieved by all persons. For the infant, failure of this need occurs if his family is unable to show love for him. There are shy, aloof adults or those with psychiatric disturbance who are not able to feel loved by anyone. They also are frequently unable to feel love for others.

Esteem Needs

The need for self-worth, positive self-image, and self-acceptance is universal. This need develops in the child as a result of the approval he receives from his family. In the adult, these needs can be classified into two parts: a desire for a sense of competence about oneself and a desire for a good reputation. The positive outcome of these needs depends first on the person's valuation of himself, his worth to his family, and the community at large. Satisfaction with his work is an important aspect of esteem needs. Many adults are unable to move beyond this level because of a lack of self-confidence or a feeling of dissatisfaction about their role in life.

Self-actualization Need

The need to develop to one's *full* potential is the self-actualization need. This need is one that is experienced as an unspecific discontent with one's life. For example, Gail Sheehy (1976) has dis-cussed the midlife experience of persons who want to develop new skills or new life styles. Maslow believes that a person *must* be what he *can* be (Sheehy, 1976; Kaplan and Sadock, 1981; Maslow, 1970).

It is important to remember that many people experience such feelings but are restricted by their life circumstances and unable to pursue their dream. Take, for example, the bright young black person in the ghetto who is scorned by family and peers because of his educational and social aspirations and lacks anyone to support him emotionally or financially, the car mechanic with four children who dreams of being able to go to college at night to become an engineer, and the woman whose children are in school and who wants to return to her former profession but whose husband will not allow it.

The goal of achieving full actualization is believed by Maslow to be a constant drive in humans. Once survival-oriented needs are fulfilled, the human being can move on toward growth-oriented needs. The goal of achieving full actualization or full development of one's potential is viewed as a major life force or drive. Maslow believes it is the motivation behind all human behavior.

Conclusion

These theories of personality development are important to you in understanding your patients' responses to illness because personality dynamics are never static; they are constantly changing. The forces that operated in a person when he was a child continue to operate in him as an adult. In addition, when the stress of illness occurs, a person will normally regress to earlier levels of personality development. By being aware of these earlier levels of development, you may be able to identify maladaptive regression or other evidences of maladaptive response to illness.

As a young child develops, he learns that some of his behaviors are accepted and approved of by the important people in his life. He also learns that certain of his behaviors are not acceptable to them. When 3-year-old Tommy throws his toy truck at his baby brother because the baby's crying annoys him, he learns quickly that this is unacceptable behavior.

The motivation that caused Tommy to throw the truck was his aggressive drive. When he felt the angry urge, he obeyed it. His mother's displeasure taught him that she would not accept his lack of control. Remember that one of Tommy's greatest needs is to have his mother love him. If he makes her unhappy with him, he feels the loss of her approval. After many similar experiences, Tommy eventually realizes that if he follows his original urge to do something that his mother disapproves of, he will probably get spanked and she will not be nice to him for a while.

He internalizes the restrictions of his home environment. When he begins to do something "bad," something inside his head warns him, "Maybe you'd better not do that." Whenever there is conflict in a normal person between what he wants to do (the libidinal or aggressive id drives) and what he believes he should do (the watchfulness of the superego), the result is an unpleasant feeling called *anxiety*. Anxiety is the emotion experienced when the id drives and the superego are in disagreement. Anxiety is experienced in the ego. Chapter 2 discussed the fact that the healthy ego is a person's very good friend and ally. It attempts at all times to protect itself from unpleasant anxiety-producing feelings and urges. This ever-watchful protectiveness results from automatic devices that the ego uses to defend itself. These automatic devices are called *defense mechanisms*.

A defense mechanism is an unconscious device used by the ego to protect itself from the feelings of conflict and anxiety that result from the impulses and drives of the id. It also will be called an *unconscious mental maneuver* or *mental mechanism*. In all instances these terms refer to the continuous monitoring by the ego of a person's feeling state or of his reaction to the environment; the ego is constantly alert to events that can cause dysphoric feelings in order to buffer or eliminate them. *Dysphoria* denotes any unpleasant feeling. The average person is usually unaware that these mechanisms are in use; because they are used by the ego to defend itself, the ego accepts them as natural.

4

The Use of Defense Mechanisms in Physical Illness

As mentioned earlier, all observations about a person's internal and external world are perceived in the ego. It quickly evaluates anything that it perceives. It is as if the ego has a receiving area that examines things before it admits them to its awareness. Anything that is compatible with the ego is allowed to enter the awareness of the ego. When ideas or impulses are acceptable to the ego, they are called *ego-syntonic.* When ideas or impulses are unacceptable to the ego and could potentially cause it to feel anxiety, they are called *ego-dystonic* (Hinsie and Campbell, 1977). When the ego senses an ego-dystonic occurrence, whether it is an internal impulse or external awareness, it unconsciously prepares to shut it out entirely, forget it, or distort it in some way so that it is not so unacceptable or anxiety provoking.

One of the main functions of the ego is to mediate and be the peacemaker between the id and the superego or the id and the environment. Another way that it defends itself is by shutting out painful external reality. A good example is that of a high school student taking College Board examinations. He or she could become overwhelmed by anxiety and not test well. A better possibility is that the ego may defend against some of the anxiety so that it is brought down to a more normal level and the test results accurately reflect the student's ability.

In the examples described above, the ego is defending itself from unpleasant feelings. Chapter 2 described several important functions of the ego. One of them is to form defense mechanisms so that unpleasant feelings can be avoided.

Carson (1979) has identified the various situations that cause the ego to respond with a defense mechanism. Whenever the ego begins to feel anxious or threatened, it quickly reacts to protect itself. The conditions that cause the ego to defend itself are as follows:

An increase in instinctual drives at puberty

Stimulation from without (the environment) that stirs the instinctual drives (a highly stimulating festive occasion or a seductive relationship)

External events that impair ego functions (extreme stress, such as the death of a loved one)

Physiologic impairment of ego functions (alcohol, fatigue, illness)

Ego deficits secondary to emotional stress during the formative years (neurotic illness or personality disorders) [p. 67].

The Importance of Recognizing Patients' Use of Defense Mechanisms

The ego uses defense mechanisms *whenever* it senses any unpleasant or *potentially* unpleasant feeling. The ego is determined to protect itself. The final result of a defense mechanism is that the unpleasant feeling is either eliminated completely or is minimized. If the ego is not strong enough to defend itself fully, there will be an underuse of defenses; the result will be anxiety or depression (Cassem, 1978; Sheehan, 1978). When the patient's ego either overuses or underuses defense mechanisms, the possible outcome is maladaptation.

Some patients *never* overcome the negative effects of the less mature types of defense mechanisms that develop during their hospitalization. As a result of this maladaptation, they *and* their families may be subject to major changes in the quality of their lives. These life changes occur for many hospital patients. The clues that the patient is not adapting well can be seen by the astute observer while the patient is still in the hospital. These "clues" are actually the patient's unconscious underuse or overuse of defense mechanisms, which can undermine his overall coping ability. When the patient is described as "not coping well," it means that his defense mechanisms are failing and are not being used, or that his defense mechanisms may be blocking out or distorting the reality of the situation.

As described in Chapter 1, the nurse may be the best person to observe these clues because of the amount of time he or she spends with the patient. Another important point to be aware of is that the patient may be responding appropriately to his illness or hospitalization but one or more of his family members may not be. Remember that although the patient is coping well in the hospital, when he is discharged he will reenter the family system and will be detrimentally affected by maladaptation in his family. If a wife views her husband as an invalid, for example, and develops acute anxiety or depression about his situation, it will seriously affect the man's own adjustment. Again, the nurse's observations and intervention with the family can be highly important during the hospitalization period. Your sensitive observations and appropriate intervention can have a definite effect on a patient's well-being *after* discharge.

Is There a Difference Between Coping and Defense Mechanisms?

Various textbooks provide many definitions for and sometimes distinguish between *coping* and *defense mechanisms*. In order to simplify your understanding of these terms, they will be clarified in this chapter. Defense mechanisms are used by the ego as a means of dealing with reality or with unpleasant feelings. They operate beyond a person's conscious awareness.

The following definitions of coping and defense mechanisms appear in Hinsie and Campbell's *Psychiatric Dictionary* (1977):

> Coping. Adjusting; adapting; successfully meeting a challenge. Coping mechanisms are all the ways, both conscious and unconscious, which a person uses in adjusting to environmental demands without altering his goals or purposes [p. 163].
>
> Defense mechanism. The means by which the organism (human being) protects itself against impulses and affects [p. 182].

These definitions indicate that coping mechanisms are all of the mental maneuvers that the ego uses to protect itself from unwanted reality in the external world or environment. Defense mechanism is the term used to describe one type of mental maneuver the ego automatically uses to protect itself against internal reality: what the person is feeling *inside* vs. what he is perceiving *outside* of himself. The following case example may shed some light on what may initially seem confusing:

Case Example

Tom is a 42-year-old married father of 3 children. After experiencing some warning symptoms, he was admitted to the hospital for a cancer workup. Within only a few days he had abdominal exploratory surgery, and metastatic carcinoma was discovered. When his surgeon told Tom the diagnosis, he developed the mechanism of denial because he was unable to cope immediately with the devastating news of his prognosis. This was an unconscious defense mechanism.

The term *coping* is used to describe the ways that the ego attempts to maintain intrapsychic stability during times of increased stress. They include conscious stress management devices such as talking out a problem, jogging, and so on. The other major coping strategy is the unconscious use of defense mechanisms. Because unconscious defense mechanisms can be the greatest ally of the ego in defending itself from severe anxiety or depression, they have a strong effect on a person's adaptive capacity. When they are maladaptive, however, they can result in coping failure. A broader view of coping and its components will be presented in Chapter 9: Stress: Its Implications in Physical Illness.

Development of Defense Mechanisms

Defense mechanisms develop as a protective response to the unacceptable drives or impulses of the id. The ego of the young child uses certain basic defenses. If he grows up in a positive environment, these early defenses gradually yield and give way to more mature ways of coping. The ego is a creature of habit as it pertains to defense mechanisms. Once the ego uses a certain way of dealing with stress, either an internal or external stressor, it usually continues to defend itself in the same way.

When the ego experiences relief in a stressful situation, it usually will try the same approach in another stressful occurrence. For example, when Tommy felt the original angry urge toward his brother, he threw a toy at him. After he was spanked he learned that his mother would not tolerate his actions. The next time he felt angry toward his brother, his superego warned him not to do it again or he would be sorry. But, what happened to his anger? It must have been uncomfortable for Tommy to be so angry but not be able to anything about it.

The peacemaker ego, which wanted to help Tommy feel better, devised a way of reducing the unpleasant feeling (anxiety) that was the result of his anger (id drive) being in conflict with his mother's wishes (internalized in his primitive superego). The mechanism that his ego used provided immediate relief because it eliminated the angry feelings and the anxiety that they aroused in him.

One day later, he dug up his mother's tulip bulbs while making tunnels for his toy cars in her garden. When his father came home after a very tiring day, he lost his temper with Tommy and lectured him very harshly. After the lecture,

Tommy experienced the same feelings of anger that he had felt toward his brother. He also experienced the same urge to retaliate in some way. He went to his room to get his crayons and then went to the hall closet to scribble on his father's briefcase.

As he was ready to draw on the case, he remembered the consequences of his anger and actions of the day before. His ego automatically used the same defense mechanism it had used successfully the day before. It will typically continue to use the same response in similar stressful situations until the child grows older and masters the various developmental hurdles described by Erikson and Freud; then the ego will cope in a more mature manner. It may come as a surprise to you to learn that the defense mechanisms that adults automatically use were well established by the age of 6 years (Fenichel, 1945; Freud, 1946). These defenses form the basis of the way that people respond to all types of stress and also the way that they relate to others. In essence, they determine a person's personality style and the way he is viewed by others.

Levels of Defense Mechanisms

Four different levels of defense mechanisms have been described (Kaplan and Sadock, 1981): narcissistic, immature, neurotic, and mature. The following list of defense mechanisms is arranged in order of their development in human beings, the narcissistic level being the earliest level of defense (Kaplan and Sadock, 1981; Usdin and Lewis, 1979; Vaillant, 1977):

Levels of Human Defense Mechanisms

Narcissistic defense mechanisms
Denial
Delusional projection
Distortion

Immature defense mechanisms
Acting-out behavior
Avoidance
Hypochondriasis
Passive-aggressive behavior
Projection
Regression

Neurotic defense mechanisms
Displacement
Identification

Isolation
Reaction formation
Repression

Mature defense mechanisms
Anticipation
Sublimation
Humor
Altruism
Suppression

The remainder of the chapter will present the various defenses used by *normal* persons as they cope with stress. As described above, the defenses have been classified according to their appearance during a person's psychological development. While taking a psychology course a student learns about defense mechanisms and reads descriptions of the various defenses. These descriptions tend to be classic examples, but they may be described in a manner that omits their underlying dynamics or are explained in complicated and confusing terms.

In this book the defenses will be explained using actual case examples from the hospital environment. In each case, some of the characteristics of the specific incidents have been changed so that patient confidentiality is maintained. The defenses have been classified according to their appearance during a person's psychological development; early defenses give way to later, more mature defenses.

The use of defense mechanisms that nurses observe in patients will depend on each patient's previous experiences with stress and conscious ability to cope actively with illness as well as the ego's use of unconscious defense mechanisms. For example, a 70-year-old man may be admitted to the hospital with his first exposure to major illness. It may tax his ability to cope far more than it would affect a 30-year-old man who is chronically ill and has been hospitalized on several occasions. These concepts will be more fully presented in Chapter 9: Stress: Its Implications in Physical Illness, Chapter 13: Psychosocial Nursing Assessment and Diagnosis and Chapter 15: Crisis Intervention With the Maladapting Patient.

It is important to remember the function of a defense mechanism; it is used by the ego whenever it senses danger. The main purpose of a defense mechanism is to relieve anxiety. All types of defense mechanisms can potentially be used by the ego in its attempt to adapt to an unpleasant internal or environmental awareness. Defense mechanisms are *always* adaptive because they help a person to cope with an otherwise difficult situation. If the defense mechanism either fails or is very rigid, however, it can result in negative and moderate to long-lasting changes in the person's intrapsychic and interpersonal functioning. At that point, the *original adaptive mechanism becomes maladaptive.*

It is essential to understand the difference between an adaptive outcome and a maladaptive outcome in the use of a particular defense mechanism. The clinical examples described under the defensive functions include behavioral characterstics of both adaptive and maladaptive defensive reactions to the stress of illness and hospitalization. Some of the defense mechanisms are intrinsically pathological, however. Accordingly, there will be no examples of positive adaptation.

Narcissistic Defense Mechanisms

The defenses used by the ego start very early in life. The first defenses, which occur unconsciously, begin in the first year of life. These *narcissistic defense mechanisms* are commonly used by children under age 5 and give way to a higher and more mature level of defense at that time. They are used by the ego when external reality is too threatening.

The normally well-adjusted adult may regress to this early level for a brief period during very acute stress or during dreaming or periods of fantasy (Lewis and Levy, 1982; Vaillant, 1977). These mechanisms, when used by persons with severe psychopathology, form the basis for psychosis.

A *psychosis* is a mental disorder in which a person loses touch with reality for varying periods. The intellectual, feeling, and perceptual spheres are affected. As a result, his relations with other persons are impaired, and he is dysfunctional during the psychotic episodes (Kaplan and Sadock, 1981). There are two main types of psychosis. Those caused by physiological disruption of the brain are called *organic brain syndrome.* They will be described in Chapter 11: Organic Brain Syndrome. The other group of psychoses are caused by functional failure of the psyche. They include schizophrenia and manic-depressive illness. These dysfunctional illnesses will not be covered in this book because they are well described in most psychiatric nursing textbooks.

The psychotic person has lost touch with reality. To the observer he seems to be in his own world. Persons who routinely display the symptoms that represent these defenses have psychiatric illnesses that include active psychotic stages: schizophrenia, manic-depressive illness, acute organic brain syndrome, and acute psychotic depression (*A Psychiatric Glossary,* 1975). The defenses in this category are denial, delusional projection, and distortion.

Denial

Denial is a mechanism that the ego uses to shut out external reality that is too frightening or threatening to tolerate. The person sees, hears, or perceives the event through any of the senses but refuses to recognize it consciously. The memory of the threatening reality is stored in the unconscious, however.

The two types of denial are explained below.

Case Examples

Adaptive denial. A 28-year-old-mother of one child was admitted to the hospital because of an undiagnosed lower abdominal mass. During exploratory surgery a malignant tumor of the uterus was discovered, and a total hysterectomy and oophorectomy were performed. The physician saw the patient that afternoon to tell her what he had found. When she saw him again the following morning, she had no memory of seeing him the day before nor any memory of her diagnosis. Later that day when he spoke to her, she was able to comprehend the meaning of his words. Her original denial prevented her from being overwhelmed with anxiety. The next day denial gave way to awareness, when she was able to acknowledge the situation.

Maladaptive denial. A 45 year-old-man was discharged from the hospital after coronary bypass surgery. He was properly instructed on all aspects of his discharge program, which involved 3 months of progressive increases in his activity. During his hospitalization and after his discharge he rarely thought about the changes in his life that his heart disease and bypass surgery would cause. Despite many overtures by his wife to find out how he was thinking and feeling, he refused to talk about his illness. Five weeks after discharge he played tennis on a warm afternoon and then went out with his friends for some cold beers. The next afternoon, when his wife was at work, he was bored and decided to move an old washing machine in his basement.

Delusional Projection

Delusional projection is a mechanism by which the ego develops a false belief that is abnormal for the person's intelligence and cultural background (Kaplan and Sadock, 1981). In delusional projection the person believes that someone is "out to get him." This mechanism has a persecutory basis. In severe psychopathology it forms the basis of paranoid psychosis. Examples of delusional projection are presented below.

Case Example

Adaptive delusional projection. Delusional projection is not an adaptive mechanism in adults.

Maladaptive delusional projection. A 54-year-old man was admitted to the intensive care surgical unit after open-heart surgery. Twelve hours postoperatively, with no precipitating event, he suddenly pulled out his endotracheal tube and all of his lines and other tubes. When the nurses tried to restrain him, he severely hit one of them because he thought she was trying to choke him. On the next day he returned to his preoperative mental state and reported that his greatest fear, since he was a child, was of choking and having something caught in his throat so that he could not breathe.

This patient had been extremely apprehensive preoperatively, and, despite efforts by nursing staff to help him discuss his fears, he was unable to do so. This deep fear was compounded by the effects of anesthesia and many drugs, which relaxed the normal defensive functions of his ego. *Decompensation,* the breakdown of his higher level of defenses, then occurred, and psychosis due to organic brain syndrome resulted.

Distortion

Distortion is a mechanism that the ego uses to reshape external reality to suit internal needs. The ego twists and distorts the aspects of reality that it cannot tolerate. It is the basis for hallucinations and nonparanoid types of delusions (Kaplan and Sadock, 1981).

Examples of distortion are presented next.

Case Examples

Adaptive distortion. Nine-year-old Timmy is a terminally ill youngster hospitalized with leukemia. His parents live 40 miles from the hospital, and both of them work. One of the nurses resembles Timmy's mother. When he is semiconscious and sees her face, he believes it is his mother. He feels safe and secure when the nurse is at the bedside.

Maladaptive distortion. Henry is 32. He weighs 350 pounds and is five feet nine inches tall. He has hypertension. After a medical examination, his physician told him that he had to lose weight in order to maintain a reasonable level of health. He was told to start dieting. The physician reviewed with him the number of calories he should eat in a day and the amounts and types of food he would be restricted to. During the discussion, Henry asked if it were possible that he had a "gland" problem that caused him to gain excessive weight. His physician said that he doubted it. After he left the office, Henry ignored the recommended diet, believing instead that his obesity was caused by some type of glandular problem that he could not control.

Immature Defense Mechanisms

The second level of defenses are called *immature defense mechanisms.* They operate unconsciously. They begin to occur around the age of 3 years and are seen in healthy children and adolescents until the age of 15 or 16 (Usdin and Lewis, 1979; Vaillant, 1977). They should be replaced in mid-adolescence by a more mature level of defenses and not be used by the adult ego unless it is under moderate to severe stress. If these mechanisms are not relinquished and are routinely used by the adult ego, the result will be a person with major character flaws (Vaillant, 1977). These major character flaws form the basis of disabling personality disorders (see Chap. 5) and borderline states (Fenichel, 1945). The immature defenses are acting out, avoidance, hypochondriasis, passive-aggressive behavior, projection, and regression. There are no adaptive uses for many of these defenses.

Acting-out Behavior

Acting-out behavior is the outward manifestation of an inner need. The inner need causes feelings that the person cannot tolerate, making him impulsively act them out (Vaillant, 1977). This inner tension that develops is not dealt with; instead, it is acted out behaviorally in an impulsive-appearing and immature way.

Examples of acting-out behavior follow.

Case Examples

Adaptive acting-out behavior. John is a 16-year-old who was diagnosed as a diabetic 3 months ago. At various times he describes feeling angry about the restrictions that his illness has imposed on his young life and his future. Whenever his level of frustration becomes uncomfortable, his football coach notices that he is far more aggressive on the practice field.

Maladaptive acting-out behavior. John's friend in the diabetic clinic is 17 and feels equally frustrated at times. In fact, sometimes he says he feels like exploding. Sometimes he describes himself as feeling very confused. He was diagnosed 7 months ago. Since that time, he has become verbally abusive to all his family members and is not doing well in school. He frequently gets drunk on weekends, although he never did so before his diabetes was diagnosed. He is abusive to himself as well.

Avoidance

Avoidance is a defense mechanism that may seem similar to denial. Using this mechanism a person unconsciously shuns any situation, object, or activity that might arouse any unwanted sexual or aggressive impulses (Hinsie and Campbell, 1977). It is also unconsciously used to avoid any encounter that will result in unpleasant and undesired emotional reactions. It differs from denial in the following way: with denial, there is an unconscious refusal to recognize a traumatic reality. With avoidance, there is an unconscious refusal to encounter a traumatic reality because it would provoke too much anxiety. The person is never aware of the reason for the change in his motivation.

Examples of avoidance follow.

Case Examples

Adaptive avoidance. Alice, a 55-year-old woman, was admitted to the hospital for a breast biopsy because of a nontender mass. The biopsy revealed cancer of the breast. A simple mastectomy was performed. Alice ac-cepted the diagnosis and subsequent surgery with no acute emotional distress. She was able to talk about it with her nurse. Two days postoperatively she unexpectedly suffered a stroke of moderate severity and developed paresis of one side. Although she was able to talk, she did not discuss her breast surgery or cancer diagnosis. When her nurse asked general questions about them, the patient focused instead on the effects of her stroke.

If Alice's avoidance of awareness of her breast surgery and cancer diagnosis continues beyond a few days, her potential for maladaptation is increased.

Maladaptive avoidance. Marian is a 32-year-old married woman who has no children. Her mother took the drug diethylstilbestrol (DES) when she was pregnant with Marian. As a result, Marian is at risk for cervical cancer. She has had two positive Papanicolaou tests during the previous 5 years and has had a cone biopsy of the cervix. Her gynecologist cautioned her that she should return for 3-month checkups because of her high susceptibility. Marian is highly anxious about the future. She knows that she will not be able to have children if a hysterectomy must be performed. During the previous year, she was lax in making appointments at 3-month intervals and, in fact, cancelled one of them when she was asked to substitute in a tennis match.

Hypochondriasis

Hypochondriasis is a mechanism used by the ego when it has real or imagined aggressive, critical feelings toward others and finds them unwelcome and disturbing. Self-reproach may also be experienced when these feelings result from loneliness or unresolved grief. This resentment is turned back on the ego and is experienced as guilt. The guilt is transformed into physical complaints. The unconsciously motivated development of these symptoms frequently occurs when the person experiences anger because his need to be cared for is not being met (Usdin and Lewis, 1979; Vaillant, 1977). By complaining about physical ailments, the social system may respond by giving the person more care and attention.

This attentive response by others is unconsciously and consciously what the person has been looking for. It is called *secondary gain*. He seeks either attention or the satisfaction of his need for love, which was never completely met during the first years of life (Hinsie and Campbell, 1977).

An example of hypochondriasis is discussed below.

Case Example

Maladaptive hypochondriasis. Sue, aged 35, is admitted to the hospital with chronically recurring abdominal pain. Her physical history reveals that she has had three major abdominal surgeries: An exploratory laparotomy at age 24, a cholecystectomy at age 27, and a total hysterectomy at age 31. The surgeries were performed by different surgeons. Her physician in this admission is yet another surgeon. The pathology reports of the removed organs revealed no demonstrable pathology. Sue has three children. Her firstborn died 14 years ago at birth. She talks about her as if she has died recently and were actually a recent member of the family. Her husband is a salesman who is away from home for prolonged periods. Whenever Sue has had previous surgeries, he has taken leaves from work to be with her.

Passive–Aggressive Behavior

Passive-aggressive behavior is the outward manifestation of anger that the person is not able to express directly toward another. Instead, it is expressed passively in ways that are frequently self-defeating (Hinsie and Campbell, 1977).

An example of passive-aggressive behavior follows.

Case Example

Maladaptive passive-aggressive behavior. A woman of 68 with myasthenia gravis of 4 years' duration was admitted to the hospital because of worsening symptoms. She was depressed and discouraged. She reported that her husband had been her sole caregiver since she had become more incapacitated during the last 2 years. She required diapers at home because of urinary incontinence. Because of weak muscles, she depended on him heavily for her mobility. She reported that he had always been very helpful and "like a saint" until the previous 4 months. During that time, he increasingly ignored her calls for help and, at other times, delayed coming to her for longer and longer periods when she asked him for help. He frequently used profanity, which she was unaccustomed to hearing from him, and it offended her. He had previously been talkative

and open with her but recently had become uncommunicative. She was afraid to go home with him and believed that it was his negative behavior that had precipitated her hospital admission.

Projection

Projection is a less pathological form of delusional projection, described above. Its basic dynamics are the same, but the ego uses it in a less disturbed way. It occurs when a person is unable to acknowledge thoughts or feelings in oneself and attributes them to others (Vaillant, 1977).

Projection is described below.

Case Example

Maladaptive projection. Anna, a 32-year-old woman with lupus erythematosus, belongs to a support group. During the group meetings she frequently asks questions such as "Mary, aren't you worried that you may become an invalid?" or, "Tom, aren't you afraid that your family is going to give up on you?" When the group leader asks Anna if these questions might pertain to her, she replies that she knows that the remission is going to "hold" and that her husband and children have been "wonderful." Actually, Anna is deeply concerned about these issues, but her ego fears being overwhelmed by the anxiety that would occur if she were consciously aware of them. These projections are outward signs of her own unconscious fears. It is as if they were slipping through cracks in her ego's defensive armor.

Regression

Regression is a mechanism used by the ego when it is severely threatened by environmental stress or when there is internal psychic stress during a particular stage of personality development. As a result, the personality functioning returns to an earlier level (Vaillant, 1977).

An example of regression follows.

Case Example

Maladaptive regression. A 29-year-old woman was admitted to the hospital with symptoms of low-grade fever, bleeding from her gums, petechiae, and an enlarged liver and spleen. After 3 days of diagnostic testing, chronic myelocytic leukemia was diagnosed. Shortly after admission, the patient became quiet and increasingly uncommunicative. She never expressed her thoughts or feelings.

Once the diagnosis was certain, she began to sleep more and more often during the day. The nurses noted that she slept in a fetal position. Her physical condition deteriorated rapidly during the next few days. Despite every type of diagnostic test, her doctors were baffled by the cause of her worsening condition. Within a week she was moved to the intensive care unit in a coma. She died within 3 days. At the time of her admission to the intensive care unit, it was learned from her family that she had been an unusually active member of the state leukemia society. Two years earlier her favorite female cousin had died after a prolonged, difficult course of leukemia. Five years earlier her younger brother had died of the same disease.

Nurses know that the effects of psychological stress can result in physiological changes as a result of action by the autonomic nervous system (Selye, 1979). Is it possible for intense psychological stress to cause death? If this woman's caregivers had known her psychosocial history, would psychiatric intervention have been appropriate once the diagnosis was determined and a maladaptive response was noted? Do you think that such intervention could have made a difference in the final outcome?

Neurotic Defense Mechanisms

The next level of defenses begin to occur at approximately the same age as the immature defenses. The difference between them is that, although classified as *neurotic defense mechanisms*, they are used by "healthy" adults throughout their lifetimes. They are seen as quirks in otherwise normally adjusted human beings. They are used to deal with stressful situations (Vaillant, 1977). If one or more of these defenses are heavily used and affect the person's capacity to enjoy life, they cause a *neurosis*.

A neurosis differs from a psychosis in that the neurotic is not as seriously disturbed as the psychotic. In *neurosis*, only a part of the personality is affected and perception of reality is not grossly affected; the quality of life is usually affected, however. In psychosis, most of the ego functions are disturbed. The quality of reality of the

psychotic person is changed markedly (Hinsie and Campbell, 1977). Psychiatric conditions in which the overuse of neurotic defenses occur and become crippling are obsessive-compulsive behavior, phobias, hysteria, anxiety, and depressive neuroses (Freedman and colleagues, 1976). The neurotic defenses include displacement, identification, isolation, reaction formation, and repression. They are used unconsciously by the ego (Usdin and Lewis, 1979; Kaplan and Sadock, 1981; Vaillant, 1977).

Repression

Repression (not to be confused with *regression*) is considered to be the main mechanism that the ego uses to defend itself. When the ego uses this mechanism, it unconsciously excludes awareness of thoughts, feelings, urges, fantasies, and memories that would be unacceptable or threatening if they were conscious. Anything that the ego perceives as dangerous may potentially be repressed. Its concept of "dangerous" results from early childhood experiences. Later events that seem entirely unrelated may result in anxiety, which causes the ego to respond by blotting out the current thought or feeling. As a result, the ego does not discriminate in a logical way when it uses repression to defend itself (Usdin and Lewis, 1979).

In some cases, the defenses of repression and denial are confused with one another. The difference is that denial is the mechanism used to defend against painful or unpleasant external reality: events occurring in the environment *outside* the person. Repression is the mechanism used to defend against painful or unpleasant internal reality: feelings or thoughts occurring *inside* the person. In each case there is an initial awareness that the ego instantly recognizes as dangerous or very unpleasant, and it shuts the awareness away into the unconscious.

In order to clarify the differences, think of a patient who hears that she has multiple sclerosis. She finds the diagnosis so threatening that she initially denies it. She used denial to shut out a painful *external* awareness. A few days later she is able to tolerate the diagnosis, and her denial fades. A week after discharge she may begin to experience anxiety as the full awareness of the future effects of the disease become known to her.

Because her ego is unable to tolerate the anxiety, which is a distressing *internal* awareness, it is repressed. It is no longer in her conscious awareness. As she is better able to cope with the changes the illness will cause in her life, the repression will gradually lift. She will move through the normal bereavement process as she becomes aware of the losses the illness will cause in her life. (See Chaps. 6 and 19 for more information about responses to loss and the normal bereavement process.) She will make the necessary adjustments in her relationships and life style. This is an adaptive response. If, on the other hand, the repression continues for a prolonged period and she develops an unresolved grief, maladaptation is the outcome.

Examples of repression follow.

Case Example

Adaptive repression. A 58-year-old woman had a stroke that left her partially paralyzed. She had been a very active woman, and the stroke was going to change many aspects of her life. As she thought about these changes she originally felt overwhelmed, but her ego shut away these negative and frightening feelings. Her energy and hope were invested in constant efforts at rehabilitation.

Maladaptive repression. A male cancer patient of 43 with terminal disease knew that he had cancer, but in conversations with care-givers there was strong evidence that he continually repressed certain aspects of his awareness that it was terminal. Before his illness he was a successful tax attorney who took pride in controlling all aspects of his family's finances. His wife, who was quite a dependent person, supported his repression with her own; she was unconsciously terrified of being left alone to raise their children. Other members of the family and his close friends were concerned because the two of them were not discussing the location of his will, insurance policies, or stock certificates. She had never been advised of their existence, let alone their location. She was unprepared to take over the family finances.

Identification

Identification is a mechanism that causes a person to accept the circumstances of other people as though they were actually his own. This acceptance can pertain to others' thoughts, attitudes, feelings, or particular experiences (Usdin and Lewis, 1979).

Examples of identification are presented next.

Case Examples

Adaptive identification. A pregnant woman attended childbirth education classes and was prepared to have natural childbirth. Her two sisters had had natural childbirth and had reported that it was a joyful experience. Their labors were uncomplicated and proceeded well. Before entering the hospital, the young expectant mother had a very positive outlook about her delivery based on the experiences of her sisters. In the delivery room, despite a very prolonged labor, she did well and never seemed to be experiencing unusual distress. She produced a 10½-lb baby boy to the amazement of all.

Maladaptive identification. A 58-year-old man was hospitalized with terminal carcinoma of the lung. The disease had been arrested by chemotherapy, but because of an unusual complication of chemotherapy, there had been heavy scarring of the alveoli; the patient was thus unable to breathe properly. His condition was similar to that of advanced emphysema. He was short of breath, and his level of anxiety was near the panic level. No amount of emotional support or sedation could decrease his panic. He did not know what was causing it, according to his nurses and physicians.

On psychiatric liaison consultation, it was learned that the patient's wife had died 5 years earlier of a pulmonary embolism and severe pulmonary hemorrhage resulting from rupture of an old pulmonary tuberculosis lesion. He had a constant image of his wife's death and was certain that he would die in a similar way, "choking on my own blood." He identified strongly with his dead wife. Once the source of his anxiety was discovered, he was able to understand an explanation that his lung disease was not like that of his wife and that it would be unlikely for him to have the same problem. He was given unlimited time to talk about his fears. His anxiety decreased markedly in only one 30-minute session. For further reinforcement, a second session was scheduled in the afternoon, with positive results. The patient's rate of respiration had slowed to a more comfortable level, and his terror was replaced by a more tolerable level of anxiety.

Isolation

Isolation is a defense by which the ego separates the normal feeling associated with a particular thought or idea. It then represses either the feeling or the idea so that only one of them remains. Usually, it is the thought content that remains. The affect or feeling associated with it is repressed. Other names for this defense are *rationalization* and *intellectualization* (Kaplan and Sadock, 1981; Vaillant, 1977).

Examples of isolation follow.

Case Examples

Adaptive isolation. Marjory is a 22-year-old single woman with a history of Crohn's disease. Since she developed her illness at age 13, she has experienced several exacerbations. Her physicians have told her that she will need an ileostomy within the next year. She is intellectually aware of the implications of ileostomy, especially for a young person, but has never experienced anxiety, feelings of discouragement, or fears of rejection by others in connection with the anticipated surgery. (Eventually, before surgery, Marjory should begin to experience an emotional response that is appropriate. If the isolation persists during the preoperative and postoperative period, it would then be considered a maladaptive response.)

Maladaptive isolation. John, a 48-year-old man, is awaiting repeat bypass surgery for repair of three coronary arteries. It is his second operation in 3 years. Since his first surgery he has been unable to work. His wife reports that he has been depressed since his last surgery. His surgeons are not optimistic about the outcome of surgery. His mortality risk is many times greater than normal, and, if he survives surgery, his cardiac surgeon believes that his rehabilitation potential is poor. His nurses are concerned because he discusses his upcoming surgery and quotes the statistics of his survival in a very neutral way. Despite his nurses' attempts to zero in on his feelings about surgery, he insists "Yes, I am concerned, and my family is worried," and is unable to describe his feelings. His mood is bland, and his face and eyes demonstrate no emotion.

When a patient consistently demonstrates such strong isolation of his feelings in the face of an ominous operation, it is wise that nurses not probe beyond a reasonable level for unacknowledged feelings. Instead, the patient's continuing inability to experience feelings should be pointed out to the physician with an accompanying question about the possible need for psychiatric consultation.

Displacement

Displacement is a defense used by the ego to redirect feelings about one object to another. Although the feelings are shifted, the instinct or motivation behind the feelings remains the same.

Examples of displacement follow.

Case Examples

Adaptive displacement. Kenneth, a 15-year-old boy, has hemophilia. Because of his illness and the danger of hemorrhage, he is unable to participate actively in his school's sports program. Accordingly, his aggressive impulses cannot be released by increased physical activity. When Kenneth was a high school freshman, he became interested in his school's debating team. As a result of his outstanding performance, at the end of his sophomore year he was chosen to represent his school in a regional debating contest. During his first 2 years on the team he demonstrated an unusual dedication to his research preparation for all debates and was without equal in his forceful oratorical presentation, no matter which perspective he was defending.

Maladaptive displacement. Tom, a 29-year-old single ex-construction worker, was injured in a construction accident 2 years ago and is paralyzed below the waist. Despite being a patient at an excellent rehabilitation center, he was poorly motivated and unpleasant to other patients and staff members. Despite opportunities in group meetings to share his feelings about his injury, he remained silent. Although physically rehabilitated, he never seemed to accept his new situation mentally. He has never consciously acknowledged to himself his fury and rage at his paralysis. He is currently living at home with his parents and a single sister. He is working in a factory on an assembly line. At home he is highly critical of his family members and erupts in anger at the slightest provocation. He is avoided at work because of his bad temper and unpleasantness.

Reaction Formation

Reaction formation is a defense used when an impulse or feeling is unacceptable to the ego. As a result, the ego unconsciously does a complete turnabout of the original impulse or feeling. An exact opposite impulse, feeling, thought, or behavior results (Kaplan and Sadock, 1981; Usdin and Lewis, 1979; Vaillant, 1977). The defense of reaction formation is sometimes known as *compensation* (Kreigh and Perko, 1979; Stuart and Sundeen, 1979). Anger or hostility is frequently the underlying impulse or emotion that is being guarded against (Topalis and Aguilera, 1978).

Examples of reaction formation are presented below.

Case Examples

Adaptive reaction formation. Tom's father has chronic arthritis. When Tom was a child, his father frequently had bouts of pain that, Tom believed, he used as a way of getting out of work. His father frequently complained about his pain. Whenever Tom's mother sat down to read or do some leisure activity, it seemed as if his father would frequently ask for some special request that caused her to jump up to meet his needs.

Tom played football in high school. He frequently incurred muscle strains in practice of games. He did not experience any desire to discuss his discomfort with his family.

Maladaptive reaction formation. Arlene, a 34-year-old woman, had a radical mastectomy 3 days ago. At an unconscious level she feels deep rage and anxiety about the removal of her breast. When caregivers enter the room, however, she is cordial, without complaint, and unusually cheerful. She denies any negative emotions about the results of surgery.

Although this response may seem adaptive, it is not. The delay in response may eventually lead to a maladaptive grief response, which is more difficult to resolve.

Mature Defense Mechanisms

The classification of the highest level of ego defenses is the category of *mature defense mechanisms.* They begin to be used around the age of 12 by well-functioning persons at all but the most stressful times. The mature defenses result from successful resolution of conflicts at earlier levels of personality development. They include anticipation, sublimation, humor, altruism, and suppression. The mature defenses are used by the ego either consciously or unconsciously (Kaplan and Sadock, 1981; Usdin and Lewis, 1979; Vaillant,

1977). These defenses are always used in an adaptive manner. If they appear to be used in a maladaptive way, they should not be confused with earlier, less adaptive mechanisms.

Anticipation

Anticipation is a defense by which the ego acknowledges both intellectually and emotionally an upcoming situation that is expected to provoke anxiety. By acknowledging it, some of the anxiety is worked through and resolved in advance.

An example of anticipation follows.

Case Example

Anticipation. Dick is a 19-year-old competitive skier. As the result of numerous accidents, one of his knees requires reconstructive surgery. He is nervous about the upcoming surgery, which is scheduled in 6 weeks. Instead of repressing his anxiety, he acknowledges it and works it through by several means. During the 6-week interim he called his physician and asked several questions about which he was concerned. His physician's answers eliminated some of his concerns. He also asked the physician to give him the names of two other people who had had the same surgery so that he could talk to them about their experiences. After talking to them, some of his concerns about the level of pain he would experience and worries about his rehabilitation were decreased.

Sublimation

Sublimation operates in connection with the defense of repression. In sublimation, a repressed urge or desire is expressed in a socially acceptable or useful way. As a result, the original impulse has a modified outlet, as opposed to being completely blocked (Kaplan and Sadock, 1981; Vaillant, 1977).

An example of sublimation is presented below.

Case Example

Sublimation. A recently divorced man of 41 was admitted to the hospital because of myocardial infarct. During the course of his hospitalization he was sexually attracted to many of the nurses. Instead of talking to them about his feelings, he wrote several poems about the nurses. In the poems he described the nurses' gentleness, kindness, and beauty of character.

Humor

Humor is used by the ego when it cannot fully acknowledge a difficult situation. This adaptive defensive use of humor is done without expense to the self or to others. It also is different from *wit,* in which the attention is diverted from the issue under discussion and the actual anxiety-provoking situation is avoided (Vaillant, 1977).

An example of humor follows.

Case Example

Humor. Bill is a 54-year-old whose right leg was amputated because of poor circulation caused by diabetes mellitus. He was sitting with a group of friends at a break from work, and they were discussing the high prices caused by inflation. One of the men told about his surprise at the cost of having a pair of shoes resoled. Bill replied, "At least I can save money at the shoe repair shop!"

Altruism

Altruism is a mature defense that connects the desire to satisfy one's own narcissistic needs with the desire to satisfy the needs of others. It is different from desiring to meet others' needs in order to relieve guilt feelings or meeting others' needs for other maladaptive reasons. The result of altruism is constructive and gratifying service to others (Vaillant, 1977).

An example of altruism follows.

Case Example

Altruism. Ellen had a laryngectomy at age 49. After years of rehabilitation, she has developed her speech well and is an underwriter for an insurance company. One evening a week, she works with the American Cancer Society teaching laryngectomized patients to speak. When called by ear, nose, and throat surgeons, she also visits patients in the hospital who have recently had laryngectomies.

Suppression

Suppression is a conscious or semiconscious decision to delay paying attention to an unwanted conflict or impulse until a later time. It is a commonly used coping device to postpone dealing with a normally anxiety-provoking situation until it can be dealt with properly (Kaplan and Sadock, 1981; Usdin and Lewis, 1979; Vaillant, 1977).

An example of suppression is presented next.

Case Example

Suppression. Mary's husband has been a patient for 2 months because of severe chronic obstructive pulmonary disease. His condition is terminal, but death is not imminent. Despite her grief about his expected death, she works each day as a supervisor at the telephone company. When she is at work she is immersed in her job and rarely is distracted with thoughts of her husband. On the bus ride home she frequently discusses her feelings about her husband with one of her co-workers, who is a good friend.

Conversion: An Unclassified Defense Mechanism

There is yet another defense mechanism used by the ego as a means of defending itself. It is called *conversion* (Fenichel, 1945). Conversion is seen in some hospital patients, and it is important for the nurse to be aware of it. It is not possible to classify it with the previous defense mechanisms because it is actually composed of elements of other mechanisms. It most frequently occurs in persons who are unable to express their feelings. As a result, they react with bodily symptoms to stressors and conflicts. The inability to express feelings verbally is called *alexithymia.* The word is derived from the following root derivatives: *a,* meaning *without; lex* from the Latin, meaning *word;* and *thymia* from the Greek, meaning *feelings.* The words, when combined, mean "without words to describe feelings." The defense mechanisms involved are repression (of feelings) and displacement (of conflicts and feelings) into bodily symptoms. This phenomenon is sometimes called *somatization* (Kaplan and Sadock, 1981; Nemiah and Sifneos, 1970).

Conversion is an immature mechanism by which the ego changes emotional conflict related to the instinctual pleasure-seeking-sexual drive or the aggressive drive into physical symptoms. It is used at varying levels, some of which are short-lasting; others cause severe impairment. In conversion the person may or may not be aware of the emotional conflict that is causing the physical illness.

An important clinical dynamic that is frequently observed in patients with physical symptoms that are the result of conversion is a history of loss or the threat of loss. Both the pleasure-seeking drive and the aggressive drive are affected by loss. Both the major drives, sexual and aggressive, are affected when an object that was pleasurable to a person is lost. Remember that this object can be another person or an abstract entity such as one's own self-image, a job, or a role that can no longer be fulfilled. When a person's self-image is threatened, he will react with anxiety to this potential loss. A person's ability to work or fulfill certain roles is one of the important dynamics in a positive self-image (Taves and associates, 1963). Both the sexual and aggressive drives motivate a person to work (Freud, 1927). The aggressive drive is also affected when there are deep disappointment, feelings of abandonment, and disillusionment regarding any object (Jacobson, 1971).

It is imperative that persons who are suspected of having illnesses that are psychogenic or "all in the head" have a very thorough physical workup before the etiology is identified as emotional. If the person is suspected of having a psychosomatic illness, caregivers must take care to avoid labeling such patients. Information on psychosomatic illness is presented in Chapter 9: Stress: Its Implications in Physical Illness. The patient at strong risk for such labeling is one with a history of multiple illnesses, hospitalizations, and surgeries. Another important point is that it is possible that a patient's previous illnesses may have been psychogenic but that *the current illness is genuine.* He could have a hidden tumor or some other potentially fatal condition.

Examples of conversion follow.

Case Examples

Simple conversion. A 52-year-old woman was scheduled for cardiac catheterization in the latter part of the morning. She was worried about the procedure because her physician had explained thoroughly the risks involved. Early in the morning she experienced abdominal cramping and three episodes of diarrhea.

Complex conversion. A 48-year-old Southeast Asian refugee who moved to America in 1977 was admitted to the hospital because of chest pain. Although he had a thorough physical workup, no cardiac pathology could be found. Before discharge, a psychiatric consultation was scheduled in order to determine if the cause was psychological. (Whenever a physical condition has a psychological basis, its cause or etiology is called *psychogenic.*)

During the consultation it was discovered that the man's parents had been killed by the North Vietnamese and that their family farm had been destroyed early in the 1970s. During active fighting in 1974, the man was involved in a severe conflict that resulted in 50% of his army unit being killed. His brother, who was in the unit with him, was also killed. After a truce was declared in 1975, he returned home to discover that his wife and children were not there. Despite 6 months of searching, he was unable to find them. There were mixed reports that they had all been killed when his village was overrun or that they were in a refugee camp in Thailand. They actually had left Vietnam believing that he had died at the same time that his brother had been killed.

He finally decided to go to Thailand to await immigration to the United States, where his sister and her husband lived. He arrived in the United States in 1977 after a difficult 2 years of waiting in Thailand. His move to the United States was uneventful. He lived with his sister, who was very kind to him. Three months before his admission his sister died suddenly. Shortly after her death his chest pains began. When questioned about his response to the loss of all his family members in Vietnam, he acknowledged that he had never felt strong grief. Instead, he felt "numb." He said, "I just had to keep on going. I had to survive." When his sister died, he did not feel any grief and did not cry.

The loss of his sister precipitated his ego to respond with the defense of conversion. His sister's death was the "final straw." His ego was no longer able to hold back the emotion attached to the many earlier terrible losses. It unconsciously feared being overwhelmed by the emotion and so automatically converted the unresolved emotional energy into a physical symptom. This was mediated by the autonomic nervous system.

• • •

Note that in this chapter many of the maladaptive examples described patients who were terminally ill. Remember that the degree of threat that is perceived by the ego will result in the use of differing levels of defense mechanisms. In terminal illness, which is one of the most threatening events a person or family can experience, there is need for more basic and stronger levels of defense. Chapters 19 and 20, the Dying Patient and the Family and

The Nurse and the Dying Patient, will describe many approaches to use with the dying patient and his family.

Conclusion

As you can tell from the preceding examples, the use of defense mechanisms can be both harmful and helpful to patients. The ego is a remarkable psychic structure. It usually is the best ally a person can have as he makes his way through life. Many patients who are hospitalized or treated for illness respond adaptively because of their well-functioning egos. In many other cases, however, the defense mechanisms used by the ego to defend against very threatening events are not given up after the crisis of illness is over. Instead, they are used in an ongoing manner that becomes maladaptive and can cause a deterioration in the quality of life of a patient and his family.

By assessing a patient's thinking, feeling, and behavioral response to illness, you will be able to identify persons in inpatient or outpatient settings whose egos are either unconsciously overusing or underusing defense mechanisms. Information about assessment of psychosocial functioning and recommendations for interventions when dysfunction is observed will appear in subsequent chapters.

In psychiatric hospitals and on psychiatric units in general hospitals, patients are frequently described as neurotic or psychotic. Within those two main categories are several subcategories of psychiatric dysfunctioning, such as schizoaffective disorder, phobic neurosis, and so on. These terms frequently seem confusing to medical and nursing caregivers in the general hospital setting. The cause of these illnesses, their results as seen in the patients, and how to take care of them and what types of approaches work best with them are often mystifying to nonpsychiatric general hospital personnel.

In order to help hospital caregivers understand their general hospital patients' personalities and responses to the stress of illness, several authors have described them and suggested specific approaches to use with each of the major personality styles (Hackett and Cassem, 1978; Jasmin and Trygstad, 1979; Kahana and Bibring, 1964; Lipkin and Cohen, 1980; Robinson, 1976; Sheehan, 1978; Usdin and Lewis, 1979). It is important to emphasize here that the majority of hospital patients fall within a broad range of normal personality styles. Most people display a few personality characteristics that fall within some of the personality styles described below. Some patients demonstrate these characteristics to an excessive degree, however, in their interpersonal relationships. Such distinct personality characteristics can cause a strain in nurses as they give care but consistently find that a patient's responses fall outside of the normal range of behavior customarily seen in general hospital patients. This can be due to a personality or character disorder or can be the result of the extreme stress that patients can experience as a result of physical illness and hospitalization.

Keep in mind that, when ill, the normal person experiences increases in the four basic needs described by Maslow (1970): physiological needs, safety needs, love and belonging needs, and esteem needs. Can you see how each of these needs is threatened by the implications of illness and hospitalization.

In caring for patients who challenge your tolerance, it may be helpful to remember that no matter what excessive traits you observe, the *basic* dynamic operating in all patients is anxiety. Patients are under stress because their basic selves are threatened. In the remainder of this chapter, each of the major personality styles will be presented so that you can understand how these styles evolve and what their major characteristics or identifying traits are. Suggestions for manage-

5

Personality Styles Seen in General Hospital Patients

ment of these patients' nursing care will be presented.

Recommendations about the best therapeutic approaches to use with the various personality styles can also be used with family members who may present problems to the nursing staff because of their response to the illness of their loved one.

State vs. Trait Characteristics

When observing the personality style of a patient, we should always ask if we are seeing the normal traits of this person or a temporary *state* brought on by acute stress. For example, there is a difference between a person who is chronically anxious, no matter what is going on in his life, and a person who is normally serene but who becomes anxious on the night before exploratory surgery for an unidentified mass.

When considering patients' emotional response to hospitalization and illness, try to determine if the patient exhibits a "state" or "trait." This can usually be determined when the psychosocial history is obtained by asking how the patient normally responds to stress or by asking him to describe himself. Needless to say, the patient or family member should not be directly asked, "Are you always this paranoid?" Tactfulness is possible by asking instead a series of questions using several personality characteristics. A nurse could ask, "Have you ever thought of yourself as being an anxious person (a depressed person, a person who has trouble trusting)?" If the patient says that he often is depressed or anxious, then what he is demonstrating is a trait. If, on the other hand, his response to illness is quite untypical of his normal personality, then a temporary state is occurring.

Personality traits are the result of the specific defense mechanism the ego used when the child's personality was developing. It is the total range of traits that a person acquires in his maturing process that determines his *personality style.*

A list of major personality styles follows (Kahana and Bibring, 1964)

Major Personality Styles Seen in General Hospital Patients

Dependent, demanding

Orderly, controlled

Dramatizing, emotionally involved, captivating

Long-suffering, self-sacrificing

Suspicious, complaining (sometimes called guarded, querulous)

Superior

Uninvolved, aloof

Antisocial

Inadequate

In using the suggestions for therapeutic approaches to the patients in each of these categories, it is essential that the suggestions be recorded on the nursing care plan so that *all* members of the nursing staff, and ideally all other caregivers, will use the same approach. If only a few members of the nursing staff use the approach, then the result will be negligible or may even increase the patient's anxiety because of the mixed messages he is receiving from the staff.

Major Personality Styles

The Dependent, Demanding Patient

Most patients become more dependent than usual when they are hospitalized. Nurses are aware of this need and usually are able to meet their patient's increased requirements for attention. On occasion, there are patients whose normal personalities are very dependent or who regress to a very dependent level. The patient is clingy, needy, and demanding. These traits evolve from the earliest level of development, the oral stage. The patient is unaware of his excessive demands on the nurse or is superficially apologetic about his constant requests. He has a low tolerance for frustration. This patient has an underlying fear of abandonment that motivates much of his behavior. While caring for this patient, nurses may initially feel guilt about their own annoyance with the patient. Evenutally, most nurses avoid going near the patient's door. This patient may have an increased tendency toward addiction (Kahana and Bibring, 1964). The addictive personality has strong dependency needs from the earliest years of life (Pattison and Kaufman, 1979).

Nursing Intervention
The basic need of the dependent, demanding patient is to be cared for by an interested and caring staff. When possible, anticipate the patient's

needs so that his fear of abandonment can be minimized. This patient often feels unloved and unwanted and may compensate by making excessive demands on the nurses.

When this happens, it may be necessary to impose limits on those demands that are unrealistic. When setting limits with a demanding patient, do it in a supportive way by explaining the realistic expectations of care the patient is entitled to as well as the effects on the staff when his demands are excessive. If, for example, he frequently calls for insignificant reasons, a wise approach is to tell the patient, in a caring way, that you are very much aware of his situation and will check on him every half hour during the day. Although your patience may be *severely* tried, avoid using a punitive or exasperated tone with him. Ask him if he can save his requests until you come in and then be reliable about arriving on time.

During the day, on at least one occasion, pull up a chair close to the patient's bed and sit down to talk with him rather than standing. When sitting down, nurses promote a stronger sense in the patient that they will not be "running out the door." You may be there *no longer than if you were standing,* but to the patient you seem more available and far more interested in him. During the time you are sitting with the patient, ask him how he is feeling at that particular time. Most demanding patients occupy the nurse's time with incessant requests to *do* things. The nurse is occupied rolling up the bed, getting a blanket, getting the patient's bathrobe, and so on. These are all *unconsciously* manipulative devices the patient uses to assure himself of the nurse's presence and attention. They are motivated by his anxiety about being alone. Frequently, this patient's anxiety level drops off dramatically and, as a result, so do his demands when a nurse sits and talks *with* him and asks him about *himself.*

The Controlled, Orderly Patient

The controlled, orderly personality is identified by caregivers and educated laypersons as having compulsive character traits. The nonpathological manifestation of these traits can be observed in many successful people. They are self-disciplined people who maintain a high level of order in their lives. They are usually hardworking and, in fact, may tend to overwork for the purpose of meeting their own set of frequently high expectations. Sometimes they may seem to be "driven" to achieve. This tendency toward high self-expectations may spill over and be projected onto other persons in the environment. As a result, expectations of others may be very high as well.

This type of behavior can be observed in a patient whose grooming, even when hospitalized, may be perfect. He may keep in frequent touch with his working environment to ensure that all is well. There usually is a rigidity and lack of flexibility in his personality. This is sometimes seen in an obstinate type of behavior and belief system. Spontaneity in conversation or thinking is rarely seen.

He tends to think rather than feel. His conversation is frequently intellectual; a listener may find it difficult to tell how he is *really* feeling. If he is very controlled, he may not know what his feelings actually are. His emotional reactions to situations are usually split off from his intellectual awareness of them. This is the defense of isolation, also known as rationalization or intellectualization (see p. 42).

The development of these traits came about as the result of events that occurred between the ages of 2 and 4 years. The patient either was raised in a rigid disciplined way and eventually incorporated the demands of his caregivers into his developing superego or was raised by indulgent caregivers who gave in to his every whim. With the latter possibility, the reaction formation defense mechanism can result. The ego reverses the situation into its exact opposite, and the person becomes very controlled (see p. 43). Many of these traits occur as a result of an internal voice that seems to say "I should . . . . I should" (Kahana and Bibring, 1964; Shapiro, 1965).

In the hospital, where the patient is no longer in charge of himself or his schedule, he frequently feels anxious. This may or may not be observed by the nurse. Occasionally, such patients control the outward appearance of their anxiety, and you will see an intensification of the character traits described above. As the patient's anxiety increases, his control may eventually begin to fail.

Type A Personality

A specific type of personality, with many of the characteristics of the orderly, controlled patient, has been identified in many cardiac patients. It is called the *Type A personality.* The typical traits seen in Type A personality are aggressiveness, anxiety, repressed emotions, hyperactivity, competitiveness, intense work involvement, high level of discipline, and involvement in a dominant and socially acceptable occupation (Poncheri and colleagues, 1978; Rosenman, 1971). Nursing care approaches with persons who demonstrate Type

A personality characteristics are the same as those recommended for the controlled, orderly patients. Nurses who work in cardiac intensive care medical or surgical units, step-down units, or cardiac rehabilitation settings frequently find that many of their patients have personality traits that fall into this category.

Nursing Intervention

The most important point to remember in caring for the controlled, orderly patient is that he needs to feel in control of himself at all times. Any event that threatens his sense of control will provoke anxiety. Examples of such events are entry into a hospital setting where the employees and hospital schedule are bound by usually inflexible rules and surgery of any type. Surgery provokes anxiety for two important reasons: anticipation of loss of consciousness while under anesthesia and inability to oversee the actions of the surgeon. Cancer or any other type of disease that is subject to unpredictable exacerbations and recurrence also provokes anxiety, as does any other type of chronic illness because of its unrelenting duration.

When caring for such a patient, you may find that he asks many questions about his illness, the medication he receives, and any procedures performed on him. You may even feel exasperated and think, "What difference does it make?" To the orderly, controlled patient, it makes a big difference. The best way to relieve this type of patients' anxiety is to answer all these questions. He needs to know *what* is going on and *why* in order to feel that he has even a little control.

Whenever you must perform a procedure for any patient, it is important always to explain *in advance* what will be done and why. With this type of patient, it is especially important that he understand in advance what will be happening. Explain the procedure step by step. This is very important, especially in intensive care units, even with semiconscious or semisedated patients who are suspected of having a controlled type of personality. Remember, too, that even when you treat the controlled type of patient at night he will always react better when given an explanation, even if he is only semiawake.

All patient teaching should be done by sitting with the patient and explaining in detail the many aspects of his illness. He may question certain aspects of his care. Positive, firm reassurances, once you have answered his questions, may promote his sense of security. Another very important intervention with this patient will be to allow him, whenever possible, to determine his bath schedule, medication schedule, and any other aspect of his care that will not be compromised if his ability to make choices is permitted. Such an approach strongly enhances his feeling of control (Kahana and Bibring, 1964; Robinson, 1976).

The Dramatizing, Emotionally Involved, Captivating Patient

The dramatizing personality is another type of patient you may see in the hospital. One of the characteristics seen in this patient is a more emotional response to events than is customary. This type of patient, quite opposite from the orderly patient, seems to feel feelings more intensely and not be able to verbalize them in an intellectual ("thinking") way. In other words, he may tend to feel more than he thinks. He may, for example, say "I feel *awful!*" but may not be able to explain why. Emotion seems to flood his intellect. The patient's increased emotionality presents itself in all ways, positively as well as negatively. He usually becomes quickly engaged with caregivers and also has a warmth and appeal that can be described as "captivating."

If these traits appear on the pathological end of the continuum, then they are described as hysterical or histrionic (*Diagnostic and Statistical Manual of Mental Disorders*, 1980). Some of the early movie heroines displayed strongly hysterical traits. They are typified by the seductive type of woman. You will rarely observe the latter traits in hospitalized patients; instead, you may find patients who respond to you in a warm, personal, and eager way. These patients may be somewhat dramatic in their statements and behavior; their behavior may, at times, seem to be attention seeking. These patients may initially seem like the dependent type of patient, but they can be differentiated by their emotionality, dramatic behavior, and engaging personality. These personality traits evolve from incomplete resolution of the Oedipal or Electra complex around the age of 4 or 5 years (Kahana and Bibring, 1964; MacKinnon and Michels, 1971; Shapiro, 1965; Usdin and Lewis, 1979).

Nursing Intervention

The most important point to remember in caring for the dramatizing, emotionally involved, captivating patient is that his emotional response to stress may be strong and exaggerated. The intellectual, detailed explanation type of approach you would use with the controlled type of personality should be avoided; it could actually increase this patient's anxiety. Instead, give a simple, calm, straightforward explanation. This type of patient may even say, "I don't want to know a thing. Just do it. Tell me when it's over." When such a patient feels a great amount of stress, you may not be able to reason with him.

The uncomfortable feeling of anxiety that these patients experience as a result of explanations or teaching cause their egos to respond with the defense mechanism of repression. Consequently, you may find that these patients forget what they are told. Whenever you are teaching such a patient, it is important to check his comprehension and ask him to repeat the instructions. It is even more important to make sure that he understands. When necessary, repeat the instructions in a calm reassuring way in order to allay his normally anxious response.

Whenever possible, ask the patient how he is feeling about his illness. His feelings tend to build up quickly, and, when he is particularly anxious, it may seem to him that he is going to be overwhelmed by them. The opportunity to talk about his feelings will have an effect similar to releasing steam periodically from a pressure cooker. He will feel relieved, and his anxiety level may decrease markedly. On occasion, this patient, because of his captivating qualities, may appear to have some manipulative tendencies.

If you are unwillingly "caught up" by such a patient, it is important to set *caring* but firm limits on the patient's demands. Many nurses unknowingly become overinvolved with this type of patient because of their normal desire to help. Some patients take advantage of this quality in nurses. Do not become angry with the patient or withdraw and avoid him, since this will only increase his anxiety; his maladaptive traits may become more pronounced, and you may eventually feel even more manipulated and resentful.

The Suspicious, Complaining Patient

The suspicious patient who questions caregivers' intentions or constantly complains about many aspects of his care may eventually undermine the best intentions of nursing staff members. One of the greatest fears of this patient is to be in a vulnerable position, physically or mentally. The main defense mechanism he uses is projection. As he becomes more anxious, he may begin to find fault with hospital policies, medical and nursing staffs, various aspects of care, or his food. The fault finding projected onto the environment is actually a reflection of his own internal anxieties and self-dislike. He may harbor grievances about real or imagined failures of the hospital support system (Kahana and Bibring, 1964). When these characteristics increase to the pathological end of the trait continuum, this patient is called *paranoid*. The fixation that results in these character traits occurs between the ages of 1 and 3 years.

The truly paranoid patient is usually not observed in the general hospital setting. It is not uncommon, however, as illustrated in an earlier case example, for an organic paranoid psychosis to be precipitated by the multitude of drugs given in intensive care units. These are usually transient but terrifying experiences for the patient as well as for the nurse.

Nursing Intervention

Although the severity of these symptoms may vary in some suspicious, complaining patients, the same general approach should be used with them. Remember that they fervently believe the statements they make. If you attempt to reassure them that the physicians are good or that the hospital policies are reasonable, how are they likely to respond?

How do *you* respond when you fervently believe something and someone tries to dissuade you in a calm and placating way? Do you become impatient, frustrated, and angry? This type of approach will increase the patient's anxiety and lack of trust. On the other hand, if you agree with him in order to halt his unceasing complaints, you may only increase his anger because this adds credibility to his statements. For example, if a nurse agrees that another nurse is unpleasant, an intern is never available, or that the food is terrible, the patient's cycle of complaints is strengthened.

The best approach to use with this type of patient is to acknowledge his beliefs but do not offer an opinion about them. If you offer either a positive or negative opinion, the situation will still be at an impasse. If you say, "I know how you feel, Mr. James, that your roommate and his family are thoughtless about your comfort, but he is paying for his bed just as you are," or "they just don't know any better" will only give him more fuel for his counter argument. *You* may even end up being more fed up and frustrated.

The most important point to remember is that if you acknowledge the patient's feelings in a way that mirrors them in words similar to his own, injecting no opinion, you will at least be letting the patient know that you understand. And just knowing that someone else understands a problem can be comforting.

The process of simply acknowledging this type of patient's feelings will usually make him feel more understood, and his anxiety will decrease. On occasion, if you further ask for his patience about these unpleasant situations and then reinforce the overall benefits of the hospitalization vs. the negative experience he is describing, he may become more amenable to care (Kahana and Bibring, 1964).

If the patient's problem is fear and suspiciousness, several different approaches can be included in the care plan. Because the patient's level of trust is poor, always explain in advance what will be happening and why. This patient does not need the technical, intellectual approach of the controlled patient. Such an explanation would increase his anxiety because it would give him something else about which he must be more wary. Refrain from touching this patient when being emotionally supportive and avoid attempts to get close to him emotionally. He is unable to tolerate this type of closeness. Accordingly, his level of suspicion may rise uncomfortably if you persist in this type of normally supportive behavior.

When approaching such a patient, slow down when entering his room. A hurried entrance and a rushed approach may trigger fear in him. Also, if it is necessary to stand near the bed, it can be less anxiety provoking for him if you stand at the foot of the bed to talk to him. Ideally, it is best to sit rather than stand to discuss something with him. Another approach that will minimize anxiety is to always allow the patient access to the door. For example, stand on the side of the bed away from the door. A very suspicious patient can become even more so if he thinks that he cannot "escape" or get out the door because you are in the way.

Other interventions that can promote a less suspicious response in the patient are to use a primary nursing approach, maintain continuity of nurses on other shifts, and outline a daily schedule of events with the patient; nurses on other shifts can be encouraged to do the same.

The following explanation by someone who underwent cardiac bypass surgery illuminates the experience of the patient with a transient drug-induced paranoid psychosis:

When I woke up I forgot where I was. All I knew was that someone was trying to find me so that he could kill me. I had something in my throat, and I couldn't talk [the endotracheal tube]. I didn't know any of the people around me, but I had to make them understand that someone was after me. Something told me that the only way they could understand me was if I spoke French to them, and I don't know how to speak French!

The more I tried to make them understand, the more they told me there was nothing to be afraid of. The only way I could tell them was by using my hands and arms. Then they tied them down, and my feet too! [Both his hands and feet were shackled in leather restraints by intensive care personnel.] I was convinced at that point that I was going to be killed because *no one* understood what was going on!

After they took the tube out I kept trying to make them understand. They all ignored me. Finally, one nurse told me she understood and would help me. I felt so relieved! I trusted her. Shortly afterward my son came in, and he too told me that he would help me. Thank God that the two of them "humored" me along. I was so frightened before that, I didn't know what to do."

Can you imagine this patient's terror? Can you also imagine his relief when, finally, one of the nurses told him she understood? If you are working with a patient who has this level of fear (psychotic though it may be, it is still very real to him) make sure that at least one caregiver allies himself with the patient and remains available to him. Another situation in the general hospital during which this type of paranoid reaction may occur is when a patient's central nervous system is responding to the withdrawal of alcohol or drugs. This process is usually called *withdrawal* or *detoxification*.

The Long-Suffering, Self-Sacrificing Patient

The long-suffering, self-sacrificing patient has a history that appears similar to the overly dependent patient. There has frequently been a succession of illnesses or other disappointments in his life. The difference, to the observer, is in the behavior of the person as he speaks. The dependent person seems to be expecting someone to *do* something because he is so helpless. The long-suffering patient needs the listener to *feel* something. There appear to be two types of these patients: one who suffers silently, is selfless, and shows no regard for his well-being because of his need to sacrifice and do for others and the one who seems to *enjoy* relating the awfulness of his situation. Also, at the pathological end of the spectrum, there is a manipulative aspect to such a patient's presentation that attempts to win the listener's sympathy. The pathological form of these traits is called *masochism*.

The masochistic person is one whose childhood was marked by harsh discipline and strong guilt instilled in him by caregivers. The consequence of this upbringing is a bittersweet experience that associates pleasure with suffering. Because of his strong and constant sense of guilt, he has a difficult time experiencing pleasure from events that would normally be enjoyed by other persons (Kahana and Bibring, 1964).

Nursing Intervention

The basic need of the long-suffering, self-sacrificing patient is to feel loved and cared for, but he is unable to simply accept such care as offered because of his high guilt level. As a result, he must first deny himself and suffer, either silently or vocally. If the patient is a silent type of sufferer, you may hear many clues to his poor self-esteem. With this type of patient, support his own needs and sense of self-worth. He may need firm reassurances that it is *normal* to take pain or sleep medication.

Frequently, it is important to do discharge planning and teaching with his spouse. He may have a strong tendency to overdo when he goes home, reassuring his wife and family that he is feeling fine. Many of these patients have spouses and family members who have become so accustomed to such a person's overindulgence of them that they have no awareness of his needs. Accordingly, his exhaustive efforts are taken for granted and come to be expected. In teaching this patient about ways to ensure his well-being after discharge, remember that he has a very low regard for his own needs and may not listen seriously to recommendations about his health. A successful way to talk with him is to remind him that his family will be without his services for a longer period if he has a physical setback because he overdid things after discharge.

If the patient is a manipulative type who seeks sympathy, it is important to remember that although he complains about his pain, illness, and so on, he does not expect you to cure it. Instead, he needs acknowledgment that you understand his discomfort. He frequently is not as distressed as the normal patient would be in similar circumstances because the illness is accepted by him as a further "trouble"; it is acceptable, in a distorted way, because it relieves his guilt.

The Patient With Superiority Feelings

The patient who has an exaggerated sense of importance is not usually comfortable in the sick role. The development of illness is sensed as an assault against his self; indeed, his body image is under strong attack. Accordingly, he is even more threatened when the illness is severe enough to require hospitalization. Actually, his air of confidence is a defense against conscious and unconscious feelings of poor self-esteem. This patient may expect preferential treatment, may insist on care only from his attending physician, or may choose the chief of staff as his personal physician and attempt to devalue the care decisions of house officers and nursing staff. He may devalue their personal qualities as well. When the traits are extreme, this patient is described as *narcissistic*. Narcissistic character pathology is derived from the first years of life, when the child may have felt special when conforming with the wishes of his mother.

Nursing Intervention

In caring for the patient with feelings of superiority, alienation between the nurse and patient can be diminished if the nurse reflects the patient's statements and feelings back to him in a nonjudgmental way. The demonstration of negative feelings such as impatience or anger by the nurse will usually increase the patient's anxiety and cause his feelings of superiority to increase as he attempts to compensate and decrease his discomfort. If his expectations exasperate and alienate the nursing staff, it is a wise idea for the head nurse to spend some time with the patient on the staff's behalf. Frequently, such a patient experiences a decrease in his need to maintain superiority when he is able to talk with another "authority" figure. This sometimes helps him to feel he has an ally. The head nurse can acknowledge his expectations. Most important, the patient's behavior should be interpreted for him from the head nurse's own perspective, and recommendations for changes in his behavior should be made. This discussion should be carried out in a positive, expectant manner rather than in a punitive one. Follow-up discussions may have to be held daily in order to maintain reinforcement and limit-setting.

The Uninvolved, Aloof Patient

The uninvolved, aloof patient may appear distant and hermitlike and may avoid encounters with other patients as well as caregivers. He may, for example, spend long periods alone in a sunroom or unit lobby. He may rarely have visitors; this is a reflection of his remoteness and lack of relationships outside of the hospital. He appears apathetic because of his bland emotional tone. He lacks the ability to show anger or express his feelings. These personality traits result from his disappointments in early childhood in trying to establish loving relationships with the important persons in his life. When these traits are especially dominant, this personality is called *schizoid* (Freedman and coworkers, 1976; Kahana and Bibring, 1964).

Nursing Intervention

The uninvolved, aloof patient's inability to establish relationships during his early childhood has resulted in a life style characterized by avoidance of all persons and situations that could potentially reawaken his early feelings of rejection and disappointment.

When hospitalized, he is forced into environmental closeness with others. This closeness raises his level of anxiety. He would be emotionally more comfortable in a single room, if possible. If it does not interfere with his care regimen, he should be allowed to spend as much time as he desires sitting alone wherever he can find privacy. In talking with this patient, be aware of his need to remain physically and emotionally distant. Avoid touching him, other than when giving direct care. During teaching or other types of discussion, accept his statements and do not probe for his emotional responses. Although he is aloof, try not to reciprocate. There is a good middle ground to maintain with him: remain available in a quiet, caring, nonintrusive way.

The Antisocial Patient

The antisocial patient is frequently the nurse's nightmare. He displays many styles of behavior that are unacceptable to nurses. Some of his traits are unreliability, manipulativeness, lack of guilt, lack of responsibility in interpersonal relations, and superficial charm (Cleckley, 1964). At times, these patients are sexually aggressive. Some drug addicts fall into this category and present a mixture of the dependent and the antisocial personality types. These patients tend to be impulsive and also have a poor tolerance for frustration. Their history often shows a lack of a positive relationship with a significant person in early childhood. The traits are

characterized by lack of superego control. Such a patient also demonstrates a lack of tension, and his anxiety level is only slightly affected in stressful situations (Kaplan and Sadock, 1981). When significant trait pathology is observed, this personality type is called *psychopathic* or *sociopathic*.

Nursing Intervention

Antisocial patients, as you can imagine from the traits describing them, can be very trying to the nursing staff. These patients frequently are young and may enter the hospital as a result of accidental injury. No matter their age, the management of these patients can be problematical if firm, *but caring,* limits are not established early in hospitalization. These limits should initially be explained by the head nurse, who is the official authority figure on the unit. The limits must be used by *all* nurses and should be carefully outlined in the nursing care plan so that they are used uniformly by all caregivers. A patient may single out one nurse who is not able to set firm limits and manipulate her into compliance in meeting his needs. If uniformity in his care is not established, he may play two groups of nurses against each other: those who are "for" him and those who are "against" him. Serious staff conflict can occur if he is hospitalized for an extended period. The process of dividing the staff into two groups is called *splitting.*

These patients usually are bright and articulate. They respond poorly to harsh rules and practices. Actually, the unfair imposition of petty rules may be an overreaction of nursing staff and may cause the patient to act out even more. When the limits are fair and explained well, they will be more effective in curbing unacceptable behavior. (See the limit-setting section in Chap. 16: Nursing Intervention With the Emotionally Complex Patient.)

Frequently, these patients, if not originally addicted, seem to rely heavily on pain medication. This issue becomes an important one for nursing staff, who have concerns about overdependence on narcotic analgesia. There are some important considerations in the care of these patients. In such patients, placebos are often discussed as a way of decreasing dependence on narcotic analgesia. If placebos are decided on, it is especially important that they not be used deceptively. Deceptive use of placebos usually results in many more behavorial complications. (See the section about placebos in Chap. 16.)

The Inadequate Patient

The last type of patient to be presented in this chapter is sometimes referred to as having an inadequate personality, which is characterized by an immature response to physical, intellectual, or emotional stress. His responses to stress are unstable and unpredictable. His adaptation to stressful events is poor, and, although he may not be dull witted, his judgment is lacking. He may react to stress with an impulsive, exaggerated response or may seem to "wilt" under pressure. The development of his personality traits is not entirely clear because he presents no clear-cut distinguishing characteristics. The development of this type of personality probably occurs as a result of emotional or experiential deprivation (Hinsie and Campbell, 1977).

Nursing Intervention

In many ways, working with the inadequate patient is similar to the experience of "walking on eggshells." Because the patient's responses are unpredictable, it is impossible to decide exactly which approach will be most effective. In working with this patient, it is important to determine exactly how his coping inadequacies are being manifested. By determining his weaknesses, you can supply extra support, which may be enough to sustain his own scarce emotional reserves.

The most common symptoms seen in this type of patient are regression, depression, overdependence, and demanding behavior. Sometimes one of these symptoms may be dominant; now and then a patient exhibits a mixed clinical picture. The most helpful approach is to anticipate spending more time with such a patient. He is emotionally needy and will feel abandoned and more anxious if contacts with him are hurried and limited only to essential physical care. The extra brief periods of time spent with him from the beginning will prove worthwhile. Without such an approach, the nurse could end up spending even more time later on giving him extra reassurance and solving other care-related problems. As the nursing member of the health care team, your liaison work with caregivers in the other disciplines will ensure a more supportive team approach. This will be sensed by such a patient as reassuring and will lessen his anxiety.

Another very important group that can be a strong support to this patient is his own family or his roommate(s), if he is not living with his family. If you instruct them and explain the rationale for the medical and nursing care the patient is receiving, they can in turn support him emotionally. In addition, they can be taught various aspects of his physical care and are usually eager to help. The patient will be comforted by their presence and concern.

If the patient seems significantly strengthened by their presence, and family members are not troublesome to the staff, the relaxation of normal hospital policies can allow someone to be with the patient and help relieve his anxiety. This could include overnight stays in the patient's room until the physical crisis is over.

While still hospitalized, once a convalescent stage of recovery is reached, the family member's presence during the critical period can be gratefully acknowledged by the nursing staff and the suggestion made to him or her that the patient is feeling better and it will be good for him to be allowed the time to rest and to become more independent. Sometimes, the family member may have a difficult time relinquishing his or her *own* need to be with the patient.

The following concepts may be helpful to keep in mind when working with family members, especially when they have an unusual need to stay with the patient for most of the day or night, regardless of the patient's condition.

1. The family member who is constantly at the bedside is potentially at risk for exhaustion.
2. When the patient returns home, the family member may be too tired to give him the extra care and time he needs.
3. The patient may become too dependent if he has someone with him all the time.
4. When the patient gets home, this type of availability may no longer be possible because of other time demands on the caregiver.
5. It is better for the patient to adjust to the lack of constant presence of a family member in the hospital rather than at home.
6. Once the patient has returned home, there is rarely a "good" time to curtail such constant attendance. The longer the patient is accustomed to it, the harder it will be for him to accept the loss of constant attendance.
7. At times, the patient's "need" to have someone with him is actually a projection of *the family member's need to be with the patient.*

Conclusion

Knowledge about personality characteristics of patients can be helpful in implementing the nursing process. Awareness of these traits during the nursing process steps of assessment, diagnosis, intervention planning, and intervention steps can give you an understanding of the dynamics that are causing the patient to respond to his illness *and* to the nursing staff in certain ways. Without an awareness of these factors, it is possible that nursing interactions can provoke higher levels of anxiety, depression, or other unpleasant feelings. Depending on the patient's personality style, nursing approaches can be planned and implemented in a way to promote psychosocial adaptation to the stress of illness.

Remember that it may prove helpful to use these approaches with family members whose personality styles can, at times, prove troublesome to their hospitalized relatives or to the nursing staff.

Have you ever been admitted to the hospital, or have you ever accompanied a family member to the hospital? Can you remember how you felt? For most people, admission to the hospital is a threatening experience. It can be an anxious time for family members as well, sometimes even more so than for the patient, who, because of his illness, may not be fully aware of what is happening.

It is not difficult to understand why patients and families are anxious about hospitalization. It is a new experience for most of them, and the outcome of the hospitalization may be uncertain. Accordingly, they may need support in coping with the stress of illness and hospitalization. In order to help them in a meaningful way, it is necessary for you to be aware that there are many underlying reasons for their emotional stress.

In understanding why people react as they do to becoming ill and being admitted to the hospital, think about the various personality theories covered in the preceding chapters. Ideally, all people pass through the stages of personality development with no problem. Realistically, no one does. That is what makes each person unique. The personality traits that a person carries into adulthood are the result of conflicts during earlier stages of development.

It is because of these unresolved conflicts that a patient has the potential to react maladaptively to illness. The level of maladaptation will depend on the degree of intrapsychic conflict he experienced during earlier stages of development, the way in which the hospitalization reawakens those conflicts, the way in which the hospital care system responds to him, and the defensive ability of his ego to help him cope with these experiences.

For example, a patient whose personality development was influenced by frustration at one or another important stage may, on admission, appear quite normal. If his illness is one that can be easily treated, if his hospitalization is brief, if his family is supportive, if the hospital care system is able to meet his physical and emotional needs, and if his ego is able to cope with these events, then this patient should have an uneventful hospitalization and adaptation should be ensured.

On the other hand, if any one or more negative situations occur, such as a life-threatening illness, a complicated hospitalization, a demoralizing family, or an indifferent hospital care system, then the risk of maladaptation rises proportionately. It is as if the underlying and normally unobservable personality conflicts were cracks in the foundation of a house. The cracks may never be a problem under normal conditions, but if the house is subjected to the stress

6

Major Psychosocial Issues of Patients With Physical Illness

of an earthquake, it may be seriously affected. So, too, can a normal person be seriously affected if the intensity of the stress he experiences as a result of physical illness is severe.

Major Developmental Issues

The unresolved old conflicts referred to above occurred as the person's personality developed. These conflicts are left over from the major developmental stages of personality development. The developmental theories of Erik Erikson were introduced in Chapter 3. He believed that there are major development hurdles that one must work through in order to proceed to the next level of personality development. It is possible that there can be varying degrees of frustration in working through each of these stages. The process of development will not stop when these partial blocks occur. Instead, the personality proceeds to the next stage of development. The fixation remains, however, and may influence the succeeding developmental stages. When a stressful event occurs and, because of its similarity to an earlier event reawakens the original conflict, the psyche may have trouble in adapting to the new conflict. It is stressful to be ill, obtain medical attention, be admitted to the hospital, recover from illness, and adjust to the family's response. All these events occur as the illness continuum is in process. This process has the potential of awakening unresolved conflicts from earlier stages of development. The seriousness of the current conflict will depend on the seriousness of the earlier unresolved problem. The potential areas of conflict that I believe present challenges in adaptation for the patient are trust, self-esteem, control, loss, guilt, and intimacy. In working with both inpatients and outpatients I have found that the cause of maladaptation can usually be traced to one or more of these major issues

Two of the most common manifestations of maladaptation are depression and anxiety (Cassem, 1978; Sheehan, 1978). It is important to be aware, however, that anxiety and depression are also adaptive processes when they are not prolonged. They can motivate the patient to take action to resolve the underlying conflict causing the unpleasant feelings. When severe forms of these symptoms occur in a patient, it is important to alert the attending physician. The physician may then request a formal psychiatric consultation. If they are not severe, you may be the person best

able to intervene with the patient and promote a more positive outcome.

In order to work successfully with a patient, it is necessary to be a good detective; understanding the nature of the patient's problem is essential. By understanding the basic personality theories of the earlier chapters, the use of defense mechanisms, the normal personality styles, and the important underlying issues that confront the patient, you have many important aids to developing insight about the dynamics involved.

These issues are described in the order of their appearance during normal psychological development. The dynamics of each of these developmental challenges will be presented in this chapter. Examples of patients' problems in each of these major areas of development, and interventions that can support the patient and promote adaptation, are included. You may be able to think of several other ways in which patients' adaptation can be further challenged by illness.

Trust

When an adult has a problem trusting other people or new situations, the roots of his distrust lie in his first year of life (Erikson, 1963). Although it may seem surprising to think that an infant's first year can have such a profound effect, it exerts a very strong influence.

The child's first experience with trust is the way in which the environment responds to him. He does not know specifically who is doing something to make him feel good, but during the first few months of life he needs food and physical comfort, which includes being held and feeling loved. In fact, the two needs are inseparable in his mind. If those needs are consistently unmet, the result is that the child feels unsatisfied; something is not right. His brain is unable to reason, but the effect is that an adequate level of trust in the environment is never established. Caregivers, one hopes, try to meet the needs of infants. Sometimes, because of their own inability to give love or because of an unusually high level of demand by the infant, the caregiver is not able to meet those needs of the infant necessary to achieve an adequate level of trust (Chess and Chess, 1980; Brazelton, 1973).

Erikson has described the developmental challenge of the first year of life as the achievement of *trust*. If it is not fully attained, the child will develop with a sense of distrust, lack of hope, and lack of drive (Erikson, 1963). Mahler (1974) describes the developmental process of the infant's establishment of trust in her studies of the first 2 years of life (see Chap. 3). The major hurdle of the infant in this process occurs during the differentiation stage of 5 to 10 months of age. One of the most important issues of this stage is the infant's ability to trust his mother. If the child feels comfortable with his mother, he will generalize these feelings to the environment at large.

When a person is hospitalized, his adaptation is challenged because he is repeatedly thrust into situations with which he has no experience. He has to trust the various people in his environment with his physical well-being. In many instances he places his life in their hands, despite the fact that he does not even know them.

In today's world of medical subspecialties, the patient's physician may be a specialist who is assigned to him. Think for a moment what this means to a patient admitted for major surgery. The physicians in charge of his case perform many vital functions. They direct his overall care, although the patient really does not know how competent they are. They prescribe medications. The patient is watched over while he takes pills, the contents of which may be unknown to him. He does not know the competency of the physician who orders them, the pharmacist who prepares them, or the nurse who administers them. The attending physician also asks other physicians to consult. The patient once again must trust the physician's judgment.

The patient must also trust his body's ability to get well. Most people rarely think about their body functions; they are taken for granted until they fail to work. In addition, the patient must trust himself, to cope psychologically with the stress of illness. When the nurse gives care, the patient's ability to trust again is challenged. The nurse performs many procedures on the patient and in his body. The patient really cannot be certain that the nurse knows his or her job. How does a patient feel when a nurse says, "Roll over to the edge of the bed. Don't worry, I've got you."

Another common example of a patient's uncertainty about trusting arises in the care of surgical patients. When you tell the fresh thoracotomy or laparotomy patient that he must cough, look at his face. You will see distrust. He is frightened that his stitches will come loose, and yet you are reassuring him that they will hold. The patient's ability to trust you is difficult at this time. He is feeling very vulnerable. The same difficulty is experienced when he must ambulate for the first time.

A third area in which the patient's ability to trust is threatened is when he is receiving care by other caregivers, for example, the recent stroke patient being supported by a physical therapist. She knows that if he lets go she will fall and injure herself. Other examples are those of the patient with arthritis who is twisted into uncomfortable positions and left alone on a cold table in a dark room while the x-ray technician takes films and the patient in acute respiratory distress who is entubated or has a tracheotomy with an automatic breathing device; he may apprehensively watch technicians and therapists manipulate dials and change his oxygen intake.

When a person is admitted to the hospital, there is little opportunity for gradual adaptation to the abrupt change in environment. Some hospital departments provide orientation programs for patients before they are actually admitted to the hospital. For example, pediatric surgical patients and cardiac bypass surgical patients are frequently taken on a tour of the areas where they will be cared for as a way of reducing anxiety during hospitalization. In most other instances, the patient is suddenly thrust into a dependent situation. For example, if he is admitted without warning for major surgery, his coping abilities may be severely stressed. He has lost the safety and security of home. The availability of known and trusted family members is interrupted. All patients potentially can be at risk because of difficulty in trusting. If a patient has good defense mechanisms that assist his coping ability, there will be no outward signs of increased stress due to problems in trusting.

The person who is most at risk is the patient with a suspicious personality style. If the continuum of suspiciousness approaches paranoia, then the patient will require strong support from the care system in order to tolerate the stress of hospitalization. The nursing care approaches described in the previous chapter should be used with patients whose adaptation is at risk because of distrust. Conversely, the patient who usually has few problems with trust is the dependent patient. His trust may seem to border on personal irresponsibility if he unquestioningly accepts *all* the treatments his caregivers propose.

Self-esteem

Self-esteem is an essential issue that affects all hospital patients. The personality characteristics that result from the other major issues discussed in this chapter remain fairly constant in the personality once they are formed in childhood. Self-esteem is more subject to temporary changes because of the patient's sensitivity to the reactions of others in his family and larger social system.

These reactions combine with his own view of himself and can cause his self-esteem to fluctuate.

The development of self-esteem begins shortly after birth. The infant gradually becomes aware of his body, and this helps to form the basis of his self-perception (Morgan and King, 1966). The most important influence on the way that a child perceives himself is the way that his parents and other important persons interact with him (Blanck and Blanck, 1979). As he grows to toddlerhood, the way he behaves or appears influences the reactions of those around him. The child's ego develops as a result of his relationships with these important "objects." The way that he will relate to other people as an adult depends on these early object relationships.

If his family and friends are loving and approving, he will incorporate their positive opinions of him, and these opinions will develop into positive self-esteem. Accordingly, if they do not value him and are critical and rejecting, this can lead to negative self-esteem. *Self-esteem* is the way that a person feels about himself. It is the way he values himself; it is a self-measurement of one's worth.

Self-esteem is described as "being on good terms with one's superego" (Hinsie and Campbell, 1977, p. 690). In addition to containing moralistic judgments about one's actions, the superego also contains one's own "positive stroking" ability. This enables a person to value himself even when other people are criticizing him.

When people are able to do this for themselves, they are described as having good *narcissistic supplies*. These are internal, intrapsychic sources of positive self-worth; they are primarily acquired during the first several years of life. The term is derived from Narcissus, a young man in Greek mythology who fell in love with his own reflection in a pool and was unable to love others because of his exaggerated self-love. *Narcissism* in toddlerhood is a normal and healthy occurrence. The child values himself very highly. His behavior serves his own needs, and he is quite unaware of the needs of others (Blanck and Blanck, 1979). It gives way to normal give-and-take social relationships as he grows older. When narcissism persists into adulthood, it is considered pathological (Blanck and Blanck, 1979).

It is necessary to understand the differences between *being* narcissistic and *having* good narcissistic supplies. The former is a negative personality style in adults. The latter helps to maintain self-esteem and is a desired ability. When a person's psyche is functioning properly, these supplies are usually present.

Self-esteem is maintained in two ways. The first, discussed above, is from one's own intrapsychic narcissistic supplies. The second is from the social environment. Are the drawbacks to the second source of self-esteem maintenance evident? What if no one in the environment is giving positive feedback? It is ideal if all persons have family, friends, co-workers, and so on who are kind and complimentary; however, this is frequently not so. If a person lacks his own internal ability to nourish his esteem, he then becomes dependent on the people in his environment to do it for him. Actually, this can impose a burden on those relationships. Think of acquaintances who are frequently "fishing" for compliments. They need to obtain from the environment what they lack in themselves. Unconsciously, they are trying to build up their self-esteem to a more comfortable level.

Self-esteem is not a constant thing; it can change daily. There are usually not wide swings in self-esteem in the same person; however, external events, if seriously damaging to a person's sense of worth, can temporarily undermine a normally good level of self-esteem. Narcissistic supplies, if strong, are usually able to help the person adapt to such an occurrence.

Patients with any type of illness experience such a challenge. Remember that *any* type of illness is a threat to the self. The result can be a change in the way a person feels about himself. Patients with many types of physical conditions often experience a *temporary* change in their feelings about themselves and an accompanying decrease in their self-esteem. Some of these conditions are myocardial infarction and cardiac surgery, cancer, amputation, chronic disease of any kind, stroke, diabetes mellitus, peptic ulcer, colitis, colostomy, skin disease, and burns. Think about how self-esteem is affected in each of these cases. If adaptation does not occur, think also of the consequences. Doubtless, you have had days when you feel totally negative about yourself. Think what it would be like to be stuck with a constant feeling of worthlessness. Unfortunately, this is what happens to some patients. The consequences for them and their families are serious. If patients do not overcome this negative self-esteem, they may never be able to participate fully in life. Poor self-esteem is one of the main dynamics in depression (Jacobsen, 1971; Mahler, 1974). Unless a person is able to achieve a more realistic view of himself, a chronic depressive state may result.

Arieti (1967) has written that the unconscious

or conscious need to maintain or improve one's self-esteem is the basic motivating force in human beings. This tells us that the need to protect self-esteem is a powerful force in man's behavior. The theory of Abraham Maslow presented in Chapter 3 describes the drive of a person to achieve his full potential. The ability to pursue full development of oneself is closely associated with maintenance of self-esteem. Accordingly, the nurse's ability to detect the clues of poor self-esteem in patients is important. Positive emotional support from the nurse may provide external stability for the patient's self-esteem until his own resources return.

Gates (1978) has conceptualized self-esteem by dividing it into four separate components:

1. The *body self*. This component contains both the body image (how a person's body looks, feels, and functions) and a person's thoughts and feelings about being able to perform basic functions.
2. The *interpersonal self*. This part of self-esteem contains a person's thoughts and feelings about the way he relates to others in both intimate and casual relationships.
3. The *achieving self*. This section includes a person's thoughts and feelings about his ability to obtain his goals in his family, work, and school environments.
4. The *identification self*. This aspect of self-esteem contains abstract feelings and behaviors that are involved with moral and spiritual concerns.

By considering the impact that a specific illness can have on one or more of these components, we can better understand the threat of illness to the self-esteem of patients and their families.

Some manifestations of poor self-esteem in hospitalized patients include the patient who is *too* compliant; he asks *no* questions about his care. Because of his poor self-worth, he complacently accepts all recommendations for treatment without being fully informed or understanding the justification for them. The patient seems to view himself as a nonperson in the presence of authority figures.

Another example of a collective form of poor self-esteem is the family with a patient who is too ill or too young to become involved in his own care. For example, a service patient with a very unusual disease may be subjected to excessive tests or procedures that will provide little benefit, yet his family does not question his caregivers about them. Another instance could be a terminal patient

in severe pain whose caregivers' highest priority is to avoid addiction (although the patient is close to death). The family members may not act to defend their loved one from an impersonal care system. Fortunately, most hospitals have caregivers who will promote the patient's rights if they see abuses by one or another different subgroup of caregivers. As discussed earlier, this role of patient advocate is frequently and unofficially filled by nursing staff members.

The last example of evidence of poor self-esteem in families can probably be attributed to lack of knowledge about how to negotiate in a hospital care system. It is compounded by less than optimum self-esteem. On occasion, when an acutely ill patient is not fully conscious or is too young to understand the aspects of his care, there is little or no communication between the attending physician and family members about the patient's current clinical condition and short-term treatment plan.

Usually, when there is no opportunity for communication in the hospital, the attending physician will make arrangements to call the senior family member at a prearranged time to bring the family up to date on the patient's condition. Some attending physicians will sidestep this responsibility, assuming that the family members can discuss these issues with house officers or nursing staff.

It is important to remember that family members have a right to obtain this information directly from the attending physician. They are paying him or her to care for the family member. Occasionally, you may have to listen to irate family members who are angry that the attending physician is not informing them of the patient's condition. When this occurs, avoid being embroiled in the problem by refraining from making frequent excuses for the attending physician; instead, promote the family's right to obtain this information directly from the person who is overseeing all aspects of the patient's care. Obviously, there will be exceptions when families, because of their anxiety, make unrealistic demands of the attending physician several times a day as a way to reassure themselves of their loved one's well-being. You will be the best judge of the reasonableness of a family's need for information from the physician. Remember, however, that it is not *your* responsibility to defend an attending physician who is avoiding his responsibility to provide information about the patient's condition to his concerned family.

While caring for patients, be especially aware of the potential short- and long-term damage to self-esteem that a patient's illness can cause. The following case example describes a difficult and tragic situation involving self-esteem:

Case Example

Nancy is a 14-year-old girl who was admitted to the hospital because of toxemia of pregnancy. She had dropped out of school 3 months earlier and was staying with an aunt in a neighboring community. Because of incest, her father is the father of her child. Her sense of shame within the family is acute. She also feels intense guilt. She had expected her secret to remain within the family. Two days after admission, she learned that her younger brother had told one of his friends in their junior high school. She expected that all the school would learn not only of her pregnancy but also of her involvement with her father. Her self-esteem was not able to combat her feelings of shame and worthlessness. By the evening of that day she decided that the only way out of her awful situation was to commit suicide. She was able, with psychiatric help, to overcome this crisis. A few days later she was walking through the main corridor of the entrance to the hospital when she spotted three young friends from the school. Joy registered in her face as she started to call out to them. Suddenly she realized that she could not talk to them without revealing her condition. She shrank back into a corner.

The cause and effects of this pregnancy have had and will continue to have a serious effect on this young girl's self-esteem. It will strike at the very core of her feelings and beliefs about herself. Psychiatric intervention consisting of support for the girl and family therapy with all members of the family, including Nancy, is essential if short- and long-term adaptation is to be achieved. This example illustrates the devastating effect that an event can have on a person's self-esteem.

If a person has had positive self-esteem, and, because of illness and a resulting change in self-image, his self-esteem becomes poor temporarily, there are many opportunities for the nurse to promote adaptation. By giving the patient the opportunity to talk about his feelings about himself, he may be able to talk out his own doubts and resolve some of his concerns. By giving *honest* responses to his doubts and also by describing other patients who have successfully overcome the same conditions, you may help him to feel more confidence in himself. Remember, you cannot *make* a patient feel good about himself. Instead, by your simple acceptance of him as a person, you are saying to him, "You're OK." *This can be far more reassuring than any specific words.*

Body Image

Body image, which is closely related to self-esteem, is the way that a person thinks and feels about his body as a whole, the various parts of his body, the functions of his body, and the internal and external sensations associated with it. It also includes his perceptions of the way that others see his body. It is possible that the early awarenesses of the infant about his body cause the ego and all its functions to begin development (Nagera, 1964). Body image development occurs in a complex, lifelong process and is closely entwined with the development of his identity. In fact, it is impossible to separate the two. Body image theory is of great interest to nurses because it deals with the patient's view of his body and its functioning at every point of the health-sickness-regaining of health continuum. Many theories have been combined to form this section (Blanck and Blanck, 1979; Brown, 1977a and b; Engel, 1968; Erikson, 1963; Fenichel, 1945; Freedman and colleagues, 1976; Freud, 1933; Hackett and Cassem, 1978; Mahler, 1974; Norris, 1978; Usdin and Lewis, 1979)

Like self-esteem, body image begins to develop shortly after birth. The newborn infant is not aware of any separation between his own body boundaries and the environment around him. In his infancy he becomes aware of where *his* body ends and, for example, where his mother's body begins. This forms a sense of separateness. The infant also is unconsciously aware that his mouth helps his body to feel pleasure because of his full stomach. (This is a basic awareness that remains throughout life in most people.) A very important factor in the child's development of positive body image and self-esteem is the amount of touching he receives from caregivers. It is essential to remember that the need to be touched continues throughout life. Hospitalized patients have deep unconscious needs to be touched caringly.

As he develops coordination during the second half of his first year, the infant becomes aware, again unconsciously, that he has a degree of control over his body. This awareness increases through his toddlerhood. It has both conscious and unconscious elements.

There is strong interaction at this point between the child's body image and his self-esteem. Each depends on the other and helps to bolster both positive body image and positive self-esteem if the social environment approves of the young child's efforts at body control. Some of these efforts are sphincter control, walking, running, and manual dexterity.

Another important aspect of body control at this age is the reaction of authority figures—parents and relatives—to the child's exploration of his body. The child has insatiable curiosity about his own body and those of others. These are normal and healthy wonderings. As he feels the inside of his nose or discovers that it feels pleasant to touch his genitals, he is in the process of developing his body image.

If the social environment is sternly disapproving, the child develops a sense that something is "bad" about his own body. On the other hand, if no gentle constraints are placed on him, his ability to develop a sense of respect for his body and self-discipline will be distorted. If he is allowed to stand in the middle of a supermarket aisle picking his nose for 5 minutes, he will sense disapproval from the other shoppers without understanding why

The child of 3 to 5 years is very aware of the physical differences between the sexes. Children are very curious about who has and who does not have a penis. Little boys worry that they might lose their penis; little girls worry because they do not have one. The acceptance and approval of the parent of the opposite sex is important to the child's overall body concept. The comfort of the same-sex parent with his or her own body is also very important to the child's overall body concept.

The school-age child continues to be aware of sex differences but predominately in a social way. Children's mastery of skills that were formerly stereotyped by sex helps them to feel good about their bodies. Cooking, ballet dancing, and figure skating were examples of typically female-role activities. For young boys, baseball, football, and ice hockey were and continue to be popular activities. Because of government mandates, all schools and public recreation programs today must offer equal opportunities to girls and boys. As a result, the opportunities for young girls to exercise actively and develop a healthy and confident sense of their bodies have increased markedly. With these changes in formal and physical education, there is an opportunity for children of both sexes to be exposed to many types of activities regardless of their gender identification.

The adolescent's body image continues to develop with his opportunities to master skills and feel that he can trust his body and that it is competent. His body image development faces many challenges: his body suddenly begins sprouting, his normally clear complexion begins to develop pimples, his facial and body hair is growing too quickly or too slowly and he feels different from his friends (girls share similar comparison types of anxiety about their breast development), and changes in his genitals remind him that sexual activity is possible; his sexual drive is on a collision course with the values of his superego and authority figures.

All these changes cause an increase in self-doubt as his image of himself alternately is pleasing and then unacceptable. He may be accepting or rejecting, love or hate, or take for granted or be anxious about his body functions or overall appearance.

If a person of any age loses a body function that has always been taken for granted, it is quite common for him to go through a grieving process similar to that outlined in Kübler-Ross (1969). The stages remain the same for the person adjusting to a change in his body: shock and denial, anger, bargaining, depression, and acceptance (Kübler-Ross, 1969). These stages are described in this chapter in the subsection on loss. Patients who experience this process include those with burns, cancer, cardiac disease, chronic illness, glandular disturbances, renal dialysis, hysterectomy, amputations, and many more. If one part of the body is not functioning properly, it can color a person's feelings about his total body concept. If his image about only one part of his body is poor, it can also spill over and affect his self-esteem:

A case example follows.

Case Example

Jack is a 38-year-old former interstate trucker whose routes covered the East coast. He enjoyed his work. He is a single man who lives with his married sister. Because of his transient life, he has few other permanent social contacts. He enjoyed meeting women in the cities that he visited and liked to take the women to night spots, where they would dance and drink until the place closed. With little warning, he experienced a myocardial infarct. He was hospitalized for 4 weeks and discharged home to await cardiac bypass surgery. He became depressed while waiting for surgery and was still depressed when he reentered the hospital.

After surgery, he felt "different." His weakness bothered him, and he became afraid that he would rupture his incision. He became anxious with every new sensation in his chest. Despite encouragement from his sister and her family, he felt unable to walk and was unable to gradually build up his strength. Before the myocardial infarct he had always perceived his body to be strong and indestructible. Now, at age 38, his body seemed to have failed him. He doubted that he could ever regain his strength to handle his truck again. He also feared the extra exertion of dancing, and, because of the required diet change, he knew tht he could never again sit and drink several beers. He was certain that his sexual enjoyment would never be the same. He also feared the rejection of his former women friends when they learned of his cardiac illness.

Jack's normal body image has suffered a sharp blow. He anticipated many negative changes in his body's ability to perform. One of the most important factors in his adaptation will be the integration of a new concept of his own body. Realistically, can Jack do this alone?

With a patient like Jack, psychosocial assessment, nursing diagnosis of his major problems, and a comprehensive nursing care plan are important during his myocardial infarct admission. These steps in the nursing process would alert a sensitive nurse to his potential problems in adaptation. He is at risk for maladaptation. It is important for him to be able to talk about his concerns with someone who can correct his misperceptions, give him anticipatory guidance, and listen to his plans for the future. These types of discussions should occur during the original admission *as well as* the cardiac surgical admission. Many patients develop misperceptions preoperatively and dwell on them. The resulting depression may then become a major complication in the preoperative and postoperative states.

Another important concept in body image is a person's reaction to the aging process. The average person retains the appearance of youth until his mid-thirties. After that, subtle changes in appearance and sensation signify that the aging process is underway: a few gray hairs, shortness of breath on exertion, joints that are not as limber, and muscles that ache after heavy exercise. There is a gradual loss of connective tissue; even a thin person develops a mild degree of flabbiness. There are changes in menstrual or sexual function. Wrinkles and other changes in appearance occur.

These different awarenesses require adjustment to a new image. This is another example of loss that requires adaptation. If the person's investment in his younger body image was strong, his reaction may resemble a mild grieving process. Chapter 19: The Dying Patient and the Family, and Chapter 20: The Nurse and the Dying Patient, discuss the grieving process more fully.

If a person maladapts to a major change in body image and develops low self-esteem, the result can be depression. One of the main dynamics in the depression is the unresolved grief about this major change. This type of depression may begin in the hospital setting and can perhaps be averted by perceptive caregivers who allow the patient to talk about his concerns (Surman, 1978). When the patient develops moderate to severe depression in the hospital as the result of a major change in body image, the nurse should suggest psychiatric consultation to the physician in order to help the person resolve his conflict.

Some patients are discharged home with no sign of depression, but it may develop as they become more aware of the loss of their normal functioning or appearance. Nurses who work in outpatient clinics, visiting nursing agencies, or physicians' offices should be observant of clinically depressed patients and perform psychosocial assessment to determine the level of emotional dysfunction. If indicated, they should recommend psychiatric referral.

Control

The ability to control what happens to oneself is important to most people. For a normally independent adult, it means that he knows what he wants and how to obtain it. Control also implies a certain sense of dominance over the environment. When a person is hospitalized, many of these functions give way to the dictates of the institution and various caregivers. The patient may be at risk for maladaptation because of his lack of control over what is happening to him.

Control becomes a major issue for the child between the ages of 2 and 3. At that time he is gaining mastery over his sphincters. A conflict occurs between the child and mother. The child wishes to maintain his own feelings and control of his urine and bowel movements. The needs of his mother and the environment at large are that he should conform to social expectations. The way that his mother ultimately wins the conflict will have a strong effect on the child's future perception of his control in new situations (Engel, 1963).

Locus of Control

Whether a person senses that events are under his control or are outside of his control has been called *locus of control.* Locus, from the Latin, means place. The term *locus of control* actually indicates the place where a person attributes the cause and control of events in his life. Some persons have an *internal locus of control*. They perceive events as being within their control and believe that they have some power over their own response to events and that they have at least some ability to modify environmental situations. On the other hand, the person with an *external locus of control* perceives events as being outside of his control and as being "the result of fate, luck, chance, or powerful others" (Johnson and Sarason, 1978, p. 206). The latter type of person believes that things are beyond his control. He tends to be more of a passive participant, believing that there is little he can do to change a situation.

Which type of person will be more at risk because of feeling that he has relinquished control? The internal locus of control person who normally believes that he has control over events in his life is potentially at risk because he has very little control in the hospital. His diagnosis, prognosis, and outcome of hospitalization and the actions of his caregivers are all unpredictable. Think of the following aspects of hospitalization in which the patient relinquishes control over many aspects of himself:

Relinquishing clothes and possessions

For some people who are particularly class conscious, clothes and possessions are very important. Having to wear a hospital gown is a sudden unexpected "leveler." They are unaccustomed to doing without this controlling factor. Remember that the way a person dresses often exerts a controlling influence on others' reactions to him.

Complying to new schedules

The hospital system is notorious for disregarding people's normal schedules. The clock seems to control many aspects of a patient's care: when to eat, sleep, urinate, and defecate, when one can or cannot have pain medication, visitors, meals, and so on.

Being subject to the orders of others

The patient is subjected to diagnostic tests of all kinds. Unless caregivers are sensitive to the patient's needs, the patient may be ill prepared for these events. He may not know what to expect from the many diagnostic procedures he has to undergo. Imagine the reaction of a frightened elderly man to a bone marrow biopsy, a computed tomography (CT) scan, and so on.

Undergoing surgery

The anticipation of surgery is often one of the most stressful times for all patients, especially the orderly, controlled patient, for many reasons. Frequently, surgery is elective, or there are at least a few days the patient must wait for surgery to be performed. The waiting period can be very difficult. The patient is ambivalent. He wants to speed up the waiting period; at the same time he would like to forget the whole thing. The fear of going under anesthesia is a powerful one. It signifies total loss of control. For many, it masks a fear of death as well. Another aspect of fear of unconsciousness is that the patient cannot control events in the operating room. If something bad happens, he will not be awake to rectify it. Some patients worry that they may say something they should not as they emerge from anesthesia. Another realistic fear is when the surgery is exploratory or will involve a biopsy. The fear that a malignant tumor may be discovered and that while he is asleep parts of his body may be removed without his full awareness can be very disturbing to a patient.

The following case example illustrates the type of problem that the person who needs control may face:

Case Example

Mary, a 75-year-old woman, was admitted to the hospital because of a persistent ulcer on her left lower leg. She lives with her 84-year-old husband in their own home. She is a woman who describes herself as a "yankee." She has been very independent, is intelligent, and has a keen wit. After 1 week of hospitalization there was little improvement in her leg ulcer. Her surgeon decided to do a vein ligation in order to improve the circulation to the site. Discharge was planned after she had recuperated from the surgery and the ulcer had partially healed. One week after the ligation her surgeon decided that the circulation had improved enough to allow skin grafting to occur. He believed that skin grafting would ensure better healing and a better prognosis for the patient.

Mary had been growing increasingly depressed, and when she learned about the new surgery she became acutely depressed. She gave up hope that she would ever be able to return home in her former capacity. Rather than being a burden to her husband, she wanted to die. Indeed, her physical condition deteriorated. Her surgery was postponed. Psychiatric consultation and supportive therapy were initiated, and her depression lifted.

Mary's leg ulcer was grafted, and she remained in the hospital for 2 more weeks before being discharged home, fully able to walk. The 2-week postgraft period was marked by Mary's resistance to pain medication, despite a very painful 10-cm × 15-cm (4-inch × 6-inch) graft donor site and a similar-size site that was debrided and grafted. She did not want to "become an addict." In addition, despite an inability to sleep at night, which increased her daytime anxiety level, she consistently refused sleep medication, saying, "I don't want to be drugged up."

Mary's personality style caused her to need to feel in control. Mary had never been in a hospital as a patient. Admission to the hospital and being a participant in so many uncontrollable events caused Mary's normally good coping abilities to fail. If psychiatric intervention had not occurred, and, despite her acute depression, surgery had been performed, Mary's prognosis would have been poor.

The supportive treatment used with Mary was to allow her to talk about her fears, correct her misperceptions, ask her how she would feel about her husband if he were in the hospital (this helped her gain objectivity about her illness), use humor to rekindle her sense of humor, and introduce discharge planning early in her convalescence to promote a sense of hope.

Mary's reluctance to take sleep medication was respected. Her anxiety became severe at the thought of taking any type of sedative. Her resistance to these medications was actually a manifestation of her need to maintain control. She finally was able to accept pain medication, "but only because you want me to take it!" However, the anxiety and fear that were generated about taking sleep medication outweighed the potential benefits of the hypnotic. The acquiescence on the part of caregivers and respect for her wishes about this point increased her confidence in them.

Another aspect of control that a patient loses is the control of his own body boundary: the place where his body begins and the environment ends. When his normal body boundary is invaded, it can seem as if there no longer is a distinct sense of where his body begins; the tubes and other objects normally found in the environment are actually *in* his body. They are inserted through his skin or the various natural or surgical openings in his body. Examples of these invasive lines are intravenous fluid and hyperalimentation, nasogastric and tracheal suctioning, endotracheal tubes, central venous and arterial blood pressure lines, chest tubes, drainage tubes from various sites, gastrostomy and ureterostomy tubes inserted directly through the abdominal wall into internal organs, cardiac and other radiographic catheters, indwelling urinary catheters, indwelling rectal temperature probes, and so on.

Stop and think for a moment. How would it feel to have an endotracheal tube such as those used during the first 12 hours after cardiac surgery down *your* throat? Even if it felt *awful*, remember, *you would have no control and could not take it out.* Here is another example. Perhaps a patient has read that if air is injected into a vein, it can kill. How do you think he feels when, lying in his bed, he observes a large air bubble entering his vein being pushed through by the fluid above it! How would you feel in the same situation? How would it be if you had just returned from surgery, were helpless, and could not reach your call bell to notify someone that an air bubble was going into your body and you believed that it would kill you?

Some patients feel an uneasiness and insecurity about the entrance of such materials and substances into their body. It is important to be aware of the cause of this type of uneasiness. If you work in an intensive care unit, for example, and suspect that this problem may be contributing to a patient's anxiety, take the time to explain the reason for the various tubes. Be prepared to ask physicians for any appropriate level of sedation if the patient maintains a high level of anxiety. Without relief, this level of anxiety can develop into overwhelming panic or, occasionally, a paranoid psychotic reaction. In either case, the physiological state of the person is more seriously compromised.

Being aware of the patient's need to control at least *some* of the aspects of the hospital environment can help him to accept his dependent status. If the patient has a "controlling" type of personality, your sensitivity to his anxiety over loss of control can make an important difference in whether adaptation or maladaptation to illness occurs.

Loss

Loss is one of the most important issues that any person has to adjust to during his lifetime. Earlier in the book you read about object relations. The emotional energy that is invested in an object originates in the id with the libidinal and aggressive drives. For the young child, his original objects are his parents or other important caregivers. He forms affectionate bonds and attachments with them. As he matures, he is able to form relationships with others based on his ability to form attachments with his parents. His basic personality is organized around his experiences with his parents (Bowlby, 1980).

The strength of a person's attachment to an object will determine his reaction to the loss of that object (Bowlby, 1980). The human being's normal goal is to establish bonds. Accordingly, the behavior of the infant, the child, and the adult is directed toward the goal of forming, maintaining, and defending against the loss of relationships.

Psychoanalytic theorists believe that only human beings can be classified as "objects." The energy invested in another human being, the ability to relate to the other person, and the quality of that relationship are object relations (Kanzer, 1979). In addition to loss of other human beings, some patients also experience loss of valuable entities, such as intact body image, role within the family, and ability to achieve their life goals. The impact of illness causes these entities to be taken away or lost. For example, a person can invest emotional energy in a job, a body that responds normally, a well-functioning heart, hair, a perfect baby, unmarked skin, working kidneys, ability to talk, and so on.

In any case, whether the emotional investment is in another person, an aspect of one's self that is concrete or abstract, a job, or any other important entity, the actual or threatened loss will cause a reaction in a patient:

> The goal of attachment behavior is to maintain an affectional bond; any situation that seems to be endangering the bond elicits action designed to preserve it; and the greater the danger of loss appears to be the more varied and intense are the actions elicited to prevent it [Bowlby, 1980, p. 42].

The subject of loss has been described by many authors. Two other terms, *grief* and *bereavement,* are closely related to loss, and sometimes the terms are used interchangeably. For clarification, definitions of each term will follow. *Loss* is a change in status of a significant object. The loss can be actual or threatened; either way, the personality will organize itself to defend against the effects of the loss. Carson (1979) defines loss as "any change in the person's situation that reduces the probability of achieving implicit or explicit goals" (p. 78). These can be abstract, such as being able to marry, obtain a promotion, or have a well-functioning, attractive body.

Grief is the emotion experienced when a *loss* occurs. It is the affective result of a loss. It is the sadness that a person feels when he *anticipates* losing something special or after he loses the valued object. The word *mourning* is sometimes used to refer to grief. It, too, means sadness in connection with a loss (Kaplan and Sadock, 1981). *Bereavement* is the actual process a person goes through after he experiences a major loss. It includes the various stages involved in the adaptation process of resolving the loss.

The reaction to loss is an important process for nurses to be aware of from the viewpoints of the following persons:

1. A dying patient who is going through the process of accepting his *own* death
2. The family of the dying patient
3. A patient who must resolve the loss of a body part, such as the uterus, or accept a change in normal body functioning, both of which involve accepting a changed body image
4. The family of the patient who is adapting to the loss of a body part or a change in normal functioning, since *their* image of the patient has also changed and must be worked through so that they can accept their changed loved one

Whether you work in an acute care, extended care, or outpatient setting, you will be able to observe the effects if this resolution does not occur. Your ability to perceive that the reaction to loss is maladaptive can be very important to patients and their families. Without appropriate intervention by you or by a referral you place in motion, the patient's and the family's quality of life can be seriously affected. Suggestions for appropriate nursing interventions when maladaptation is observed appear in Chapter 18: The Coping Challenge of Chronic Illness, and Chapter 19. Many of the interventions presented in the chapter are appropriate for patients and family members who are responding to any type of loss.

The process of *adapting to loss* is one that can take a few days or a lifetime, depending on the meaning of the loss to the person experiencing it. If the loss is a significant one, such as a spouse or a body part, it may take up to 1 year for the pain of the loss to be resolved. Bowlby (1980) has described bereavement as a normal response to the loss of a significant object. For many, the process is slowed and the quality of life of the grieving person is detrimentally affected beyond the 1-year period (Parkes, 1972). When this occurs, it is called *unresolved grief* or *pathological bereavement.* These concepts will be further explored in Chapters 18, 19, and 20.

The best-known theory of the bereavement process is that of Elisabeth Kübler-Ross (1969). Her original book, *On Death and Dying*, describes the stages that a dying person ideally goes through before he finally is able to accept his own death. Remember that he is actually facing the loss of himself, that is, the loss of his own being. The stages are denial, anger, bargaining, depression, and acceptance. Although her book is written about the dying patient, *these stages are the same for any person who is either anticipating or has already lost a valued entity or a valued object.* This can be a woman reacting to the loss of a breast, a man who is adjusting to a severe myocardial infarct, an adolescent with diabetes mellitus, or parents whose child has died.

Family members each will experience the loss in their own way. Accordingly, their process through the stages will usually be different. They will not be in the *same stage* at the *same time* as their husband, wife, or child. This dissimilarity of feelings can provoke serious coping problems for the family. These will be discussed more fully in Chapter 8: The Family as a System, and Chapter 15: Crisis Intervention With the Maladapting Patient, as well as in Chapters 18, 19, and 20.

In the *denial stage,* the person is shocked by his prognosis, and his ego protects him with a cloak of denial. Within a few days he should move into the *stage of anger.* The anger may be rational; it can have a specific reasonable focus. It can also be irrational and nonspecific, and the patient may verbally strike out at anyone for any reason. People in this stage may unleash their anger at a "safe" person, one whom they trust not to retaliate against them. Frequently, nurses are the subject of this type of anger because they spend a great deal of time with the patient.

The next stage is *bargaining.* In this stage, the dying or grieving person actually is trying to postpone his dying or, in the case of someone who is responding to loss, his acceptance of the loss. He is not ready to accept it just yet. The bargaining person will, for example, make "deals" with God. If God will allow him to live, he will make amends with his long-lost brother or will change his life. In another manifestation of bargaining, he may also take risks in order to test the effects of his illness on his body. The bargaining stage is also marked by frequent mood changes and ambivalence.

Depression is the fourth stage. It is as if all the defenses of the earlier stages have failed. The patient or family member feels overwhelmed by the loss. Its full impact hits him. He may be responding to losses he has already experienced with the current illness, or an old unresolved loss may surface once again. He may also be responding to anticipated losses. A dying woman may never live to see her daughter married. The amputee will probably never ski again. The recently blinded man will never see his first grandchild's face.

The final stage is *acceptance.* The person finally feels at peace about the loss. This stage involves a final "letting go." The emotional ties to the lost object are loosened, and the person is able to invest in a new object. The dying patient is able to say goodbye to his family and is ready to accept the peace of death. For the person responding to loss, he is able to allow a new object to replace the old one with no guilt. In order to visualize this concept, imagine that you are holding a ball in your hand. It is impossible to catch another ball while you are still holding the first one. Unless you let go of the first ball, you will be unable to catch the second. The following case example illustrates this concept:

Case Example

Ellen is a 28-year-old woman who has been admitted to the hospital with hyperemesis gravidarum. She is 4 months pregnant. Two and a half years ago she delivered a nine-pound baby boy who aspirated meconium. He lived for 7 days. She and her husband have had a very difficult time accepting the loss of their child. In fact, for a brief period they separated because of the high level of conflict that developed in their marriage. Ellen reports that she and her husband have finally accepted the loss of their baby, yet her mood is depressed and she begins to cry each time she mentions the infant who died *and* the infant she is expecting.

Ellen is intellectually saying that she has accepted the loss of her baby, yet her emotions demonstrate that she has not resolved the loss of her first baby. She has not worked through the ties that are still holding on to her lost child.

Guilt

Another major issue of patients with physical illness is guilt. The ability to feel guilt develops when the superego is formed around the age of 4 or 5 (Fenichel, 1945). As a result of a strict and demanding superego, some persons experience uncomfortable levels of guilt in contrast to the guilt level felt by persons with normally or poorly developed superegos. *Guilt* is felt when a person violates his own conscience or moral code (Perley, 1976). Erikson (1963) has described guilt as the negative balance of initiative in the early childhood stage of psychosocial development. Initiative is the amount of direction and purpose that a person has. It is the outward and positive manifestation of the libidinal and aggressive drives.

During adolescence the superego may initially be harsh, but gradually, as the adolescent matures, it softens and becomes more self-accepting. When this does not occur, the result is an adult who excessively displays some or all of the following behaviors: expresses guilt, rationalizes and intellectualizes, makes apologies when none are due, is depressed, denies sexual pleasure with resulting sexual dysfunction, uses avoidance behaviors in order to avoid guilt feelings, lacks realistic concern for the self (*e.g.,* masochistic behaviors), blames himself for events that are beyond his control, and is hypersensitive to others' comments (Perley, 1976).

These manifestations of excessive guilt feelings may be observed in the following hospital situations:

1. The excessively apologetic patient who finds it hard to let caregivers do anything for him
2. The patient who refuses pain medication but displays pain behavior
3. The patient who views his illness as a form of punishment

When you observe signs of excessive guilt in patients, remember that the patient's psyche has been operating in this way since he was a child. You will be unable to change his severe self-expectations. Attempting to decrease his guilt with strong counter arguments will only *increase* his anxiety. Instead, for example, ask him to talk about why he will not take pain medicine. You can listen and then respond that you have known other patients who have felt the same way but then were relieved when they took the medication. You can be gently persuasive.

You should also be aware of evidence of normal guilt in the hospital environment. Frequently, family members experience guilt when a choice must be made about whether their loved one should have a cardiac alert or rush (each hospital has its own name for its response to a cardiac arrest) or whether the patient should be categorized as "no cardiac alert" and the patient allowed to die if an arrest occurs. This is another example of a time when caregivers, the physician in

this case, can make a recommendation to the family, rather than arousing the family's guilt by leaving the entire decision to them.

The young patient in an intensive care unit whose brain death has been verified also poses a poignant dilemma for family members. At times, physicians will favor discontinuing life support systems, and the family has a difficult time agreeing with the physician's decision. Usually the family needs a day or two to live with the gravity and hopelessness of their loved one's condition before they can accept the finality of the situation and make a decision. The nurse can encourage ventilation about their guilt with an opening comment such as, "This must be a difficult decision for you." Gradually, most families are able to work through this guilt, and their decision can be made.

Another guilt ridden time for some families occurs when a relative needs constant care because of physical or mental infirmity. The decision to place their loved one in a nursing home or other institution can produce strong feelings of guilt in some family members who believe that the person *must* be cared for at home. Other members of the same family may believe that, because of the effort and strain on the remaining members, the nursing home is the most realistic alternative.

Serious family conflict of a long standing nature may arise at this time if all family members are not in agreement. The family member(s) who takes the elderly person into his or her own home may eventually feel "used" by other family members who do not have the responsibility. Later on, resentment may occur and be directed at the other members. Although this type of family conflict rarely is referred to a family therapist, it frequently causes permanent splits in relationships between families of the same generation and has far-reaching consequences into subsequent generations (Guerin and Guerin, 1976).

Many losses are experienced in this conflicted family cut off process. Ideally, this and similar types of conflicts should be referred for professional assistance in mediation. The underlying dynamic that precipitates many of these family conflicts is guilt. Another cause of conflict often appears to be jealousy of other family members. One of the basic dynamics of jealousy is guilt (Freud, 1924).

When guilt becomes a problem for patients and family members, be aware of the possibility that you may be working with someone who has a tendency to place himself into situations in which he feels oppressed. Encouraging such patients to talk about *why* they cannot take pain medication or why they cannot relax and let others help them may give you the opportunity to present a more realistic perspective than their own. As mentioned above, they may need permission that it is normal and acceptable to take pain medication and treatments that relieve pain.

Some people maintain their suffering behavior no matter what approach is tried with them. In fact, they seem to enjoy the hovering effect it has on their families and other visitors. For such patients, it is advisable not to reward their behavior by your increased attention. By withdrawing such increased attention, the patient's behavior may return to more normal limits.

Intimacy

Intimacy is another important issue of hospitalization that may present problems in adaptation for some patients. In the progression of personality development, intimacy is the major developmental hurdle of the young adult (Erikson, 1963). In Western culture, the word *intimacy* often has the same meaning as sexual closeness. This is only one aspect of intimacy. Actually, the young adult needs to be able to tolerate closeness interpersonally. He needs to be able to be emotionally close to people. Closeness is the ability to be open and honest, to trust, and to take risks in a relationship. Mature intimacy means knowing the other person interpersonally: his dreams and hopes, what gives him joy, what makes him sad, his positive side, his negative side, and *who* he really is and allowing one's self to be similarly known.

In his book *The Transparent Self,* Jouard (1971) writes that "no man can come to know himself except as an outcome of disclosing himself to another person" (p. 6). He also writes that self-disclosure requires courage, not only the courage to be and to do, but also the courage to be known as one knows himself to be (pp. 6 and 7).

Some examples of types of close, trusting relationships are those between a parent and child, a childhood or college friend maintained through a lifetime, a husband and wife, or people who work in the same environment. These types of relationships are mutually supportive and enriching. The emotional give and take in the dyad may be uneven at times but is equal over an extended time.

The ability to form intimate relationships is considered an essential aspect of full personality development. Psychiatry has described this essential quality as the ability to form good object relations (Blanck and Blanck, 1979). The foundation of intimacy is derived from the young child's experience in trusting others. The ability to trust is the building block of the ability to form an intimate relationship.

The capacity to form an intimate relationship is essential to a meaningful sexual relationship. Patients' sexual functioning is often affected when serious or chronic illness occurs. The subject of sexuality was generally avoided, until recently, in the curricula of many nursing and medical schools. In addition, it is a sensitive subject for many caregivers to talk about with their patients. Accordingly, although it may be of concern to a patient about to return home, the subject may not be discussed.

Chapter 16: Nursing Intervention With the Emotionally Complex Patient, includes recommendations that can be helpful in discussing patients' sexual concerns. In addition, Chapter 17: Psychosocial Aspects of Specific Physical Conditions, and Chapter 18: The Coping Challenge of Chronic Illness, contain information on sexuality in several types of conditions or illnesses.

Some patients have never had a close relationship with another person. When such a person is admitted to a hospital, suddenly all aspects of his privacy are invaded, and he may be very threatened and find it difficult to cope. The physical surface of his body is felt, examined, pushed, prodded, washed, rubbed, shaved, pricked, and incised.

An artificial closeness may suddenly be thrust on him by innumerable caregivers whom he has never met before. Questions are asked about many aspects of his functioning—social, physical, sexual, emotional—and about history of substance use—medications, alcohol, illegal drugs. He is asked about the cause of death of family members. He is told to take off all his clothes. His sense of body modesty seems violated by the body positioning required for proctological, urological, or other procedures.

An aspect of intimacy that can be troublesome for the very shy, aloof, or suspicious patient is the type of social history taking that may occur in some settings. Remember that this patient is very uncomfortable revealing intimate information to anyone, even his own family members. Accordingly, he will probably have difficulty confiding personal information to his primary caregiver if intimate questions are asked about his functioning. Sometimes caregivers who repeatedly ask for such information forget about the emotional impact they have on the patient. These questions are often experienced by such patients as an invasion of privacy. Although these questions may be important, they can be asked in a supportive manner so that the patient's embarrassment is accepted and empathized with. Frequently, it is helpful if you explain how you will use this information in designing his care. If he understands the beneficial effects of his disclosures, his discomfort may be decreased, and his motivation to share this information will be more positive.

Conclusion

As explained in this chapter, the issues of trust, self-esteem, control, loss, guilt, and intimacy are important underlying dynamics in a patient's capacity to adapt to illness. When maladaptation occurs, usually one or more of these issues can be implicated. The success of a nursing intervention plan designed to resolve or lessen a crisis can depend in part on the nurse's ability to identify a major underlying issue and its dynamics. When a nursing diagnosis is established, the underlying dynamic should also be described if it can be identified. The specific issues addressed in this chapter are applied in Chapters 17 and 18. By referring to those chapters, you can develop a deeper understanding of the challenges they present to psychosocial adaptation.

One of the most important concepts in this book is that human beings are constantly affected by events occurring within themselves and in their environment. Physical illness is a significant event for patients and their families. The human being consists of two main subsystems: physiological subsystems, such as respiratory, cardiovascular, neurological, and so on, and an intrapsychic subsystem, through which the person perceives, thinks about, and responds to internal and external stimuli and stressors. Man is himself a subsystem of other social systems: the family, the work group, other reference groups such as a religious community, clubs, sports groups, and so on, and society at large.

As you read, picture man as a figure suspended by a string in a large hanging mobile made up of many other figures that represent his various physiological and psychological subsystems, the separate roles he plays within his family, work group, and so on, and the multiple events that affect him in society at large. Now, imagine that you are touching one of the figures with your finger. What will happen to the whole mobile? All the figures will move in response when just one of those figures moves. Remove one of those figures. What happens then? The mobile is unbalanced.

The development of physical illness has a similar, multiply disturbing impact on the patient and the family system. Man is a dynamic being, constantly interacting with multiple internal and external events. He responds to them; they respond to him. The context in which they occur is never static. By envisioning man as a complex entity made up of many elements and as a part of many complex social groups, we are viewing him both as a system made up of many subsystems and as a subsystem or element of many larger systems. In fact, we can call a large system a supersystem.

What Is a System?

The word *system* is defined as follows:

> An orderly combination or arrangement of parts, elements, etc. into a whole . . . . An assemblage of organic structures composed of similar elements and combined for the same general functions: the nervous system . . . . The entire body taken as a functional whole.*

It is also described as "a group of units so combined as to form a whole and to operate in unison." Another description of a system

*Definition abridged from FUNK & WAGNALLS STANDARD COLLEGE DICTIONARY. Copyright © 1977 by Harper & Row. Reprinted by permission.

7

General Systems Theory in Clinical Practice

is that it is "a complex of interacting components" (Bertalanffy, 1968, p. 91).

The essence of systems theory is that *any* action, whether social or biological, causes a reaction within its own environment. The action also changes the relationship of that thing to all the other things in its environment. These changes or adjustments alter the overall system to which they belong. Using these definitions, think of some things that can be classified as systems. Is a television set a system? Does it have a series of parts that operate together and cause it to be a television set? Is a family a system? Does it have a series of parts that cause it to be a complex unit? Is a human being a system: What kinds of parts go into a human being? Your first answer will probably be his anatomical parts. Are there any other parts? What about his psychological functioning, that is, his ability to think and feel? A person can function psychologically whether alone or with someone else. Another very important part of a person is his social functioning. Can a person function socially when alone? No. He must interact with others. Once he interacts with others, he opens himself to many opportunities as well as risks.

Man belongs to many types of systems, some of them social: a family, work force, social clubs, friendships, and so on. He is also a part of the ecological supersystem of the environment. He is a vital link in the earth's biological chain. For example, he inhales oxygen produced by the photosynthesis of the earth's greenery. After his body uses oxygen, he exhales carbon dioxide, which is essential to the same plants and trees in their production of oxygen. His body is a large system made up of many smaller physiological subsystems, each of them essential to the functioning of the total body equilibrium. Optimally, they operate in unison to support the integrity of the entire body.

All living things and all social groups are dynamic. The word *dynamic* used in this manner is related to the branch of physics that concerns itself with the production of motion due to various forces. It also deals with the effects of these forces on bodies in motion or at rest. When used as a noun, *dynamics* (within the context of psychosocial functioning) are the multiple and ever-changing forces or factors that are behind the actions of human beings (Hinsie and Campbell, 1977).

Systems theory is an exciting concept that can help nurses to be far more aware of the impact of multiple factor relationships *everywhere:* in the body, in intrapsychic psychological functioning, and in all types of social relationships.

Types of Systems

All systems can be generally classified by the amount of contributing factors or input that have the potential to cause change. They fall into two main categories, open and closed, as described below:

Open system. An open system is one that has an unlimited number of ever-changing dynamics. A normal family can be called a relatively open system because all its members are subject to change. The openness in a system comes from the vast number of subsystems that exist within the overall system. In a family there are various members or components, each of whom brings his or her intrapsychic, physical, and social subsystem components. Each component has the potential to change the dynamics in that person, as well as those in each of the other members, because of the constant interaction that occurs in a family. The more that openness exists in a system, the *less* predictable is the outcome of any change in the system.

Closed system. The closed system consists of specific variables that react with a *predictable* outcome. While it is possible to change the number of variables in a closed system, prediction of a high degree of probability differentiates the closed from the open system [Abbey, 1978, p. 20].

Within the body, an example of a closed system could be any of the main body subsystems. It is important to keep in mind that none of them is *ever* static. They are all subject to change based on the external or internal stresses they are subjected to. The amount of change is not infinite, however. There is a normal range of variation beyond which the subsystem, and eventually the entire body system, would fail. For example, a body temperature of 94°F to 106°F will continue to sustain life. If prolonged below or above this range, most body systems would soon fail. Body temperature adjustment mechanisms are fairly rigid. Once exhausted, they stop working. They cannot tolerate an infinite range of temperature variation. The temperature-regulating mechanism is a moderately closed system.

All the physiological subsystems that may initially seem distinct and separate are interdependent. One cannot live without the others. If the gastrointestinal system lost its blood sypply, its tissues would die. It would also die because it would have no way of eliminating toxic wastes. All the tissues in the other body systems would fail because of lack of carbohydrates, fats, proteins, minerals, vitamins, and water, which are the end products of digestion.

Until now, I have discussed only the concrete subsystems of a human being. Other important types of systems influence him and his actions. Even when man is asleep, the intrapsychic subsystem never ceases its dynamic process. It is constantly affected by external events and its own reaction to them. It also responds continually to neurotransmitters and other biochemical substances of the physiological subsystem. These subsystems operate interdependently. None of them operates in isolation.

General Systems Theory

History

Although all types of systems have existed since the beginning of the world, the formal idea of systems theory was not conceptualized until the late 1920s, when the biologist Ludwig von Bertalanffy described his *organismic viewpoint*. This simply means that all organisms are organized things. In studying the metabolism, growth, and biophysics of organisms, von Bertalanffy was struck by the interdependence between one biological system and another. He was the first to describe the concept that, rather than being distinct and separate systems, biological systems were actually a part of a still larger system (1968). He called them subsystems of the larger system.

As von Bertalanffy's theory emerged in the early 1930s, scholars from many disciplines discovered that the concept of general systems theory applied equally well to their own fields, such as chemistry, physics, and the social sciences. The application of general systems theory to psychiatry was helpful in conceptualizing the development of personality.

Application to Personality Development

The development of the psyche is an abstract process occurring within the human being's emotional system. It is affected by many factors. Brazelton (1973) has theorized that the infant is born with an inherited set of unique personality characteristics. Thomas and Chess (1980) have written that the "fit" of the parents' personality characteristics with the unique characteristics of

the child can subdue or cause a marked increase in the strength of those characteristics.

Catecholamine research has demonstrated that greater or lesser amounts of biochemical neurotransmitters—substances known to be in the physiological realm—affect the emotional realm (Hillenbrand, 1980; Iverson, 1979; Snyder, 1980). In fact, the two major drives of human beings, the libidinal and aggressive, are inseparable from the endocrine subsystem. The ego develops defense mechanisms in order to defend itself against the anxiety caused by its inability to tolerate the conflict of these internal id drives with the internal demands of the superego and the external demands of the social environment (Carson, 1979). Here we can see a multiple interaction relationship between a physiological subsystem and an abstract psychological subsystem. Remember, too, that external influences such as infection, trauma, or natural disaster can also have a profound impact on these internal subsystems.

The emotional stress of physical illness can result in increased stress on an already impaired physiological subsystem. The increased stress that the family experiences during hospitalization of one of its members also affects the ill member. In general, the more open a system, the more tolerance it has for stress and the less likely psychosocial or physiological dysfunction will occur. For example, a family may have a father who has maintained "iron" rule over his wife and children. The wife and children have always adhered to his authority. Their functioning in the family and in their roles outside of the family has always been in line with the father's expectations. This family demonstrates "closedness." There is little flexibility. If this father were to become seriously ill or die, the remaining family members would be at far more risk for dysfunction because of their own lack of development as independent beings.

So too with body functioning. Although the physiological subsystems operate within ranges that are required to sustain life and can be classified as closed systems, there can be differences in the range of closedness. For example, a person who has chronic obstructive respiratory disease complicated by frequent infections has a more closed body system than a healthy person. Both the emotional and physiological stresses of illness have a greater potential to promote dysfunction in the person with a more closed body system.

Thinking in terms of systems is an important concept for nurses to remember. It can be applied to *all* patients. It is essential for you to be aware of systems theory and the complex impact that a set of circumstances can have on several aspects of a patient's life. Major illness, for example, affects not only the patient's physiological and psychological subsystems but also the familial and extrafamilial supersystems. The effects are similar to the ever-widening set of ripples set off by a stone tossed into a pool. When you use systems theory in designing and implementing your care plans, you will deliver more holistic, realistic, and compassionate care than nurses who view the patient as a sick being with an acute medical disease who is temporarily isolated from all other aspects of existence.

Application to Nursing Practice

A person with any type of illness, chronic or acute, is affected by many factors, including what the illness means to him, how it affects him physically, how it affects him emotionally, the quality of medical care available to him, the quality of nursing care available to him, and how his family and friends react to his illness. Look back at these factors. Is any one separate and distinct from the others? Is it possible that the effect of one of these factors can influence one of the others? Is it also possible that one of these factors can influence *all* the others?

To illustrate the interrelationship of factors and how one of them, depending on the degree of its impact, can cause a varying response in the others, let us examine the factors listed above.

What the illness means to the patient

Imagine that a patient has been admitted for a hemorrhoidectomy. As a nurse, you may classify this illness as nonthreatening. Remember, that is *your* perception. The way the patient perceives *his* illness may be quite different.

The hemorrhoidectomy patient may be someone who is normally fearful in a new situation. Let us say that this patient is a woman with a very low pain tolerance who has never before been hospitalized. She does not respond well to stress; her coping ability during stressful periods is poor. Her physician has cautioned her that the pain from the surgery may be severe for the first few days. She has had chronic constipation for years; the idea of moving her bowels after surgery already frightens her. In addition, her cousin died many years previously while undergoing anesthesia for a minor surgical procedure. She fears that she too could die during surgery.

In assessing this patient's perception of her illness, we find that her illness is very threatening to her. Many of her perceptions are based on accurate cognitive awarenesses. She has definite reasons why she is fearful.

In evaluating the effect of the meaning of illness to a patient on the various factors above, we will examine them one by one. An asterisk will mark each instance in which one factor is capable of setting off a response in another subsystem and triggering a series of changes in other subsystems.

Will the patient's high level of fearfulness have an effect on her physically?

Think of this patient's potential postoperative response. Will she be unusually tense and frightened?* Will this psychic tension and alarm trigger her adrenals?* What are some of the effects of adrenalin on vital signs* and on the musculoskeletal subsystem?* Will this affect *all* her muscles?* Could her vital signs be altered as a result of her high level of muscle tension?* Perform the following exercise:

Make a fist with your right hand. Tense the muscles in your right arm and squeeze your fist. What effect do you think this tenseness has on your pulse, blood pressure, and respirations? In this example, the patient's vital signs are already affected by the adrenal response to her fear. The accompanying muscular tension heightens and aggravates the already stressed cardiovascular and pulmonary systems.

Will she possibly need more analgesia than a normal hemorrhoidectomy patient? Could she require frequent analgesia? Will this analgesia alter her other physiological responses?* Will her first bowel movement be complicated by an unusually tight anal sphincter (gastrointestinal subsystem)?* Could there be bleeding complications as a result (cardiovascular subsystem)?* Will she ambulate well (musculoskeletal subsystem)?* If not, could venous or pulmonary complications be precipitated (cardiovascular and respiratory subsystems)* if she is inactive due to her pain and level of fearfulness?

Will the patient's perceptions of the seriousness of her illness affect her emotional functioning?

Because of her high level of anxiety, do you think this patient will be fully receptive to preoperative teaching (affective and cognitive-intellectual parts of intrapsychic system)?* Actually, her fear may cause her to blot out your words. Her ego is prepared to protect her from hearing *anything* that may overload and overwhelm her (affective and ego defensive parts of intrapsychic system).* As a result, when she awakens in the recovery room, she may be unprepared for the experience, and her level of anxiety may be high.*

After returning to her room, she may not comply with the normal postoperative precautions of turning, coughing, and deep breathing.* Her emotional response to pain* and her level of fearfulness* about the anticipated bowel movement may even cause her to require sedative medication.* Her anxiety may also cause her to be demanding and difficult with the medical* and nursing* staff and with her family.*

Will the patient's perceptions of the seriousness of her illness have an effect on the quality of medical care available to her?

The quality of medical care available to a patient can differ from institution to institution and, within one institution, from physician to physician and from nursing unit to nursing unit, as well as from nurse to nurse. Ideally, physicians should respond with a caring and professional manner to all patients. Because they are human, however, they can be affected by a patient's response to his or her illness. A compliant, noncomplaining, respectful, and friendly patient will promote a positive physician-patient relationship. A patient with an inappropriate level of fear who lacks trust in his physicians and questions them about all aspects of his care may invite a negative response.*

Nurses may complain to the physician about the patient* with comments such as, "She's constantly ringing and asking for pain medication," or, "When she had her first bowel movement yesterday, she had to have someone stay with her the whole time. Every time the nurse would start to leave she would become nearly hysterical." These comments further reinforce the idea in the physician that his or her patient is a nuisance. He or she may be inclined to interact with the patient as briefly and superficially as possible.*

The frightened patient then perceives the physician's abruptness as impatience with her (and she may be right.) and becomes even more anxious.* Unfortunately, she may have contributed to this changed impression without being aware of it.

Will the patient's perceptions of the seriousness of her illness have an effect on the quality of nursing care available to her?

Nurses who care for this patient during an 8-hour shift may eventually become exasperated and impatient if her "negative" behavior continues.* They may begin to withdraw from her because she is difficult to be with and because they want to avoid losing their tempers.* They may eventually respond less promptly to her requests for pain medication after the first few days* if she asks for more medication than they believe is necessary for a 2- or 3-day postoperative hemorrhoidectomy patient.

Will the patient's perceptions of the seriousness of her illness affect the reactions of her family and friends?

The patient's reaction to her illness may be one that demonstrates that she is in great pain. Accordingly, she may arouse much sympathy in her family.* They will frequently approach nurses about being more attentive to their wife's or mother's needs.* Friends also may respond with much sympathy to the patient and, by doing so, may cause a prolongation of pain behavior* because of the secondary gain the patient derives from their attention. They eventually may become tired of her need for attention.* *Secondary gain* is "the obvious advantage that a person gains from his illness, such as gifts, attention, and release from responsibility" (Freedman, 1976, p. 1328).

• • •

On the other hand, the patient may be one whose pain experiences encourage her family to defend her actions with the nurses and her physicians.* If, for example, the patient senses the rejection of caregivers because of her negative response to her hospitalization, she may cause her spouse or her children to admonish the nurses for their "poor" care,* to report the nurses to the physician* or, in some cases, to the hospital administration,* to report house officers or attending physicians for their "poor" care,* or to complain to persons in the community about the "poor" care available at the hospital.* These comments, if convincing, may influence their acquaintances' attitude toward the hospital.*

• • •

This example of a patient's response to illness points out the many effects that just one factor can have on only five of the many other factors that affect overall hospitalization. It is clear that one component of illness can begin a whole series of responses. Each of those responses can then trigger another whole series or chain of events, some physical, some emotional, some affecting hospital personnel, some affecting the family's emotional and social response, and some affecting the hospital and the community at large.

Conclusion

The use of a general systems approach in the nursing process involves the assessment of all aspects of a patient's functioning: physical, psychological, and social. When an event occurs in any one of these realms, it will affect the other two. For example, if a person has a severe headache, the cause is due to a physiological disequilibrium, but psychological functioning will also be affected

Intellectual functioning will be dominated by the intrusion of thoughts about the pain the person is experiencing. Will his feeling state be affected as well? Does a person with a severe headache feel happy even in the middle of a joyous occasion? How do you think his interactions with others will be? Picture this person at a wedding. Will he fully participate in the experience with others in the same way as he would have if he did not have a headache?

All the categories of nursing diagnosis (which will be introduced in Chapter 13: Psychosocial Nursing Assessment and Diagnosis) are strongly influenced by general systems effects. Understanding of general systems effects in the assessment, planning, intervention, and evaluation steps of the nursing process can help you to understand more fully the effects of a particular illness on a particular patient and family. By using this type of holistic framework, your nursing care can promote an adaptive response in the patient and family.

8

The Family as a System

Systems theory has been applied to a special type of social group that is essential to the development of all human beings: the family. The family system is one that is ever changing and is constantly affected by the larger social order as well as by events that have an impact on each member. The intrapsychic reaction of each family member to a specific event will determine his or her actions with *each* of the other members. These reactions are based on many dynamics within the family group: the role that each member fills within the family, who has the real power in the family, the unwritten rules of the family, and so on.

Theories about family functioning have been proposed by psychiatric researchers who wanted to discover the roots of psychopathology in patients with severe psychiatric disturbance. A patient's entire family was admitted with him, and methods of communicating were closely observed (Bateson and colleagues, 1956). Eventually, the many types of relationships and communication styles that exist between family members in well-functioning as well as in poorly functioning families were described (Ackerman, 1966; Bowen, 1971, 1974, 1976a; Fogarty, 1975, 1977; Framo, 1965; Guerin, 1976; Haley, 1971; Jackson, 1967; Menuchin, 1974; Satir and associates, 1975).

Nurses should understand family systems functioning for many reasons. One reason is that most patients are members of families and have certain roles in their families that are disrupted by their illnesses and hospitalizations. The loss of a person in his or her normal family role results in shifts in functioning in all other family members. For example, if a mother is admitted to the hospital, her husband and children usually assume some of her responsibilities. In addition, because of their worry about her illness and prognosis, all members may become more emotionally needy. Because *all* the members need support, they may be unable to satisfy these emotional needs within the immediate family. Accordingly, they may turn to extended family members, friends, or professionals. If the family member is normally shy and aloof, he may be unable to ask for emotional support or unable to receive it, even if it is available. If the emotional stress of a family member is severe and is unrelieved for an extended period, then physical or emotional illness could be the outcome (Engel, 1962).

During the process of emotional adaptation of each family member, the ill member, the one who is actually *causing* the emotional stress of the other members, is going through an emotional process of his own. Because of the different dynamics in each member, adaptation processes are not occurring at the same rate; the opportunity for a shutdown in communication in order to protect one another may occur. Conflict is another possibility. Many families find it difficult to maintain open and empathic communication among all members during a time of acute stress.

Another very important aspect of family systems theory is that it can be generally applied to nursing groups and most other social groups; baseball teams, social clubs, school classrooms, and so on all operate within the theoretical framework of family systems theory.

These concepts will have a strong impact on you as you work in any nursing setting. They can be applied to a visiting nurse agency, a general hospital unit, a nursing faculty group, or any other working environment in which there is a group of people whose membership and leadership remains fairly stable. By using these concepts, you can better understand the "rules" that will have a strong effect on your relationships within that social system.

Family Systems Terminology

Some of the following terms may already be familiar to you. In case they are not, they will be defined in order to clarify the ways they are used in this chapter.

Family of origin. The family of origin is the family into which a person is born. It includes the immediate family members (mother, father, siblings, *and* any other person who is a *consistent* member of the household). Any person, by living permanently in the home, influences the overall dynamics of the family.

Nuclear family. The nuclear family is a new family that is created by a husband and wife. It consists of the mother and father (each of whom has a family of origin and an extended family) and their children or the children they might bring from a previous relationship.

Extended family. The extended family is the family network beyond the family of origin. It includes grandparents, aunts, uncles, cousins, nieces, nephews, and grandchildren. It also includes dynamics that are passed on from one generation to the next. For example, if a grandmother has a tendency toward multiple illnesses with much secondary gain, this pattern will often be repeated in succeeding generations in her niece, granddaughter, and so on.

Differentiation of Self

Before the family can be examined as a group, and before there can be an understanding of the patient as he relates with other family members, we first must understand the functioning of the patient. A concept proposed by Murray Bowen (1976) is differentiation of self. *Differentiation of self* is the degree to which either a person's intellect *or* his emotions control his functioning. It "defines people according to the degree of fusion or differentiation between emotional and intellectual functioning" (p. 65). An example of good differentiation is the response of a nurse who is told by his head nurse that he should spend less time talking with his newly admitted patient. Instead of being overwhelmed by feelings of guilt or anger toward the head nurse (emotional fusion), his emotions do not take control of him. Instead, his intellect dominates and he says to himself, "Mrs. Ames doesn't know that this new patient is being admitted directly from being at her husband's funeral. The patient is very upset and needs me. I'll explain it to Mrs. Ames later." This nurse's intellect is well differentiated. A distinct boundary separates a "feeling" response from a "thinking" response.

Bowen believes that this concept is so universal that all people can be categorized on a single continuum. There are people whose emotions and intellect are so inseparable that everything they do is dominated by their emotions. They are at the fusion level of the continuum. Their life energy is devoted to avoiding feelings of displeasure, unhappiness, guilt, anger, jealousy, and so on. Their intellect is totally dominated by their feeling state. Their lives are governed by their feelings. Few persons are totally controlled by their feelings, but many dependent persons and a number of persons who develop chronic illness as an unconscious means of avoiding the demands of adulthood fall on the first 25% of the continuum (Bowen, 1976).

Another aspect of Bowen's theory is that of *undifferentiated ego mass.* An *undifferentiated ego mass* operates in a family when one person feels anxiety. One or more other members of the family automatically begin to feel the same anxiety. They are not able to differentiate their own feelings from those of their family member. They are not able to maintain their own feelings if they are different.

If Bowen's theory is correct, then it is possible to see that two like-minded emotional people will raise their children in an environment that fosters emotionalism. When a person with a low level of differentiation is admitted to the hospital, he may flounder because he has lost the highly charged emotional setting in which he is comfortable and accepted. Instead, the hospital system is cool and clinical and is unable to tolerate lack of emotional control in patients. Frequently, hospital staff members attempt to confine emotionalism by being authoritative, using an intellectual approach, and withholding their acceptance. This will increase the patient's level of anxiety and may cause his already minimal coping ability to be even more threatened. By understanding the patient's normal level of functioning, you can then design a care plan that encourages stronger emotional support from caregivers. Kind and caring limit setting can help the patient as he attempts to retain a level of emotionalism that is tolerated by the staff and that will not cause them to abandon him.

What Is the Self?

Before explaining the difference between the low levels of differentiation of self and the higher levels, it is necessary to understand the concept of self. Bowen has described two ways in which people function in regard to their beliefs about themselves. The *solid self* is the beliefs that a person has about himself and his environment. They result from his life experiences since birth. The *pseudo self* is the self that a person presents to the world. (Pseudo is derived from the Greek *pseudes,* meaning false.) It is the result of the emotional pressure applied by a person's social system to conform to specific role expectations. For example, a female lawyer can fill each of many roles. She may behave differently in each one based on the expectations of others *and* her level of self-differentiation. These roles may include:

A woman

A girlfriend or wife

A mother

A daughter

A parttime college professor

A high-level professional (within her professional role she may relate differently to other lawyers in her firm who rank above or below her, secretaries and paraprofessionals, janitors and other maintenance workers)

Ideally, if the level of solid self is high, people should behave according to their *own* beliefs, rather than demonstrating changes in behavior based on the particular role they are filling at the time.

If the level of pseudo self is high, the person presents himself differently in each of his social relationships. He is never really *himself.* For example, a man may be an unresponsive husband, a demanding and insensitive father, a passive, acquiescing son, a bully type of foreman, a "good old boy" bowling-team member, and a "tough guy" neighbor. Actually, this man does not appear to have a "down deep" type of self. The hospital system and the outpatient care system tend to encourage patients to suppress or deny their own needs and conform to the care system's expectations of appropriate patient behavior. The individualist with a strong sense of solid self may have a difficult time if he clashes with physicians or nurses who have other expectations of him. It is wise for us to remember that our main objective in caring for patients is *to help them to return to their presickness state.* Requiring them to change their normal level of interpersonal behavior may help *us,* but it may be detrimental to the patients.

The Levels of Self-Differentiation

The concept of level of differentiation is an important one for you to understand as you evaluate the patient's response to his illness and the hospital care system (Fig. 8-1). It is also valuable in assessing the patient's presickness level of emotional functioning, his adaptation potential in the hospital system *and* his adaptation potential when discharged into his normal family system (both of which may be quite different and impose different expectations), his emotional reaction to his illness, his family's emotional reaction to his illness, and his reaction to his family's reaction to his illness.

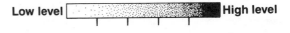

(feelings in total control)   (intellect in total control)

Figure 8-1. Differentiation of self continuum.

The latter factor may sound confusing until you think of a cancer patient who has a low level of differentiation of self. On her own, in the hospital, she might be able to achieve a reasonable level of psychological adaptation. If she is discharged into a family with an undifferentiated ego mass, and they feel helpless and hopeless about her cancer, then their feelings will overwhelm her and she will be unable to maintain her own feelings and beliefs.

When the stress of illness occurs, it is important to remember that the patient's normal level of functioning may regress to a lower level. Viewed within the context of the stress of illness, the level of differentiation is indicated by the degree of dysfunctioning that occurs when a person or a loved one is seriously ill. The level of dysfunctioning that occurs and the time it takes to regain equilibrium depend on the level of differentiation in the person as well as in the family group. For example, the person or family with poor differentiation is more likely to become emotionally overwhelmed by illness. The person and family with a moderate to high level of differentiation will be more likely to maintain control and cope adaptively. Another important point is that one or more of the patient's family members may regress to a lower level of functioning because of the emotional stress they experience about the illness of their loved one. What change do you think this can bring about in intrafamily relationships and communications?

Low Level

At the low level of differentiation of self, the intellect and its ability to reason and analyze situations is dominated by feelings. Feelings tend to govern the intellect most of the time. Such people have a strong need to keep relationships in harmony as a way of avoiding anxiety. Accordingly, the solid self submits almost entirely to the pseudo self. The avoidance of anxiety, guilt, and other negative feelings has a strong influence on the person's actions and the choices he makes in his life. He and other members of his family do not integrate easily into the world at large. They usually remain close-knit. Relationships outside of the immediate or extended family are not strongly encouraged. If a member of the family attempts to separate from the family, strong pressure is exerted on him by other members to conform to their expectations.

When working with patients in this category,

and especially when doing inpatient discharge teaching or planning or outpatient work of any kind, it is essential to include one or more family members in the process. Unless someone in the patient's family shares the experience and understands the treatment recommendations, the family's expectations of the patient after discharge may cause him to sway from his prescribed plan. The inclusion of other family members in the steps of nursing process is important. Assessment of highly anxious family members includes identifying their specific fears. During the planning and intervention steps, there is significant value in talking with them. In doing so, their anxiety, which was probably due to an unknown cause, may be narrowed to a definite fear. Once their fear is identified and talked about, their level of anxiety usually decreases.

Moderate Level

Persons with a moderate level of differentiation fluctuate between behavior governed by both intellect and feelings. Their lives are relationship oriented. They are more open and honest in expressing feelings than people on the lower level of the continuum. Their relationships and communication are largely pseudo self in expression because of their need to meet others' expectations. This type of person usually adapts well to the hospital environment. He and his family are able to understand the expectations of the hospital and those of their caregivers. They rarely have difficulty in conforming.

High Level

The person with a high level of differentiation demonstrates strong evidence of solid self. He judges his own value systems to be safe and does not feel any need to meet others' expectations. He enjoys relationships and is free to be himself rather than feeling a constant need to meet others' expectations of him. He remains independent when he so chooses. The highly differentiated person is fully aware of himself as a person. Bowen (1976) writes, "They are remarkably free from the full range of human problems" (p. 73). Note, however, that the highly differentiated person is not rigidly cold and controlled. The highly controlled person actually has a strong need to avoid his own affect, and many of his emotions may be repressed.

Other Concepts of Family Systems Theory

In order to evaluate fully a person's level of psychosocial functioning, there are other family systems concepts that will help to determine his in-hospital level of functioning as well as provide an indication of how he will function after discharge. Remember also to apply these concepts to your own social system of family, working environment, relationships with roommates, or classmates or to any other social group to which you belong. They can be very helpful in understanding the dynamics in a particular group or setting.

Boszormenyi-Nagy believes in viewing families within the context of their extended family environment. He believes that families are always attempting to maintain balance and fairness within their unit. This requires giving and receiving on the part of all family members. Although there may be members within the family who appear unable to give, they are aware of their indebtedness to the family system. All members carry an *unconscious* awareness of the balance "ledger" (Boszormenyi-Nagy, 1965). The development of physical illness within the family presents a dynamic that can temporarily unbalance the ledger as roles shift within the family. However, this can have a positive as well as a negative effect. For example, one family member may have been primarily on the "receiving" end in the family. If the ill member has been a giver, it is possible that the "receiving" person can temporarily move into a giving role. Accordingly, his view of himself and of other family members can become more positive, and the potential for his change to a contributing member within the family system is enhanced.

Subsystem

As described in Chapter 7, a subsystem is a working unit in a larger structure called a system. Each person in a family is a subsystem who belongs to many systems. He is a subsystem within his own family, and he is a subsystem in each social group to which he belongs: his working place, his social support network, and his nuclear and extended family, in which he functions differently depending on his role as husband, father, son, nephew, grandson, and so on. In each of these roles he has different levels of power and different functions (Minuchin, 1974; Minuchin and colleagues, 1978). "Subsystems can also consist of more than one individual such as a dyad of husband and wife or a dyad of mother and child" (Jones, 1980, p. 63). Subsystem dyads can also occur in other combinations, such as two persons within a family who share the same interests, are of the same sex, serve the same function (for example, two brothers-in-law), or even share the same illness.

Sibling Position in Family of Origin: Application in the General Hospital

The understanding of systems theory is important to nurses for many reasons. One of these is a concept that is not widely known, yet is very helpful in understanding why patients behave as they do. It is the idea that the particular role occupied by a child in his original family exerts an influence on his interpersonal functioning in his adult life. No matter where he is or what his social situation, he will continue to demonstrate many of the traits that developed and were tolerated by his parents and siblings.

> This does not mean to imply an inescapable determinism, but recent and contemporary influences should not be overestimated in view of the early experiences that have been having their effect for much longer. . . . They appear in sentiments and attitudes, in basic wishes and interests of which the person may be partly unaware. They do affect his social behavior, and, to be sure, they often do so more strongly, the less conscious they are [Toman, 1976, p. 6].

Although initially this idea may seem foreign, think of the following case example of a 61-year-old lathe operator who was admitted to the hospital because of lower extremity vascular insufficiency caused by diabetes.

Case Example

Henry was the youngest of six children. As the youngest child his needs were met, frequently before he became aware of them, by his mother and his next three closest siblings, who were sisters 2, 3, and 5 years older than he. He enjoyed their attention to his needs, and they enjoyed taking care of him. He lived at home until he married. As he approached his mid-twenties, he imagined marriage to various young women he knew. Those who seemed passive and seemed to be quite dependent did not particularly appeal to him. Instead, a very motherly, nurturing young woman who seemed capable and self-assured became his bride. In their marriage she was the dominant partner. She enjoyed her dominant role in the home, and he found it pleasant to be catered to.

Within 2 weeks after his hospitalization, his surgeons decided that bilateral, below-the-knee amputations were unavoidable. A few days after surgery the nurses who were caring for him began to encourage self-care during his bath and other activities. Henry refused to participate in his own care, claiming that it was too tiring. Each morning, shortly after the nurse left him with a wash basin and other items for morning care, his wife appeared and gave him a complete bath. The frustrated nurses soon discovered that as soon as they left him with instructions to complete as much of his care as possible, he telephoned his wife who lived near the hospital and asked her to come and help him because the nurses were not doing their jobs.

In this example, it is possible to see the effects of this man's upbringing on his choice for a mate and also as they relate to his hospitalization. In order for the nurses to succeed in motivating such a patient to become more independent, they would first have had to assess the type of social system this patient was accustomed to. This is one of the most important steps in psychosocial assessment.

Because temporary emotional and intellectual regression is normal in adaptation to illness, this patient did not respond to the nurses' intellectual reasoning. Instead, he circumvented them in order to receive the type of nurturing he needed, both emotionally and physically. It was important for the nurses to identify this situation as a problem stemming from his social system. His nurse, acting on her own, was not going to be able to modify this patient's self-defeating behavior. Instead, his wife, his children, and the other nurses on the unit all needed to modify their behavior to him and maintain a systems approach to him. A *systems approach* is a *unified* approach in which all caregivers are consistent in their caregiving style.

Before rehabilitation could be promoted, it was important to ask his wife to come in to talk with the nurse. When she came in to give Henry a bath, she was responding in her usual way, without realizing the negative effects of her caring. The nurse explained the importance to *her* and her husband of his ability to be independent.

One of the best ways to persuade people to do something is to point out the positive advantages to *them* if they follow your recommendation. By pointing out the advantages to yourself or to someone else, their compliance may not be as complete or as long lasting. In this case, Henry's dependence on his wife was encouraged by her constant attendance to his needs in the hospital, and he could become a permanent invalid requiring her constant presence and care. After he returned home, *her* quality of life as well as *his* would be affected.

In the case example above, the nurse asked the wife to support her in her insistence that Henry do as much for himself as possible. When the nurse explained to the wife that she understood that the wife wanted to help him and that withholding her help was untypical, the wife began to understand that she would actually be prolonging her husband's illness if she continued coming every time he called her. It was also a relief to her, she admitted, because she was becoming very tired.

As part of a general systems and family systems approach, the nurse asked the wife to be present when she explained to the patient the importance of his caring for himself. When the three of them were together, the nurse explained to the patient that she had talked to his wife about not coming in when he called to ask her for help. His wife told him that she would come in to visit but would no longer give him his bath or feed him. The patient's self-care program was listed in detail in the nursing care plan so that all shifts would support his rehabilitation in the same way.

Family Rules

Within a family there are certain rules that are unwritten and may also be unspoken. These rules have been passed down from generation to generation. When a man from one family marries a woman from another family, they combine their respective rules into expectations of their own functioning and that of their children. Most commonly a person will choose a spouse whose inherited rule system or values are comparable to his or her own.

These rules can be modified based on the effects of education and enlightenment; however, the importance of family rules cannot be discounted because of the enlightened younger generation's ability to establish different rules. Within an extended family, the majority of couples in the younger generation retain most of their families' expectations. Those who establish different rules are often ridiculed or encouraged in more subtle ways to conform.

When adolescent and adult children break markedly from family rules and expectations, this is often a source of serious conflict between generations, the brothers and sisters of the older generation and the younger generation, and all other sets of relationships in the family (cousin vs. cousin, aunts and uncles vs. nieces and nephews).

If one person's rule does not combine well with a rule of the spouse, then one or the other will assert himself or herself or compromises will be agreed on. The rule that emerges will govern the family's expectations. These expectations usually are discussed and decided on before a couple decides to marry.

Religious beliefs are an important aspect of family rules. After the marriage, other family rules will be decided on as the need arises. For example, at what age will a daughter be allowed to date or to get her ears pierced? Decisions about family rules usually are determined by the parents' own experiences and beliefs about their own families of origin.

Some examples of times when family rules may form the basis of conflict in the health care system are decisions about the care of elderly, infirm relatives or the care of children or adults with severe handicaps (home care vs. institutionalization), moral choices about an unwed daughter's pregnancy, sterilization, choice of treatment of specific illnesses, and so on. When one branch of an extended family chooses a form of care that conflicts with the family's "normal" rules, the result can be conflict with one or more other branches of the family. Depending on the lack of differentiation in the family, the conflict can extend into the entire family and result in the rulebreakers' being forced out of the family.

Boundaries

All people define themselves as they relate to others (Aponte, 1976). Within a family system, *boundaries* are the rules that keep the role of one family member separate from another. Boundaries are the unwritten principles that tell who belongs to a subsystem and how that participation is supposed to take place. Boundaries come into being because of family rules (Minuchin, 1974; Jones, 1980).

Actually, it is the development of boundaries that creates subsystems or subdivisions within the family that promote effective family functioning. For example, it is important that the mother-father dyad be able to maintain its separateness from the

children-sibling subsystem for effective relations within the family. If the father, for example, consistently functions as a child within the family and abdicates his leadership role, an elder son may move into the void to serve as an authority figure for younger siblings. This creates confusion in family boundaries and can lead to family dysfunction. The outcome of physical illness can, at times, create these types of boundary disruptions within family subsystems.

In the hospital, patients and family members may appear to be either overfunctioning or underfunctioning in their roles within their families. These may be the roles that the dynamics of their own intrapsychic and family system functioning have created for them, however. You and the remainder of the hospital care system have very little power to change these dynamics during a hospital admission. It is better to learn to work with them and design your care to include these idiosyncrasies rather than discounting them because you have counseled the family members to change their role functioning.

> Clarity of boundaries within a family provides a barometer of how well the family is functioning. To function adequately subsystem members must have contact with one another, but must not interfere with each other's functioning . . . . The two pathological extremes are disengaged (where there is no contact between family members) or enmeshed (where there is too much control) families [Jones, 1980, p. 64].

Fusion

The concept of fusion was introduced earlier as it related to the undifferentiated ego mass that can exist in highly emotional families. Another aspect of fusion exists in many families: when two or more persons consistently relate to one another on a more emotional level than they do with other members of the same family and form their own subsystem. Minuchin and colleagues (1967) have called this phenomenon *enmeshment*. These relationships can be either positively or negatively charged. They can be dominated by feelings of closeness *or* of conflict. The fusion between two or more members implies that there is "tight interlocking" in the relationships (Minuchin and colleagues, 1967). This is essentially a problem caused by poor boundaries within a family.

Because of the system effect of a tight relationship between two or more people in a family, other members are automatically excluded. These other members may join together in a form of alliance as well in order to avoid feeling excluded. This is not generally the case, however. Instead, they remain outside, waiting for an "opening" so that they may join the fused subsystem.

Remember that fusion can exist to some degree in any normal family. It becomes a problem, however, in many families in which there is chronic physical or mental illness. There is an overreactivity on the part of one family member, often the mother, to the sick member, frequently a child. The sick role of the ill member is reinforced by the reaction of the other member.

> Their quality of connectedness is such that attempts on the part of one member to change elicit fast complementary resistance on the part of others [Minuchin and colleagues, 1967, p. 368].

In the hospital or outpatient setting, you may observe situations in which an overbearing parent, spouse, or some other family authority figure encourages sickness behavior in the ill family member. If the chronically ill member moves toward healthy rehabilitation, his efforts may be thwarted and undermined by the other member of the fused dyad, who unconsciously *needs* the ill person to remain sick.

The process of enmeshment or fusion is one that takes place during the early developmental years of the marriage and becomes more pronounced as children enter the family. Jones (1980) describes the effects of this process on a family when it reaches pathological levels:

> *Enmeshment* is essentially a weakening of the boundaries that allow family subsystems to function: the boundary between nuclear family and families of origin is not well maintained; the boundary between parents and their children is crossed frequently in improper ways: the roles of spouse and parent are insufficiently differentiated so that neither the spouse subsystem nor the parental subsystem can operate; and finally, the children are not differentiated on the basis of age or maturational level so that the sibling subsystem cannot contribute properly to the socialization process [p. 65].

The following case example illustrates this point.

Case Example

Danny is a 12-year-old boy with asthma. He has been asthmatic since age 2. He has an older brother and sister. His mother has always been overprotective of him. During Danny's elementary schooling, his mother refused to allow him to join the Boy Scouts or Little League because she feared that any strenuous activity could bring on an acute asthma episode. Danny acquiesced to his mother's wishes, gradually became introverted and isolated from his friends and more attached to and dependent on his mother. His older sister's disposition, which had been sunny in childhood, slowly gave way to sullenness as her mother had less time to spend with her due to increased attentiveness to Danny. Danny's father, an outdoorsman, had always enjoyed the camping trips that his wife and he had taken with their family. When Danny developed asthma, his mother decided that Danny and she would no longer accompany the family on the trips. Danny's father has come to resent his son's illness and his wife's decreased interest in their relationship as a couple.

If you should observe the effects of pathological fusion in a chronic care setting, a pediatric unit, a psychiatric unit, or an acute care medical-surgical unit, it will be difficult for you to approach the family about the negative short- and long-term effects of their family interactions. Remember, they have been operating in this manner for years. When fusion is present in a dyad, there will potentially be more serious implications when one member develops a chronic illness or becomes terminally ill. The process of loss involved in either instance causes a major shift in equilibrium in the relationship. In fact, the entire family system will feel the effects if the dyad becomes dysfunctional.

Being approached by one nurse who suggests that their relationship needs to change will not usually have an impact on such a patient and his family. Instead, share your concerns with the attending physician. Use your knowledge of general and family systems theory as you document the negative interactional style of the family and as you discuss the negative long-term implications if it is not modified. (For example, the patient's sick role, which may be accompanied by behavioral acting out, will be promoted by nonintervention.) You can also approach a psychiatric liaison nurse specialist or a social worker for further system support. Their evaluation will further reinforce your assessment and credibility with the physician.

Remedial work on a negative fusion process can occur in many ways, depending on the severity of the fusion, the *willingness of all the family* members to be aware of the process, and *their motivation to work on rectifying it.* These last two points cannot be overestimated. It is very important to be aware that the reason why fusion occurs, develops, and is fostered is because of underlying intrapsychic needs of all family members. The dominant persons in the fusion process will not be able to change easily.

If the process is not severe, the family can be worked with by astute medical and nursing caregivers and the outpatient care system. If the process is deeply entrenched, treatment should be done by a skilled family therapist to whom the attending physician has referred the family.

Triangles

Another concept that is important in understanding how a social system operates is the phenomenon of triangling.

> The triangle, a three-person emotional configuration, is the molecule or the basic building block of any emotional system, whether it is in the family or any other group. The triangle is the smallest stable relationship system. A two-person system may be stable as long as it is calm, but when anxiety increases, it immediately involves the most vulnerable other person to become a triangle. When tension in the triangle is too great for the threesome, it involves others to become a series of triangles [Bowen, 1976, p. 76].

As Bowen implies, the ability for a two-person relationship to remain static and "calm" decreases when any type of tension occurs. When one member of the dyad is under stress, his or her anxiety is reflected in the relationship. Unconsciously, in order to decrease the tension and restore stability, one or the other member will bring in a third member. This causes a shift in the tension so that the stress "within" the dyad is reduced. Triangling can have both positive and negative outcomes depending on the developmental maturity of each of the members. The previous case example describing fusion between Danny and his mother could also be an example of triangling if we added the information that before Danny developed his asthma, his parents' marital relationship had been deteriorating. There was increasing conflict and tension between them. Danny's mother in effect triangled in Danny as a way of avoiding ongoing conflict with her husband. Indeed, the relationship between the mother and

father now is distanced, and active conflict within the couple dyad has been rare.

Application to the Nursing Unit

The concept of a triangle may at first seem complicated and too specific for use in understanding the complex dynamics in the general hospital, but it is a concept that can help you understand the ways in which all people relate in the general hospital social system.

> In the beginning, the essence of a triangle is easy to understand. As one probes more deeply into its nature, the essence tends to become obscure. It is no longer such a simple idea. But this should not be discouraging. The very muddling around to understand more and more about triangles leads to a deeper understanding of the one (the person), the twosome (the personal relationship), and the threesome. This understanding is critical [Fogarty, 1975, p. 11].

The staff nurses who work on a particular nursing unit often relate to each other in a family style of interaction. Their peers are similar to siblings, the head nurse represents the mother, the physician, the father, and so on. The concepts presented here can all be applied to the social system of a nursing unit. Formerly confusing dynamics in a nursing staff can often be recognized by using family systems concepts. Triangles that are common in some families are also common in the interpersonal dynamics of a nursing unit. The following case example may clarify the idea. As you read, be aware of the inclusion of a third person in the various triangles that are created and the potential for escalation of conflict that is created. (Conflict is represented by the symbol X; △, △, and △ signal creation of a triangle.)

Case Example (Fig. 8-2)

Jan and Tom are staff nurses in an intensive care unit (ICU). Tom has worked there 1 year longer than Jan, who has been at the hospital for 8 months. Tom has always been protective of Jan and has been available to share his knowledge of patient care. In the past few months, Jan has become more confident of her knowledge. Instead of gradually decreasing his "mentor" role, however, Tom hovers nearby and frequently checks up on Jan's care (X).

Jan has begun to resent his overprotectiveness (X). She does not discuss this with Tom. She could have let him know she is grateful for his earlier help but wants him to

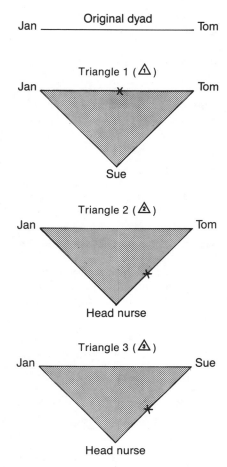

Figure 8-2.
Triangles. Based on an intensive care unit example. *X* signifies conflict between an original dyad.

accept her as more of a peer now that she is more skilled in her intensive care nursing procedures. Instead, she shared her frustration with Sue, a fellow ICU nurse (△). Sue was a sympathetic listener and, in fact, added to Jan's frustration with Tom by telling similar stories about Tom's interpersonal difficulties with other nurses in the unit (X). Sue suggested that Jan talk with the head nurse so that the head nurse could handle the problem. As soon as Jan talked to the head nurse, the head nurse became angry and decided that she would speak with Tom (△).

Sue didn't tell Jan that she has been thinking for several months that the head nurse has been "above" getting involved in the actual day to day operation of the ICU (X). Sue also didn't tell Jan that 2 years earlier she had been passed over in consideration for the head

nursing position. In this case, Sue really had a hidden motive. She wanted to "test" the head nurse's ability to get involved in and resolve the difficult situation (△).

This example points out the possible dynamics in a situation that originally existed between two people. Do you think that Jan could have spoken directly to Tom and resolved the problem? Why do you think she chose not to? Most people find conflict unpleasant. In this case, it is possible that avoiding conflict was Jan's underlying motivation for not handling it directly. Instead, it seemed "easier" to involve others.

Sometimes, when people triangle in a third person, they wonder why situations get out of hand and eventually become even more conflicted. Additional triangles are often created, as happened above. A staff can become seriously splintered and lose its sense of mutual support when this occurs. The basic reason is the tendency to bring in a third person to relieve a person's own sense of conflict or anxiety. In this example, let us examine the various triangles that were created.

In order to see the overall effect that triangling combined with lack of boundary awareness can have in a social system, read the outcome (# signifies boundary violation, and △ signifies creation of a new triangle).

Jan spoke to the head nurse about Tom and asked her to speak to him about being less critical of her. Jan also added other information about Tom that she had learned from Sue (#). The head nurse felt angry toward Tom as she listened to Jan (#). She went immediately to Tom and berated him publicly for his various "wrongs."

Tom became angry for three reasons: First, his head nurse was accusing him of doing things that he had never realized were problems to others. No one had ever come directly to him to talk about a problem with him. Second, the head nurse was emotional. Her anger caused her to be irrational. Third, she was speaking loudly in a patient care area in front of both patients (#△) and Tom's peers (#△). He was unable to reason with her about the situation.

Because he was hurt and angry about the head nurse's lack of professionalism and inability to listen to his explanation, he spoke to the supervisor about the head nurse (△). When he went home that evening, he displaced his frustration onto his wife (#△).

Do you see the potential for increased conflict and deterioration of the situation if triangling goes on unchecked? In this example, the triangling and escalation process could have been avoided if Jan had dealt directly with Tom and they had reasonably discussed the situation. When that did not occur, and the problem was presented to the head nurse, she could have wisely suggested that Jan go back to Tom about the problem. If Jan had protested, saying that she did not know what to say, the head nurse could have helped Jan to discuss ways of approaching Tom. She also could have suggested that Jan role play the approach, pretending that the head nurse was Tom. By doing so, the head nurse would not be absolving her leadership role. Instead, she would have promoted more mature interpersonal skills in her staff member. Later on, given a similar situation, the staff member would be better able to handle this problem herself because she had a new behavioral skill. If the head nurse, by talking directly to Tom, "solved" the problem for the nurse, it would have promoted a continuation of the staff nurse's helplessness and passivity in a similar situation, whether professional or personal. In the example above, the head nurse consistently violated boundaries:

1. She listened to hearsay conversation from Sue instead of discouraging extra information unrelated to Jan's specific problem with Tom.
2. She did not maintain her own self-differentiation. She allowed her emotions to overcome what could have been a reasonable, professional listening stance.
3. She did not approach Tom in a reasonable, intellectual way in order to learn what had actually happened. Instead, her feelings dominated.
4. Any type of discipline should be handled only between the persons directly involved. When it occurs with others present, this is actually a further triangling situation.
5. Nurses should not subject patients to their own interpersonal issues that are not directly related to patient care.

Awareness of the triangling process can be especially helpful to nurses in both their professional and personal lives. An underlying dynamic in many nurses is their desire to be helpful. This dynamic can unknowingly cause them to become involved as the third member of an interpersonal triangle. Patients, family members, and friends may ask a nurse for help, when, with encouragement, they have the ability to resolve the problem themselves.

Power

Power is another important dynamic in any family or unified group. In families, we normally assume that the father or mother holds the most power. Similarly, in the case of a nursing unit, we may expect that the head nurse is the most powerful figure. This is not always so. Power is the ability to do something or control others.

Within a family, a physical symptom in one member can have a strong effect on all the other members. For example, a child who is prone to asthma can ultimately control his family with his physical symptoms. If a physical symptom in one member does exert strong control in a family, it is usually because the normally expected balance of authority in the family has been temporarily or permanently disrupted. In the case of an asthmatic child, a mother may interact in a submissive way to the child in order to avoid precipitating an emotionally induced asthmatic attack. She may also insist that all other family members alter their normal responses to this child as well. Frequently, this type of change in family dynamics becomes permanent and may weaken normal family functioning.

In looking at the effects of power on a nursing unit, depending on the leadership of the head nurse, the power on the unit can be controlled by a disruptive patient. Unless the head nurse is able to maintain control of difficult situations, the staff nurses may emulate the head nurse and be unable to manage effectively a troublesome situation with a patient. A highly manipulative patient on a nursing unit has a great deal of power. Accordingly, the nurses feel angry and helpless and react in passive but negative ways.

Scapegoating

Family members often assign fixed roles to one another. One of these roles is the scapegoat. *Scapegoats* are persons who are made the "victims" of the other members of a family because of their own inability to tolerate specific aspects of their own functioning.

The scapegoat role is determined by many factors, not the least of which is a dim awareness on the part of the person filling it that playing this role is vital to the psychic balance of the family, and has its rewards and importance as well as its pains and handicaps. The scapegoat is always as much volunteer as victim, and the role is fulfilled out of love as well as fear [Skynner, 1979, p. 645].

Scapegoating is a specific type of triangling that brings in a third person when two other persons are unable to mediate the tensions in their own relationship. The scapegoated member may be a child or sick person who differs in some way from the remainder of the family. He may have a chronic mental or physical condition. By scapegoating, the parents or the entire family are able to avoid the deeper and more basic problems within the family structure (Skynner, 1979; Pierce, 1979). Scapegoating also may be common on nursing units when troublesome patients are avoided by some nursing staff members.

Family Secrets

One of the dynamics in a family that gives it ongoing momentum is the tendency of a family to have secrets. This dynamic is particularly strong in families with a high level of fusion and tightness. The following case example will clarify the concept:

Case Example

Jim is a successful 51-year-old businessman with five children. After college he enlisted in the army and served in the Korean War. While stationed there he had an affair with a female officer. She became pregnant. Both of them were dishonorably discharged. They did not marry. She had a child after they returned to the United States. He sent her voluntary child support payments until the child was 18 years old. Meanwhile, he was married a few years after he returned from the war. He told his wife of the earlier relationship and the existence of his child.

As part of their family functioning, when she became angry she occasionally raised the issue of his illicit affair and berated him for the expense of the child support payments. Their children were never aware of this family "secret." As they grew older, they wondered about the bitter tone in their mother's voice when the family was under financial strain from time to time. In addition, the mother imposed very restrictive dating policies on their adolescent children. The father, although forceful and confident in his business and social relationships, became helpless and silent about his wife's uncompromising attitude toward the social lives of their children. When they appealed to their father for help in changing their mother's harsh policies, they became frustrated and puzzled by his response, "Your mother knows best."

Family secrets cause rigidity and anxiety in families. They can be the underlying reasons for perplexing behavior and reactions that you observe in patients. Probing and questioning will not usually bring them forward unless you know the patient well. Remember that most people have spent years and sometimes decades burying these secrets. Instead, if you observe the detrimental effects of a suspected secret, recommend that the patient share the problem with a physician, clergyman, or other professional who may be able to help the patient deal with it rather than continuing to have it undermine his well-being and that of the family.

Secrets can also be used within families during times of acute family stress when there is concern about "overloading the system." The following case example can help clarify this concept.

Case Example

Linda and Gerry were expecting their second child. Their only daughter was 2 years old. During her eighth month of pregnancy, Linda was in a serious automobile accident. Although every effort was made to save her life, she died after 1 week of intensive care. A cesarean delivery performed before her death produced a son who quickly developed respiratory difficulties. He was diagnosed as having hyaline membrane disease and was struggling for life in the newborn intensive care nursery.

Grief stricken, Gerry told his daughter about her mother's death. Gerry decided that unless his daughter asked about the baby, he would withhold news of the baby's birth until the baby's health had stabilized. Gerry feared that it would be too much for the child to learn of the arrival of a new brother, only to learn later of his death.

Feedback

One of the essential qualities of a system is the relatedness of its units. The way in which each of the units relates to the other units is by feedback (Putt, 1978). *Feedback* is the communication that occurs between and among all members of a system. Feedback can occur between family members.

A physiological example of the concept of feedback is the essential mechanism the body uses in maintaining physiological homeostasis. One cell signals to another cell that it needs more or less input in order to maintain its normal level of functioning; one body system notifies another system that it needs to speed up or slow down its level of functioning in order to promote the well-being of the entire body system.

Feedback is the process by which a system maintains itself. In social systems it can be positive or negative. *Positive feedback* from one member of the system reinforces a particular action or behavior of another member and promotes similar behavior in the future. *Negative feedback* from one member to another discourages a particular action or behavior.

Homeostasis

In working with families, it is important to view the entire family as a system when you are trying to promote positive change in one family member. In every family there is a balance created by the total contributing dynamics of each family member. This is called *family homeostasis*. If change occurs in one family member, it will create a major change in the family balance. This is caused by all the differences in interactions between the patient and other family members.

This is an essential concept in designing a treatment program for patients with many types of emotional and physical problems. It frequently is the underlying reason why treatment approaches that appear to be successful while the patient is hospitalized are dismal failures once the patient is discharged into his regular family system. The family will continue to interact with the patient as a "sick" member. He will quickly fall into his original and accustomed role in the family because the family homeostasis depends on it.

Without intervention with the family, it will continue to promote the person's sickness, whether by a heightened reaction to his gastro-intestinal symptoms of Crohn's disease or to his symptoms of alcoholism. A systems approach that addresses the interactional style of the family and enlightens members about the ways they feed into and promote a continuation of the patient's problems is an essential aspect of the management of chronic physical or mental disease states.

Conclusion

Family systems are indeed complex. Most people, especially in their own families, *feel* the effects of family dynamics but often are unable to identify the specific forces that are occurring. This chapter was written for two reasons: to help you to understand the response of a family to a loved one's illness and to understand the social dynamics of your own nursing unit. (Remember that the social dynamics of a nursing unit can have a strong effect on patient care because of the overall general systems effect of a positive or negative working environment.)

Family dynamics are important in the overall response of a patient to illness for many reasons. A person is often influenced by his family's response to the stressful experience of illness. If the family system goes into crisis, the patient's ability to maintain an adaptive level of coping can be seriously undermined. This is because the ability to support a given member is one of the most important functions of a family. When the family system is severely stressed or in crisis, this essential function is seriously weakened. So, too, if the patient is unable to cope, his family will be more threatened by the illness. The anxiety of all members will be continuously interchanged. The effects of stress on families will be discussed further in Chapter 15: Crisis Intervention With the Maladapting Patient.

9

Stress: Its Implications in Physical Illness

The word stress, when pronounced, has a dragged out sound; it lingers. Both these characteristics of the word itself fit the way in which most people view the phenomenon of stress. In this age of increasing technology and increasing social pressures, the concept of stress has captured attention in most cultures. In this chapter the implications of the effects of stress will be explored as they affect a person physically, emotionally, and intellectually. As the chapter evolves, you will see that it is impossible to separate the effects of stress into the specific realms of physical, emotional, and intellectual functioning. A stressor (anything causing stress) may be perceived initially by any of these three spheres, but ultimately, because of a general systems effect, all systems become involved in the manifestation of a stress response. The *Le Chatelier principle* from the science of physics can be applied to the effects of stress on a human being:

> If stress is applied to a system, the system will readjust to reduce the stress.

Reread the sentence above. It may help you to begin thinking about what stress really is. Usually when we describe stress, we are thinking of two *different* concepts: one, an *external* state that is abnormal, results in the *internal* distress that most people describe as "stress." In order to clarify the difference between the two entities, we can call any external environment event, such as taking a final examination, touching a hot iron, almost being in an automobile accident, becoming married, or winning the grand prize in a lottery, a stressor. A *stressor* is any external or internal demand on the person (Powers and Kutash, 1980). *Stress* is the response to the demands of that stressor. It is a physical and psychological uneasiness (Snyder, 1980). It unbalances and upsets equilibrium.

The subject of stress is complex. Knowledge about stress and its effects has evolved from decades of study by psychologists, sociologists, neurobiologists, psychosomaticists, and scientists in many other fields. Accordingly, knowledge of stress involves many types of concepts. Some of these concepts are specific. They are the result of research into either the physiologic, psychologic, or social spheres of humankind. As time passes, the theories resulting from this research continue to be accepted.

An important development during the last two decades, however, has been a growing awareness that it is impossible to completely separate these three spheres of man (Reiser, 1974). Instead, many researchers and theorists believe that the human being must be viewed holistically in his response to stress. A general systems viewpoint is the basic framework that assists in evaluating the effects of stress on a person's body, mind, and social system (Alexander, 1950; Engel, 1968; Hurst and colleagues, 1979; Kimball, 1970; Leigh and Reiser, 1977; Lipowski, 1968).

This chapter will present several theories about stress. Each contains a different perspective. They will be discussed in three sections. The first section presents stress theories that evolve from a specific subsystem approach to stress: physiological, psychological, or social. The second section presents theory about the way that stress is mediated by psychosocial functioning. The third section presents a biological-psychological-social model that is compatible with the unitary man nursing model proposed by Rogers (1970) and the holistic nursing concepts of Roy (1980).

Part One: Specific Subsystem Responses to Stress

Physiological Stress

Hans Selye: The General Adaptation Syndrome Stress Response

One of the most recognized authorities in the field of stress research is Hans Selye. During his medical training in Czechoslovakia in the 1920s, he observed the following:

> Whether a man suffers from severe blood loss, an infection, or advanced cancer, he loses his appetite, strength, and ambition; usually he also loses weight and even his facial expression betrays his illness. I felt sure that the syndrome of just being sick, which is essentially the same no matter what disease we have, could be analyzed and expressed scientifically [Selye, 1979, p. 12].

A few years later Selye returned to graduate school for a doctorate in biochemistry. During that time, while studying the effects of all types of toxic substances on rats, he discovered that the rats

were changed in three ways: (1) the adrenal cortex became enlarged, (2) the thymus, the spleen, the lymph nodes, and all other lymphatic structures shrank, and (3) deep, bleeding ulcers appeared in the stomach and upper gut.

He began to realize that these changes actually were the objective manifestations of stress. They became the basis for his stress concept, the General Adaptation Syndrome (GAS). These physiological responses are the foundation of the syndrome that Selye (1974) calls "just being sick."

Selye identified three stages of the GAS. First is *the alarm reaction,* in which the body attempts with all its defensive abilities to fight off the effects of a noxious substance. After the initial shock of a stressor is met with a strong defensive response stimulated by hormones from the adrenal cortex, the body gradually settles into a less stimulated phase, during which it continues to maintain its defenses. If the stressor is severe, such as third-degree burns or severe shock of any kind, death can result. Body defenses are overwhelmed. This is the second stage: *the stage of resistance.* During this stage the body maintains its resistance until the noxious agent disappears and the body is able to return to homeostasis. If the body's defensive capability is so completely used up, it enters stage 3, *the stage of exhaustion.* If the stage of exhaustion is not reversed by removal of the toxic substance, or the body's resistance capability is not supported by medical intervention, then the result is death.

Psychological Stress and the Coping Process

Richard Lazarus: Cognitive Appraisal

Richard Lazarus, a psychologist, is one of the leading theorists in the psychological stress field. His theory, called cognitive appraisal, is described as follows:

> [It] is the cornerstone of my analysis of the emotions; and this appraisal, from which the various emotions flow, is determined by the interplay of personality and the environmental stimulus configuration [Lazarus, 1977, p. 145].

Lazarus has applied the word *transactions* to the constantly changing relationships between man and his environment. This ongoing process involves continuous feedback loops of information to a person about the many variables in his environment. Rather than independent cause and effect relationships between man and his environment, Lazarus believes that the process is circular, similar to the question "Which came first, the chicken or the egg?" Lazarus's theory is rooted to a general systems framework.

The constant evaluation and reevaluation by man about the events occurring in his life is called *cognitive appraisal*. The first step in this process is called *primary appraisal*. It involves decision making and judgments about a person's encounters with the environment. It asks the question, "Am I okay or in trouble?" (Lazarus, 1977, p. 153). There are three possible outcomes of primary appraisal:

1. The event is irrelevant . . . . It has no significance to the person and can be ignored.
2. The event is benign-positive . . . . It is beneficial or desirable.
3. The event is stressful . . . . It involves a judgment of harm-loss, threat, or challenge:
   a. *Harm-loss* refers to harm or loss that has already occurred, such as a major loss of self-esteem, changes in or losses of significant relationships or role functioning, or incapacitating illness.
   b. *Threat* differs from harm-loss in that the person fears the events described under harm-loss. They have not yet occurred; the fear is anticipatory.
   c. *Challenge* is contrasted to threat by the emotional quality that it causes. With threat, there is a negative or frightened emotional response. A challenge results in a positive response to an event. It focuses on the possibility of mastery or gain (Coyne and Lazarus, 1980, p. 151).

Lazarus's theory of cognitive appraisal is important in conceptualizing patients' responses to illness. For example, a patient who is appraising his physical illness and hospitalization customarily will not view the event as irrelevant or benign. Rather, his appraisal is most likely to fit into the third category described above; it is perceived as stressful.

The next step in a person's awareness of an environmental event is called secondary appraisal. *Secondary appraisal* occurs after the person answers the challenge of primary appraisal, "Am I okay or in trouble?" If he decides he is in trouble, he then asks, "What can I do about it?" (Coyne and Lazarus, 1980, p. 153). During this secondary stage

of cognitive appraisal, the person consciously applies coping strategies that have worked for him in the past.

He continually evaluates his response to these coping efforts and makes additional coping attempts if his level of anxiety and fear is not reduced by the original efforts. *Reappraisal* occurs when his evaluation results in changes in his original coping attempts. (Coyne and Lazarus, 1980; Lazarus, 1966, 1970, 1977). This process involves continuous feedback between a person's emotional and intellectual psychic subsystems and the environment. When a person is physically ill, it also involves transactions with the physical subsystems. Body sensations feed into his emotional and intellectual response (Coyne and Lazarus, 1980; Lazarus, 1966, 1970, 1977).

Coping is defined as "efforts, both action-oriented and intrapsychic, to manage (that is, to master, tolerate, reduce, minimize) environmental and internal demands and conflicts among them which tax or exceed a person's resources" (Lazarus and Launier, 1978, p. 311). The Lazarus model divides coping into two types: problem oriented and emotion regulation. Problem-oriented coping is an attempt to actively change one's own mental reaction to stress by conscious intellectual actions or by changing the condition in the environment that is causing the stress. Emotion regulation refers to efforts of the psyche to maintain emotional control and reduce its own distressed feeling state (Coyne and Lazarus, 1980).

Think, for a moment, of the person who is physically ill or hospitalized. He has little control over his situation. He is not able to use fully the problem-oriented method of coping because the problem is within his own body. It did not originate in the environment and cannot be resolved by leaving or changing his surroundings. Instead, his coping must, of necessity, be intrapsychic in order to maintain equilibrium.

The way that a person responds to illness or hospitalization depends on the following factors:

1. Change in cognition, which can be positive or negative, depending on the person. It can increase or decrease perceptual ability, thought, judgment, problem solving, motor skills, or social adaptation (Lazarus, 1966).
2. Coping responses initiated consciously and unconsciously in order to promote adaptation:
   a. Disturbed affect, such as fear, anxiety, anger, depression, and guilt. These form the single largest category of stress responses.

b. Physiological change, which may involve all the body systems (neurological, endocrine, cardiovascular, respiratory, gastrointestinal, and so on).

c. Motor behavior, seen most commonly as increased muscle tension (e.g., body posture, certain facial expressions, or tremor).

The sequence involved in Lazarus's theory about cognitive style, stress perception, and coping appears in Figure 9-1.

Once the person is aware of a harm-loss or threatening stressor, his coping ability will also determine the level of emotional and physical response to that stressor. Two psychological factors are most important in understanding Lazarus's coping process: the degree of threat that the person perceives and his ego strength. Ego strength is the intrapsychic and primarily unconscious supply of defense mechanisms that the ego uses to master the threat (Lazarus, 1966). Lazarus scales the ego defenses from appropriate defenses to maladaptive levels of defense (both types are discussed in Chap. 4). With coping failure, defense proceeds in a deteriorating continuum from self-control to increased alertness, fantasy, displacement, panic attacks, violent loss of control, schizophrenic breaks with reality, and ultimately death.

The most mature reaction to threat occurs when the degree of threat is slight to moderate. When the degree of threat is high, the result is usually a very primitive response because of the inability of the ego to adapt. The defense mechanisms outlined in Chapter 4 may cause the person to shut out completely the threat by denial or reduce his perception of the actual degree of threat by repression, distortion, and so on.

As you read about Lazarus's theory, keep in mind the example of a 43-year-old woman who is admitted to the hospital because of bleeding of unknown etiology in her intestinal tract. If a person is ill or hospitalized, his or her response to this stressor will depend on the following:

1. *Belief system concerning transactions with the environment.* These include intellectual resources, education, and sophistication. The degree of presence of these resources may make a person more or less prone to a stress reaction, depending on his familiarity and experience with the threat. The lack of these resources could also contribute to an incorrect threat appraisal. When a situation is believed to be threatening, a stress response is initiated. In the case of the woman patient above, let us review her belief system. She knows that blood in the intestinal tract is abnormal. She knows it could be caused by ulcers or cancer; both are frightening diseases to her. She remembers what happened to her uncle whose ulcers caused him much difficulty, and she remembers that one of her neighbor's sisters died of cancer of the intestine.

2. The *resources of a person to defend himself or herself from harm-losses or threats.* In this case the patient may have poor coping ability and be overwhelmed by fear of the situation. The patient described above may be so threatened that denial quickly shuts out the reality, and she may delay treatment to her own detriment. She may also react with an appropriate suppression of her fears and

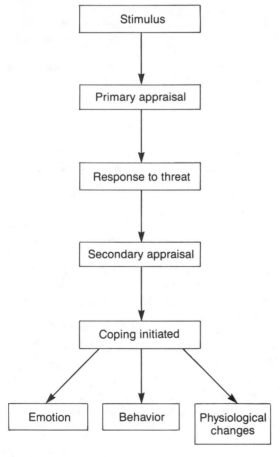

Figure 9-1.
Lazarus stress response sequence. (After Coyne J, Lazarus R: Cognitive style, stress perception and coping. In Kutash I, Schlesinger L [eds]: Handbook of Stress and Anxiety. San Francisco, Jossey-Bass, 1980)

obtain immediate treatment in a calm way. If she responds by being overwhelmed or by completely denying her symptoms, her physical well-being is further jeopardized because of inadequate and maladaptive responses. If the person is in a prolonged state of panic, there is an increased rate of physiological deterioration of the body due to the GAS in addition to the already existing disease state.

This is one of the reasons why your awareness of increased psychological stress in patients is very important. If it is undetected, no therapeutic intervention will occur that could reduce the stress level and avoid further physical weakening. In addition to the psychological stress of a threatening external stressor, unrelieved pain can produce a stress response in the body because it produces psychological and physical distress. Accordingly, nurses' sensitivity to patients' pain medication needs is important in avoiding unnecessary stress. If the psychological distress of this woman is acute, there are many options to consider to help bring it down to a more normal level. Interventions for persons experiencing high levels of stress as the result of illness will be presented in Chapter 15: Crisis Intervention With the Maladapting Patient, Chapter 16: Nursing Intervention With the Emotionally Complex Patient, Chapter 17: Psychosocial Aspects of Specific Physical Conditions, and Chapter 18: The Coping Challenge of Chronic Illness.

Social Stress

Holmes and Rahe: The Significance of Life Events as Stressors

Two stress researchers, Holmes and Rahe, wanted to know what events people considered stressful. They initially interviewed people to learn what types of life events required personal adjustment and how stressful they considered those adjustments. The researchers wanted to apply numerical values to each of the life events in order to develop a scale. They asked those interviewed to consider, for instance, the adjustment necessary in the process of getting married; a value of 50 points was then assigned to the various types of stress involved in the events preceding and immediately following marriage. They were then asked to rate the other life events as more or less demanding

than the readjustments necessary in being married (Snyder, 1980).

Holmes and Rahe called the questionnaire the Social Readjustment Rating Scale. It asked people to report the types of change they experienced in the previous year. The numerical points for each of the life events were totaled. Long-term follow-up studies of the participants' rates of medical illness revealed that the more stress a person experienced in his life in a given year, the more likely he or she was to develop physical illness. After many years of studies, Holmes and Rahe have assigned a total yearly point value of over 300 points as a positive indicator of likely development of illness. Their scale appears on the following page.*

Because a stressor is usually expected to be a negative event, it may be surprising to realize that positive events also produce stress. A promotion to a new job, for example, requires leaving comfortable relationships and entering a new social environment. There is also the stress of having to work at a higher level of functioning. A promotion may also involve a transfer to a new community. This involves the loss of known friends, home, community, and so on.

Part Two: Psychosocial Mediation of Stressful Events

Adaptation to a Major Life Event

Once a stressful life event has occurred, there are ways in which the person usually works through it and adapts to it. The adaptation process is similar for most people and contains both conscious and

---

*If you find that your own life events during the last year have been excessive, these thoughts may be helpful to you. Hans Selye has said that people respond in different ways to stress. Some are like race horses: they thrive on it. Others are like turtles and are able to tolerate only a low level of stress (Cherry, 1978).

You may find that your stress level is currently high and that you are feeling its effects. If so, it can be wise to avoid taking on any challenges in your life in the immediate future about which you have a choice. For example, moving to a new job, being married or divorced, or taking on a debt for a new car may all be postponed until a less stressful period in your life.

Holmes and Rahe Social Readjustment Rating Scale

Item Number	Life Event (Item Value)
1	Death of spouse (100)
2	Divorce (73)
3	Marital separation (65)
4	Jail term (63)
5	Death of close family member (63)
6	Personal injury or illness (53)
7	Marriage (50)
8	Fired at work (47)
9	Marital reconciliation (45)
10	Retirement (45)
11	Change in health of a family member (44)
12	Pregnancy (40)
13	Sex difficulties (39)
14	Gain of a new family member (39)
15	Business readjustment (39)
16	Change in financial state (39)
17	Death of a close friend (37)
18	Change to a different line of work (36)
19	Change in number of arguments with spouse (35)
20	Mortgage over $10,000 (31)
21	Foreclosure or mortgage or loan (30)
22	Change in responsibilities at work (29)
23	Son or daughter leaving home (29)
24	Trouble with in-laws (29)
25	Outstanding personal achievement (28)
26	Spouse begins or stops work (26)
27	Begin or end school (26)
28	Change in living conditions (25)
29	Revision of personal habits (24)
30	Trouble with boss (23)
31	Change in work hours or conditions (20)
32	Change in residence (20)
33	Change in schools (20)
34	Change in recreation (19)
35	Change in church activities (19)
36	Change in social activities (18)
37	Mortgage or loan less than $10,000 (17)
38	Change in sleeping habits (16)
39	Change in number of family gatherings (15)
40	Change in eating habits (15)
41	Vacation (13)
42	Christmas (12)
43	Minor violations of the law (11)

(Holmes TH, Rahe RH: The Social Readjustment Rating Scale. J Psychosom Res 11:213, 1967) unconscious elements. These common themes are described by Horowitz (1976):

1. Fear of repetition of the event in real life as well as in memory.
2. Shame over helplessness or emptiness. There is a sense of loss of control because the person was not able to control the event or its outcome.
3. Rage at the source. Although the anger may be irrational, a person needs to blame someone for the event.
4. Guilt or shame over aggressive impulses. The anger described above usually collides with a person's conscience and results in guilt or shame. This can include negative feelings toward a person who has died.
5. Fear of aggressiveness. A person fears that he will not be able to contain his angry impulses and may uncontrollably act them out.
6. Survivor guilt. If the event involves injury or death to others, the survivor, although he had no power over the situation, often feels guilty that he was spared or was less seriously injured. Awareness of this phenomenon in survivors of accidents or fires who are hospitalized will help you to give more sensitive care to these persons. They may not be able to verbalize their guilt. Gentle questioning of the patient may produce relief by his being able to talk about it. This guilt may also present itself in the form of nightmares about the event.
7. Fear of identification or merger with victims. This is a primitive response based on a human being's early perception that he is "one being" with his mother (see the discussion on Mahler in Chap. 3). Although the reality of this situation is not possible, it operates at an unconscious level.
8. Sadness in relation to loss. Any major life change contains elements of loss that the person must work through.

Horowitz proposes that the two mechanisms commonly present in people who are working through these eight common themes are denial of the event alternating with intrusive and unwanted repetitions of thoughts, emotions, and behaviors related to the event.

He believes that maladaptation occurs in persons when there is either excessive *or* insufficient coping as the result of the intrapsychic stress experienced. Accordingly, the stressful event is never completely worked through and resolved.

Types of Responses to Stress

All people are subject to stress. It is part of the human condition. Most theorists agree that the effects of a stressful event can be mediated by the presence of adaptive coping mechanisms (Lazarus, 1968, 1977; Mason, 1971; Snyder, 1980; Ursin, 1978). Ursin (1978) has identified the factors that determine whether a person's coping ability will be able to withstand a stressor:

1. The level of fear caused by a stressor
   a. Fear of some type of harm
   b. Fear of failure
2. The person's resources
   a. Familiarity with a preceding similar event
   b. Level of education and sophistication
   c. Availability of a support system
3. Role identification
4. Intellectual strategies
5. Defense mechanisms

The first determinant of a person's response to a threat, as presented above, is the level of fear caused by a stressor. The important, but unstated, inference is that a specific event may cause a mild stress reaction in one person and a more severe one in someone else. The response will primarily depend on the degree of threat that a stressor presents. For example, a trained parachutist looks forward to an opportunity to jump out of a plane. He feels no fear. Instead, he is exhilarated. There is very little threat present; his coping abilities are rarely called on. Now, stop for a minute and picture *yourself* 4000 feet above the earth in a small plane with a parachute strapped to your back. Imagine your response as the jump director beckons you to get ready to jump. You might have difficulty even approaching the door because of your level of fear. You may normally have a good ability to cope because of efficient defense mechanisms, but the terror of having to jump out of an airplane may temporarily overwhelm them.

Another important concept is that the way that a person copes with a stressful event is usually similar for most events. For example, if a person typically responds to stress with an angry outburst, this tends to be his "normal" response when he is under pressure of any kind. The way that a person reacts to stress as an adult relates very much to the coping patterns he used as a child. These coping patterns tend to moderate during adolescence and then remain relatively constant during adulthood.

It is also generally accepted that most people remain relatively constant in their ability to tolerate stress. If, for example, a person's history indicates that he has coped well with stressful events in the past, it is likely that he will cope well with a current or future stressful event. Accordingly, a person whose past history indicates that he has rarely coped well with the pressures of life can be expected to have similar difficulty coping with a current or future stressful event. This is an *essential* concept for you to remember as you care for patients in inpatient or outpatient settings. Part of your *early* assessment of *every* patient should be a question about how he normally responds to pressure (see Chapter 12: Counseling Techniques for Nurses). If his response indicates that he does not handle stress well, then begin *at that time* to include extra supportive measures in your nursing care plan to avoid maladaptation.

Another clue that a patient's normal ability to cope is at risk is if the patient reports a series of very stressful events during the year before he was admitted to the hospital. The major life events listed in the Holmes and Rahe stress scale are the types of events that require major adjustment. If the patient has experienced an unusual number of them, his hospitalization, even if it appears routine, may be "the straw that breaks the camel's back."

Discussion in this chapter is restricted to the many types of responses that are normal when people are adapting to stress. Concepts about the effects of coping failure and subsequent maladaptation and crisis will be presented in Chapter 15: Crisis Intervention With the Maladapting Patient.

Part Three: Biopsychosocial Mediation of Stressful Events

Experts in the fields of medical science and physical pathology frequently have viewed the development of physical disease as a primarily physiological entity. They considered that disease occurs as the result of failure of normal organ functioning due to purely physiological causes.

You have read in several sections of this book that it is impossible to separate physical phenomena from emotional phenomena. The physical subsystems are *constantly* interacting with the psychological subsystems because they are part of *one* body system. They both respond continuously to social and environmental demands.

This thought may be acceptable to you based on your own awareness of patients as well as on the many documentations to support this concept that are included in this text. During the past decade, nursing theory has developed a holistic or systems approach toward understanding of human beings and illness.

The Psychobiology of Stress Mediation: The Mind-Body Bridge

Many nursing caregivers have clinically observed a relationship between the way a person feels emotionally and his physical state. Until recently, it has been impossible for them to document a definite association between the two. Lack of high-level technology inhibited research in the psychosomatic field of study.

One of the most important concepts of a systems approach to understanding of stress is that in addition to physical illness causing emotional and social stress, *emotional and social stress can cause physical illness*. There is a constant circular relationship between all these factors (Leigh and Reiser, 1977). Effective coping *can* stop this cycle. When coping fails, there is increased stress on all the subsystems, and physical illness can result.

The following excerpt from a chapter on psychobiology provides further evidence of the mind-body interaction:

> In order for acute or chronic psychological stress to induce disease in an organ, the stress would have to be transmitted from the brain to that organ by the autonomic nervous system or by some neuroendocrine pathway. The autonomic nervous system and the neuroendocrine system are the only routes by which the brain can directly affect the activity of the internal organs. Both the autonomic nervous system and the neuroendocrine system are relatively autonomous,* taking care of the routine business of keeping the internal environment constant. However, this ordinary reflex activity can be overridden by higher centers of the brain when they sense some change in the environment and prepare the body to meet it.

*Automatic, self-governing.

Many studies have shown that the structures of the limbic system are involved with basic drive states such as fear, hunger, sexual excitement, and aggression. . . . The limbic structures are shaped like a "C," forming a ring around an even older, more basic structure called the brain stem. The brain stem contains centers which are involved in regulating basic vegetative functions. For example, the centers for temperature control, blood pressure regulation, and sleep-wake activation are located in the brain stem. The brain stem passes information to the internal organs by way of the autonomic nervous system. Thus the emotion of fear, generated in the limbic system, influences the nearby brain stem structures to alter the activity of the internal organs . . . our blood pressure rises, we begin to breathe rapidly, our heart starts to pound, and our muscles fill with blood.

The autonomic nervous system has two major divisions, the sympathetic and the parasympathetic. In general, the sympathetic system mediates the response to challenges presented by the environment. The adrenal medulla is a specialized and enlarged sympathetic ganglion. When stimulated, the adrenal gland releases epinephrine, which is also called adrenaline. The parasympathetic system is involved during periods of physiological restoration—for example, when digesting a meal . . . . Both divisions of the autonomic nervous system have been implicated in psychosomatic illness.

Besides the autonomic nervous system, the other major route by which psychological stress is transmitted to the internal organs is the hypothalamic-pituitary neuroendocrine system. The hypothalamus lies at the base of the brain and receives input from most other parts of the brain. Electrical messages from other brain areas are translated to chemical messages in special hypothalamic cells . . . they secrete polypeptide hormones. These polypeptides from the hypothalamus, also known as releasing factors, travel down into the pituitary gland via a special blood vessel network.

The pituitary, sometimes called the master gland, secretes hormones into the general circulation when activated by hypothalamic polypeptide hormones. The pituitary hormones may act directly on other organ systems, or they may stimulate other endocrine glands such as the thyroid and adrenal cortex to release hormones.

Thus, in addition to autonomic arousal, psychological stress can activate a chain of hormonal responses which eventually alters the activity of the internal organs [Sack, 1980, pp. 191 to 193].*

Sack is quoted in order to present the rationale for the relationship potential between the etiology of physical illness and psychic stress. In the quotation above there was no discussion of the impact of social and environmental factors, however. Remember that, in most instances, awareness of social or environmental stressors triggers a cognitive appraisal or physiological response that can result in the activation process described above. Accordingly, discussion of the interaction effects of stress on the mind and body cannot be isolated from the multiple social stressors (sitting for state board nursing examinations, being involved in an argument) or environmental stressors (extremes of temperature, exposure to infectious disease) to which people are constantly exposed and responding. It becomes necessary to study the effects of stress within the context of general systems theory.

Historical Development of a Systems Approach to Stress

The evolution of a systems approach to illness has been occurring for centuries. There is evidence in the Bible and in Socrates' writings that there seemed to be a relationship between hopelessness or melancholy and the development of physical illness. On occasion, similar references appeared in medical literature before the 20th century.

During the early 20th century, Cannon (1929) attempted to prove an association between the mind and the endocrine system. Because of inadequate laboratory facilities, such attempts were doomed to failure. However, his theories about the possibility of an association between the two formed the basis for those who researched this subject in later decades.

Another important theorist in the field of psychosomatic medicine was Alexander (1950). Beginning in the 1930s he and his associates spent several decades attempting to prove that persons with certain personality styles were prone to specific types of illnesses. The development of illness was believed to represent some type of intrapsychic conflict.

The diseases they studied were duodenal peptic ulcers, bronchial asthma, rheumatoid arthritis, ulcerative colitis, essential hypertension, neurodermatitis, and thyrotoxicosis. Their research focus identified three factors that they believed would result in the development of one of these illnesses. The factors were predominantly intrapsychic. They were believed to be related to the physiological subsystem by direct action on the end organs by the peripheral mechanisms of the autonomic nervous system (1950). These theories are now considered by some to be oversimplified when considered in the light of recent advances in understanding the complexity of the mind-body interaction (Reiser, 1974). Other well-respected theorists in the field continue to find them applicable (Engel, 1974).

Advances in technology have made it possible to identify neurotransmitters and their function in development of physical illness (Mason, 1974). A section on neurotransmitters and their role in neuroendocrine functioning follows. The study of the effects of stress in the development of illness continues. More attention is being paid to the effects of both physiological and psychological genetic dispositions, the personality structure developed as a result of family dynamics, the overall social system, and environmental effects because of research that has demonstrated their impact on the development of illness.

Effect of Stress on the Development of Physical Illness

Currently, stress is implicated in the development of all physical illness (Engel, 1974; Leigh and Reiser, 1977; Mason, 1974; Reiser, 1974). The effects of stress on the immunosuppressive system have been described by many researchers and theorists. They propose that there is a relationship between stress, inadequate coping, and the development of cancer (Bahnson, 1980, 1981; Greene, 1966; Hagnell, 1966; LeShan, 1966; Lewis and Phillips, 1979; Reichel, 1977; Schmale and Iker, 1966; Selye, 1979).

The Role of Neurotransmitters

All our thoughts and feelings emanate from information processing events in the brain.

Less well appreciated is the fact that virtually all this information processing seems to involve communications between nerve cells (which are called neurons) via chemicals known as neurotransmitters [Snyder, 1980, p. 69].

The most basic connecting link in the bridge between the mind and the body is the *neurotransmitter*. It is a chemical messenger that relays information between neurons (Iverson, 1979). A neuron is the basic unit of the nervous system. It consists of a body, an axon, and one or more dendrites. The axon sends impulses or messages away from the neuron body; the dendrites receive messages from other neurons (Taber's, 1973).

Neurons do not actually touch one another in the process of sending and receiving messages to one another. Instead, there is a minute space between them called a *synapse*. A message from one neuron is sent through its axon to the dendrites of hundreds or thousands of other neurons. When the cell body initiates an impulse to its axon, the axon automatically releases a neurotransmitter substance that will carry the message across the synapse to the dendrites of neighboring neurons.

Different parts of the brain contain specific types of neurons with particular functions. The neurotransmitters that they release differ chemically from those of other neurons. There are approximately 30 different types of neurotransmitters that are known or suspected to be neurotransmitters in the brain. Each of them has a different stimulating or inhibiting effect on neurons. All brain functioning, whether it involves thinking, feeling, or sending messages to the muscles of the limbs or organs, depends on these neurotransmitters (Snyder, 1980).

Neurophysiologists may have just scratched the surface in understanding the importance of these chemical substances in our bodies. By studying the effects of having too much or too little of these biochemicals in humans and laboratory animals, their specific roles in neuroendocrine functioning will be increasingly documented. In fact, some theorists believe that further research on these substances will show that they hold the key to whether people will become ill as a result of immune system failure or whether they will remain well (Locke, 1982).

The Role of Stress in Myocardial Infarct

Stress has also been suggested as a cause of atherosclerotic heart disease. Rahe and Lind

(1971), in questioning the families of persons who died from myocardial infarct (MI), discovered that the amount of life change and stress the victims experienced during the year preceding death (see the Holmes and Rahe stress scale) was significantly higher than the stress they experienced during the 2 years preceding it. The 6 months preceding death showed the highest increase of all.

One of the possible causes of the relationship between stress and the development of atherosclerosis is that stimulation of the sympathetic nervous system is known to cause the release of fatty acids and glycerol from the fat tissues. Carruthers (1969) has theorized that sympathetic adrenal medullary stimulation could repeatedly raise blood fatty acid levels, resulting, after several biochemical steps, in the buildup of fatty acid deposits on the walls of arteries (atherosclerosis). Accordingly, it is possible that both high blood pressure and the development of coronary heart disease could be precipitated by stress (Sack, 1980).

In reviewing the types of stressful events that occurred in the lives of subsequent MI patients, Hurst and colleagues (1979) discovered that different persons reported varying levels of distress about a given life event. Accordingly, they propose that it is the events that a person finds *personally* upsetting that may undermine his coronary status.

The most up-to-date theory about the relationship between stress and physical illness suggests that many factors influence the development of illness:

1. The genetic personality and physical dispositions the person inherits (see Chap. 2)

2. Effects of the environment on personality development as determined by
   a. Family dynamics
   b. Type of defense mechanisms that develop as response to the conflict between the person's needs and the family system's needs
   c. The person's overall coping ability (see Chaps. 2 to 8)

3. Mutual feedback between the mind, body, and the environment as discussed earlier in the chapter
   a. Includes 1 and 2 above and other contributing factors such as biologic body rhythms, fatigue, impact of psychosocial events, and availability of a social support system (Engel, 1974; Leigh and Reiser, 1977; Mason, 1974; Reiser, 1974).

A Comprehensive Model for Evaluating Stress

The integration of the various concepts presented in this chapter is assisted by the model proposed by Jenkins (1979). After using the traditional stress models outlined above, he wrote:

> A major weakness of most stress research has been its limitation to a two-variable research design: a noxious stimulus is introduced and a response of discomfort or disease is observed . . . defined in terms of the presence of a physical or psychiatric illness [Jenkins, 1979, p. 265].

His solution to the incompleteness that he has found in the traditional approaches to stress is to introduce five variables:

1. The person's adaptive capacity
2. The stressor
3. The alarm reaction
4. The defensive reaction
5. The pathological reaction

In addition to the psychological and biological outcomes usually associated with the stress response, Jenkins has found that a person's ability to adapt to stress also depends on his interpersonal relationships and the overall society in which he functions. By reading about the many possible responses to stress in Table 9-1, you can see the potential for negative effects of stress on patients who are unable to cope with their illnesses or their hospitalizations.

Conclusion

The effects of stress on the body are being increasingly recognized by nursing and medical practitioners as well as by scientists in many fields. In general hospital and traditional medical care settings, however, many patients continue to be treated with a biomedical model based on diagnosis and treatment of physical pathology. There may be little attention paid to the effects of the psychological and social subsystems in the development of illness. Similarly, there may be little consideration given to the interaction of these three states during the active treatment process.

Professional nursing has identified the significance of assessing the patient from a holistic perspective. The movement toward implementing nursing diagnosis as an essential part of the nursing process has especially highlighted the nurse's

Table 9-1.
A Model Depicting the Interaction of Stress and the Organism

Level	Adaptive Capacity	Stressors	Alarm Reaction	Defensive Reaction	Pathological End-State
Biological	State of physique, nutrition, vigor Natural or acquired immunities	Deprivation of biological needs Excess inputs of physical or biological agents	Arousal—hunger, thirst, pain, fatigue Changes in physiological function	GAS Physiological compensation Shifts in metabolism Changes in pain threshold	Deficiency diseases "Exhaustion" Addictions Chronic dysfunction Structural damage
Psychological	Resourcefulness, problem-solving ability Ego strength Flexibility Social skills	Perceptions and interpretations of danger, threat, loss, disappointment, frustration, or sense of failure or hopelessness Loss of self-acceptance Threat to security	Feelings of deprivation— boredom, grief, sadness Feelings of anxiety, pressure, guilt Fear of danger	Ego defenses— denial, repression, projection Defensive neuroses Perceptual defenses— wishes, fantasies, motives Planning Problem solving	Despair, apathy Chronic personality pattern disturbances Psychoses Chronic affective disorders Meaninglessness
Interpersonal	Primary relationships including family Network of social supports	Social isolation Lack of acceptance Insults, punishments, rejections Changes in social groups, especially losses	Antagonism, conflict, suspicion Withdrawal Feelings of rejection, punishment	Defensive, rigid social relating Avoidance Assuming sick role Aggressiveness "Acting out" Enlisting social supports	Chronic exploitation Becoming an outcast Imprisonment Permanent disruption of interpersonal ties Chronic failure to fulfill roles
Sociocultural	Values Norms and practices "Therapeutic" social institutions Systems of knowledge and technology	Cultural change Role conflict Status incongruity Value conflicts with important others Forced change in life situation	Communication of concern and alarm Expressive behavior of crowds Mobilization of social structures	Culturally prescribed defenses— scapegoating, prejudice Explanatory ideologies Legal and moral systems Use of curers and institutions	Alienation, anomie Breakdown of social order Disintegration of the cultural systems of values and norms

(Jenkins D: Psychosocial modifiers of response to stress. In Barrett J, Rose R, Klerman G [eds]: Stress and Mental Disorder, p 269. New York, Raven Press, 1979)

importance as the monitor of the patient's psychosocial response to illness (Kim and Moritz, 1982).

The information presented in this chapter further emphasizes the impact of the psychosocial spheres on both the development of illness and the patient's response to illness. The effects of stress and inadequate coping promote an ongoing illness potential in all people. When stress overcomes a person's ability to cope, then the potential for maladaptation or crisis in the physical, psychological, or social sphere increases. Crisis assessment and intervention recommendations appear in Chapter 15: Crisis Intervention With the Maladapting Patient.

10

The Mental Status Examination

The ability to perform a formal mental status examination is considered essential for all professionals who work in the field of mental health. A *mental status examination* determines if there are abnormalities in the *thinking, feeling,* or *behavior* of the person being "examined." It is not necessary to carry out a formal question and answer mental examination process in order to evaluate a person's mental status, however. Instead, you can obtain a good idea of a newly admitted patient's mental status by being attentive to his way of thinking, expression of feelings, and behavior during your normal nursing assessment process.

One of the challenging aspects of assessing a patient's psychosocial functioning is that the thinking process you use involves processing many nonverbal clues that the patient gives you as well as integrating other bits of information you acquire about the patient. These bits of information, which are *unique* to any given patient, when combined with the theory included in this chapter, can help you arrive at a good nursing assessment of mental status functioning.

During their basic education, many nurses are not exposed to the specific aspects of mental functioning that are assessed in a routine mental status examination. Why this has been the tradition is unclear. Without knowing the various psychological functions that are normal and abnormal, valuable clues to psychosocial dysfunctioning in patients may be missed by otherwise astute nurses.

Working with a patient without knowing the symptoms of mental status change can be compared to looking at the surface of a pond without knowing that there is anything under the surface. More important, it can be compared to looking at a pond without knowing that there is a whole *world* under the surface.

If you were to stand overlooking a pond with a naturalist, he could introduce you to the many species of life under the surface. Suddenly, where there had been nothing unusual apparent to you, you would be introduced to a myriad of water creatures and species of vegetation. You would have a different understanding of the pond in the future. From then on, whenever you viewed any body of water, you would immediately look *beyond* the surface and be looking for things you previously had not realized were there.

This analogy can be compared to our knowledge of mental functioning. If we do not know the symptoms of mental dysfunction, it is possible to overlook many clues that a person's brain is not working normally. The importance of recognizing mental dysfunction is especially important in the general hospital setting because of the possibility that changes in normal functioning can be caused by physiological factors.

The Difference Between the Symptoms of Functional and Organic Psychiatric Disorders

Earlier in this book the differences between functional and organic psychiatric disorders were presented. Because this difference is such an important one for you to remember, it will be reemphasized. A *functional psychiatric disorder* is caused by a dysfunction in the *abstract* psychic structures of the mind: the id, ego, or superego. For example, a patient's defense mechanisms may not adequately help him to cope after he has had an unexpected amputation. The defensive aspect of ego functioning may overprotect him so that his denial shuts out the actual reality, or the ego may be so overwhelmed that the patient's normal defense mechanisms fail him.

An organic psychiatric disorder, also called *organic brain syndrome,* is caused by a dysfunction in the actual anatomical structures or the biochemistry of the brain. In the latter category, it is possible that medications, infection, elevated temperature, or any other factor that affects physiological functioning can cause a change in mental functioning. Chapter 11 discusses organic brain syndrome in detail. The ability to recognize this important, yet underrecognized, syndrome is essential for all nurses.

Because of the great variety of new stressors with which hospital patients are bombarded, they are at risk for mental dysfunctioning due to coping failure *and* physiological failure. Regardless of the cause, there are usually ways of resolving the dysfunctional state. No remedies can begin, however, if the subtle clues of mental dysfunction are missed by caregivers. The types of symptoms of mental dysfunction that the patient demonstrates can be important clues in identifying whether the etiology is functional or organic. Chapter 11 explains the differences in symptoms between the two main causes of psychiatric dysfunction. Because you will be spending more time with the patient than any other health caregiver, you will be in the best position to observe his ongoing physical and psychosocial adaptation to illness.

The Importance of Mental Status Observation

Notation about the status of a patient's thinking ability, feelings, and behavior during the admission process and ongoing nursing care is an important part of a nurse's accountability. The evaluation of a patient's mental status is an essential aspect of his overall psychosocial functioning. As you obtain the patient's history with subjective data that he tells you, be constantly aware of the nonverbal data that he is giving you about his mental functioning. Your observations of his thinking style, feelings, and behavior, when based on a sound understanding of normal and abnormal mental functioning, will form a solid basis for your psychosocial nursing assessment.

These observations can be accumulated while you are giving routine nursing care. The importance of obtaining a good baseline mental status on admission cannot be overemphasized. Even more important is your notation of *any* change you observe from the mental state you saw on admission and the exact time you noticed it. If, for example, mental dysfunction is noted on the third day after admission, and the patient was normal on admission, then the contributing factor may be attributed to some aspect of hospitalization and is frequently reversible.

In order to determine if changes are occurring, the patient's current mental status should be compared to his mental status on admission *as well as his prehospitalization level of mental functioning.* This can be done in many ways:

1. Compare the patient's mental status on his first day of admission to his mental status on ensuing days.
2. Ask the patient if his current feelings, thoughts, the way he thinks, and his memory are similar to what they were before he was sick. If they are different, ask him to describe *how* they are different and *why* he thinks they are different. Frequently, we forget that the patient usually has good insight into the cause of his current physical and mental functioning. Unfortunately, we rarely ask him what *he* thinks is wrong. Accordingly, we lose valuable information that could help all caregivers in the diagnostic and treatment process.
3. If the patient is disoriented and confused, ask the family about his presickness mental functioning. For example, if an 83-year-old patient

were disoriented, *never* assume that it is the result of senility due to aging. It is possible that this patient was alert and articulate before hospitalization, and, because of toxicity due to an undiagnosed systemic infection, organic brain functioning is temporarily affected due to neurological causes. Unless you check the patient's prehospitalization mental status with the family, you and the medical caregivers could lose valuable time in correctly arriving at possible causes of the physical disease process.

4. Use any extra information about the patient in assessing his or her current status.

One of the challenging aspects of assessing a patient's psychological functioning is that the thinking process you use involves processing of many nonverbal clues that the patient gives you as well as integrating other bits of information you have about the patient by using your own social awareness. Deductive reasoning, similar to that used by a detective in solving a mystery, can help you to use your curiosity in determining a patient's current mental response to illness.

Mental status is an essential part of the patient's total psychosocial functioning. In order to clarify the difference between mental status assessment and psychosocial assessment, the former is an evaluation of the functioning of the patient's intrapsychic system. Psychosocial assessment includes an evaluation of the patient's intrapsychic system, his social system, and *the interaction between the two.* Chapter 13: Psychosocial Nursing Assessment and Diagnosis includes psychosocial assessment and diagnosis and explains these essential aspects of the nursing process.

The following case example may help to illustrate the importance of using extra information available to you:

Case Example

Mr. Menz is the 62-year-old national sales manager of a nationally known company. Four days ago he was operated on for intestinal obstruction. At 2 PM on his fourth postoperative day he is unshaved; his face appears sad, with no animation. He is wearing hospital pajamas, although his wife brought in his own pajamas and has been encouraging him to wear them. He is lying in bed, facing the wall, with the sheets pulled over his shoulders. In the admission nursing assessment it was noted that his affect seemed appropriate; no depression was apparent.

In the case described above, we know that Mr. Menz is a national sales manager of a large company. We know that a national sales manager must have a very high level of ability. He has also been a salesman himself in order to be in his current position. How do you normally picture a salesman, especially one who has climbed to a very high position in a company and can therefore be thought of as a "supersalesman"? Gregarious, confident, and optimistic might be suitable adjectives. Do these adjectives fit the current picture we have of Mr. Menz? Are we possibly making an assumption when we reason that his current mental status is probably not normal for him? No. We are using deductive reasoning based on valid information.

In the care of patients, consider your assessment process to be similar to that of a detective. Actually, it can be challenging and creative to think through the clues you have available to you. The last step in this "sleuthing" process is to check your deduction with the family. They may tell you that Mr. Menz had a positive outlook and had no apparent problems before surgery. If so, then it is possible that with appropriate nurse counseling and support, the cause of his current maladaptation may be discovered and intervention will yield positive results. On the other hand, you may learn from the family that the patient's normally positive disposition has been deteriorating over the past several months. At home, before admission, he was withdrawn and depressed. His wife was frustrated in her efforts to talk with him about what she was observing. He was unable to trust anyone with his feelings and thoughts and had insisted, "I can figure it out by myself."

When the preadmission history includes depression (or anxiety) that has lasted more than a few weeks, it is wise to remember that there are probably complex factors present of longstanding duration. In such cases, psychiatric referral of the patient should be recommended to the attending physician. When recommending psychiatric referral, it is essential to document precisely the symptoms you have observed in the patient and include the patient's observations (and those of the family if the patient is not reliable) of his preadmission emotional state.

When a preexisting maladaptive emotional state is compounded by the stress of hospitalization and recuperation, the task of adaptation is seriously jeopardized. The astute nurse's observations and patient advocacy in recommending psychiatric referral and outpatient psychiatric follow-up care can have a profound effect on the future quality of life for the patient and all members of the family system.

The Categories of Mental Status Evaluation

The many aspects of a patient's mental status are listed in the categories described below. All these categories are actually manifestations of various ego functions (see Chap. 2: The Building Blocks of Personality). Ego functioning can be temporarily changed by such effects as toxicity from drugs or infections or by the overuse or underuse of defense mechanisms (as with the patient who uses denial to shut out the reality of catastrophic illness).

In the process of obtaining the general information needed, it is possible to assess the following categories (Langsley, 1979; Solomon and Patch, 1974):

1. Level of awareness and orientation
2. Appearance and behavior
3. Speech and communication
4. Mood or affect (feeling state)
5. Disturbances in thinking process, disorganization of thought process, disturbance in content of thought (delusions, phobias, obsessions), problems with memory and concentration
6. Problems with perception (hallucinations or distortions of reality associated with any of the senses)
7. Abstract thinking and judgment

Whether these categories are actually evaluated in these exact terms can be your own choice. Noting your observations about the patient's mental status in your own words is acceptable as long as these main categories of mental functioning are assessed.

It is not intended that you memorize the psychiatric terms that appear on the following pages. Instead, they are presented so that they will be available if you want to refer to them to determine the proper terms for thinking and feeling and behavioral, perceptual, or other types of mental dysfunction you may observe in your patients. By using these terms, your notations will have a more professional tone.

Level of Awareness and Orientation

Level of Awareness
The level of awareness is one of the more observable aspects of brain functioning. This is an important indicator, especially for hospitalized patients. Usually the first sign that a patient is developing a toxic physiological state is a change in his level of consciousness and orientation. Nurses should be alert to subtle changes in these two important indicators of brain functioning. Their early observations, when presented in an articulate manner to physicians, will usually result in prompt diagnostic and treatment measures that can reverse the cause of the toxic condition that is causing an organic brain syndrome. The levels of awareness range on a continuum from unconsciousness and frank coma to drowsiness and hypersomnolence to alertness, hyperalertness, or suspiciousness to frank paranoia or mania. Figure 10-1 shows the range of levels of consciousness observable in general hospital patients.

At the opposite end of coma is a patient hypervigilant and hyperaware of his environment. Hyperalert awareness is seen in a person with a suspicious, paranoid personality style or a patient who is manic. It is most commonly seen in the intensive care units of general hospitals, when otherwise normal patients are prepsychotic from interactions between organic causes, frequently medication related; environmental factors, such as sensory deprivation and sleep loss; and impairment of normal ego functioning due to the stress of illness or preexisting personality conflicts or both.

Orientation
Orientation is the patient's ability to identify *who* he is, *where* he is, and the *approximate* date.

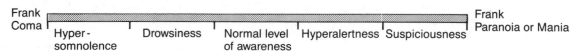

Figure 10-1.
Continuum of levels of consciousness.

These three indicators of orientation are frequently termed orientation to time, person, and place. They may be abbreviated to *orientated* × 3. The approximate date is accepted because it is quite easy for any well-functioning person who has been hospitalized for several days to confuse the date by one day. Postsurgical patients and patients with admissions extending beyond 1 week often lose the points of reference for days of the week and dates that they would normally be aware of if they were in their normal environment.

The list below (Kaplan and Sadock, 1981) contains terminology commonly used to describe level of consciousness and orientation:

Levels of Orientation and Consciousness

1. *Confusion*
   Disorientation to time, person, or place
2. *Clouding of consciousness*
   Slight to moderate disturbance in perception or thought
3. *Stupor*
   Shock-like inability to recognize or react to environment
4. *Delirium*
   Moderate to severe disturbance in perception, thought, and emotion. Accompanied by marked fear
5. *Dreamy state*
   Hallucinatory type of disturbed consciousness
6. *Coma*
   All consciousness is lost

Appearance and Behavior

A patient's appearance and behavior include any observable characteristics. They are listed by category. Following each category is a partial list of words that describe the characteristics observed (Davis and Foreyt, 1975, p. 145; Dubin and Stolberg, 1981, p. 11; Freedman and colleagues, 1976, pp. 402–403). One or more words can be used in describing each category.

A. Dress
   1. Neat
   2. Careless
   3. Eccentric
B. *Facies* or facial expression
   1. Animated
   2. Fixed
   3. Sad

   4. Angry
   5. Color of face (pale, reddened, and so on)
C. Posture
   1. Relaxed
   2. Tense
   3. Erect
   4. Sitting, lying, and so on
D. Motor activity
   1. Agitated, restless, and so on
   2. Tremors: coarse or fine
   3. Motor retardation: slow movement
      a. *Catatonic:* immobile
      b. *Waxy flexibility:* body maintains position in which it is placed
   4. *Apraxia:* inability to carry out purposeful movement to achieve a goal
   5. *Echopraxia:* mimicking the body movements of the interviewer
   6. Abnormal *(dystonic)* movement
      a. *Akathisia:* extreme restlessness
      b. *Akinesia:* complete or partial loss of muscle movement
      c. *Dyskinesia:* Excessive movement of mouth, protruding tongue, facial grimacing (a common side-effect of the major tranquilizers)
      d. *Parkinsonian movement:* fine tremor accompanied by muscular rigidity
   7. *Hypomania:* a state characterized by increased motor activity accompanied by a mild to moderate level of emotional excitement
E. Physical characteristics
   1. Unusual appearance of any part of body
F. Reaction to interviewer
   1. Friendly
   2. Suspicious
   3. Hostile
   4. Indifferent

This category requires subjective judgment on your part. You probably already go through this process with patients but have never formally identified it as part of your nursing assessment. It is not uncommon for nurses to comment to one another in the clinical setting, "I don't like the way Mr. Burnes looks today."

Nurses traditionally have not specifically verbalized what it is about a patient that makes them suspect that his condition is worsening. Actually, if you look at the list of characteristics above and recall the last time you "knew" something was wrong with a patient, you may discover that your judgment was based on sound clinical objective data. Your sensitivity in seeing the changes in these characteristics is what led you to your conclusion. Unfortunately, instead of recognizing that nurses' evaluations of patients are based on actual clinical judgment, these observations have been classified by many nurses themselves as "nurse's intuition" or "nurse's instinct."

Speech and Communication

In evaluating a patient's speech and communication, you will be observing *how* he is communicating rather than *what* he is communicating. What the patient is communicating is the content. The content of a person's speech is actually a reflection of his thought process. The thinking process is described later in this chapter. The following aspects of the patient's speaking style should be observed (Langsley, 1979):

1. Rate
2. Volume
3. Modulation and flow
4. Production

The rate of speech is usually consistent with the patient's overall psychomotor status. If a person is depressed, his speech, as well as his activity level, is usually slowed. Conversely, a rapid rate of speech usually indicates elation or, in some cases, a manic mental state. Accordingly, the *volume* or loudness of speech will range from almost inaudible in very depressed patients to loud in manic, confused, or suspicious patients.

Modulation and *flow of speech* pertain to the range of the speech. Does the person talk in a dull monotone, or is there a spirited and lively quality? There is cause for concern if you observe a patient displaying a lively speech rate that alternates with a subdued pattern within a few hours. This may be the first indicator of the development of an organic brain syndrome.

Speech production is the patient's ability to produce words. He may be mute. He may display pressured speech. *Pressured speech* is a very rapid rate of speech, usually associated with extreme anxiety or mania. His speech may be slurred; the words are then poorly formed.

Affect (Mood)

Affect is the way a person *feels* and the way he *appears* to observers. The term *mood* is used to describe the patient's subjective feelings (Hinsie and Campbell, 1977). The terms are frequently used interchangeably in the clinical setting, and this has become an acceptable practice.

The various disturbances in affect that may be observed in patients are listed below (Kaplan and Sadock, 1981; Shapiro, 1965). (Only those feelings that are considered abnormal and are indicative of mental status dysfunction are included. A list of commonly observed affects appears on p. 16.)

A. Inappropriate affects
  1. A patient who is not responding as expected in a given situation
  2. The content of a person's discussion does not fit with the emotions accompanying his statements
B. Pleasurable affects
  1. *Euphoria:* excessive and inappropriate feeling of well-being
  2. *Exaltation:* intense elation accompanied by feelings of grandeur
C. Unpleasurable affects (dysphoria)
  1. *Depression:* hopeless feeling
  2. *Grief or mourning:* prolonged and excessive sadness associated with a loss
  3. *Anxiety:* feeling of apprehension caused by conflicts of which the patient is not aware
  4. *Fear:* excessive fright resulting from consciously recognized danger
  5. *Agitation:* anxiety associated with severe motor restlessness
  6. *Ambivalence:* alternating and opposite feelings occurring in the same person about the same object
  7. *Aggression:* rage, anger, or hostility that is excessive or seems unrelated to a person's current situation
  8. *Mood swings* (also called *lability*): alternating periods of elation and depression or anxiety in the same person within a limited time
D. Lack of affect
  Blunted or *flat affect:* a normal range of emotions is missing, commonly seen in persons with depression, some forms of schizophrenia, and some types of organic brain syndrome; it also can be seen in persons whose personalities are tightly controlled (in such a case the person's feelings—indeed, his whole personality—is called *constricted*)
E. "La belle indifference"
  This French term translated literally means "the beautiful unconcern"; used to describe the lack of worry that an ordinary person would customarily feel in a difficult situation

Thinking Process

A person's thinking process is the way he functions intellectually. It is sometimes also called cognitive style or state. It is the way he thinks, the reasoning he uses about the world, and the way that he connects or associates these thoughts. When you are talking with a patient, abnormalities may be noted in the *speed of his thinking:* his thoughts may be very slow in being presented or may tumble out quickly (*racing thoughts*).

Another important observation is the *organization of his thoughts.* These are the associations or the connection between a patient's thoughts. As you listen to the patient's thoughts, you may or may not be able to understand how they relate to one another. You may find yourself with a patient whose thoughts are *so* unconnected that they remind you of a bouncing ball in a confined space. You are never sure where his thoughts are going to bounce next.

The process of thinking is ongoing for most people. The ability to think is triggered by the need to perform a task or solve a problem. Normal thinking occurs whenever a logical sequence of thoughts results in a reality-oriented conclusion (Kaplan and Sadock, 1981). When this process is abnormal, you may see any of the following disturbances (Kaplan and Sadock, 1981).

Symptoms of Thinking Disorder

A. Disturbance in thought process (also known as disturbance in associations or connections between thoughts)
   1. *Loose associations.* When a patient's thoughts are poorly connected (see below).
      a. *Circumstantiality.* A flow of spoken thoughts that results in a patient's eventually getting to a conclusion after many digressions to associated ideas. It can be compared to someone starting out on a journey from New York to Los Angeles and stopping off in Montreal, Canada, and Anchorage on the way.
      b. *Tangentiality.* A flow of spoken thoughts that results in many digressions, but in which the patient never reaches a conclusion. It can be compared to a journey that starts with someone having a vague idea of where he wants to go, but, in the process of going, he stops in so many other places that he eventually forgets his original desired destination.

   2. *Neologism.* A new word that a person makes up. It may sound like a nonsense word.
   3. *Flight of ideas.* Rapid speaking with a quick shifting from one idea to another. Unlike the process of loose associations, these ideas do have a logical connection. Frequently seen in manic patients.
   4. *Perseveration.* Repetition of the same thought or word in response to different questions.
   5. *Word salad.* Disconnected mixture of unrelated words.
   6. *Blocking.* "Sudden cessation in the train of thought or in the midst of a sentence" for no apparent reason (Hinsie and Campbell, 1977, p. 100).

B. Disturbances in content of thought
   1. *Delusion.* "False belief, not consistent with a patient's intelligence and cultural background, that cannot be corrected by reasoning" (Freedman and colleagues, 1976, p. 404). The most prevalent forms of delusions are as follows:
      a. *Delusion of grandeur.* An exaggerated belief about one's abilities or importance.
      b. *Delusion of reference.* False belief that one is the center of others' attention and discussion.
      c. *Delusion of persecution* (*paranoia*). False belief that others are seeking to hurt or, in some other way, damage a person either physically or by insinuation.

   2. *Preoccupation of thought.* When a person is preoccupied he connects all occurrences and experiences to a central thought, usually one with strong emotional overtones. For example, a patient who was injured while escaping from a fire may continue, even while safe in the hospital, to fear being trapped again. This preoccupation may be present whether he is awake or asleep.

   3. *Obsessive thought.* An unwelcome idea, emotion, or urge that repeatedly enters a person's consciousness (Hinsie and Campbell, 1977)

   4. *Phobia.* A strong fear of a particular situation.
      a. *Claustrophobia.* Fear of being in an enclosed place.

b. *Agoraphobia.* Fear of being in an open place, such as outdoors or on a highway.

c. *Acrophobia.* Fear of high places (Kaplan and Sadock, 1981).

C. Other disturbances of thought

1. *Memory impairment.* Any type of change in ability to accurately recall thoughts from the unconscious into consciousness

   a. *Amnesia.* Complete or partial inability to recall past experiences.

   b. *Confabulation.* The filling in of gaps in memory with untrue statements. This is done by the patient unconsciously because he is unable to recognize his intellectual deficits. It is most frequently seen in organic brain disease. It is common in alcoholic patients with Korsakoff's syndrome (Hinsie and Campbell, 1977). Laypersons may describe the patient as making up stories or telling "white lies." It is actually an unconscious attempt by the patient to compensate for memory deficits.

   c. *Déjà vu.* Translated literally from French, this means "already seen." A feeling that one has experienced a new situation on a previous occasion. (This can normally occur in anyone who is fatigued or under stress.)

Memory

Human beings possess two types of memory: recent and long-term memory. *Recent memory* is the ability to recall events in the unconscious that have occurred in the immediate past and up to 1 or 2 weeks previously. *Long-term memory* is the ability to recall events from the distant past: names of schools attended, dates of siblings' birthdays, the sequence of U.S. presidents, and so on. When memory fails, recent memory is the first to be affected. These memory deficits can most often be seen in patients with chronic organic brain syndrome (the irreversible senile dementias such as arteriosclerosis), acute organic brain syndrome (the usually reversible toxic brain syndromes), and depressed patients whose cognitive abilities are temporarily slowed.

Patients with recent memory deficits will demonstrate confusion about recent events but will be able to tell you the names of their grandparents, their places of birth, or who was president when they graduated from grade school. This is so because the process of memory storage

of recent events is fully or partially dysfunctional because of the presence of organic or functional pathology.

In order to test a patient's long-term memory, you can ask him specific questions about his childhood and early adulthood. With questions about recent events, it is essential that you know the correct answers in order to validate the accuracy of the patient's responses. If the patient can answer the following questions, it is likely that his mental status is within normal range. If there are many gaps in his ability to answer these questions, there is a greater likelihood that brain dysfunction due to a physiological disorder is present.

Ask the patient to tell you information about the following:

1. His present illness: when it began, the symptoms, people involved, and so on (tests for recent memory)
2. His or her past: birthdate, date of high school graduation, marriage, names of siblings, children, and so on (long-term memory)
3. Significant events in topic that patient acknowledges interest in, for example, politics, baseball, or job, during the past 5 years (recent and long-term memory)*

These types of questions can all be asked conversationally without causing the patient or you to feel as if you are "examining" him.

Perception

Perception is the way that a person views himself, the environment, and his relationship with others in his environment. Perception is derived from the senses of vision, hearing, touch, and smell. The input from the senses is mediately by the ego and its defenses. In determining whether a patient's perception is normal, you should look for any behavioral manifestation that the patient is distorting reality. If, for example, you observe a patient who appears to be picking things from his bed, his body, or the wall, there is a strong possibility that he is having visual hallucinations. (This is a common type of hallucination in hospitalized patients with organic brain syndrome. The patient thinks he is seeing insects or other objects.)

The major type of perceptual dysfunction observed in hospital patients are hallucinations. *Hallucinations* are false sensory perceptions that

*Woodhouse R: Personal communication, 1982.

do not exist in external reality. The types of hallucinations are listed below:

1. *Visual hallucination*
   A hallucination in which the person sees objects that are nonexistent (this is one of the most common symptoms of patients with organic brain syndrome caused by delirium tremems [DTs], drug toxicity, or delirium caused by any other physiological imbalance.) Visual hallucinations are rare in persons with schizophrenia or other forms of functional psychiatric disorder (Solomon and Patch, 1974).

2. *Tactile hallucination*
   A hallucination in which the person feels objects or sensations that are nonexistent. (These are also common in organic or toxic-induced psychoses and are rare in functional disorders [Solomon and Patch, 1974].)

3. *Auditory hallucination*
   A hallucination in which the person hears voices, bells, or other sounds that are nonexistent. As pointed out above, auditory hallucinations usually will help to determine that there is no physical or toxic cause to the dysfunction. Auditory hallucinations are most common in schizophrenia, manic-depressive illness, and other transient psychiatric functional states (Solomon and Patch, 1974).

4. *Hypnagogic hallucination*
   A hallucination in which a person senses any type of false sensory perception during the twilight period between being awake and being asleep. This type of experience also may occur in normal people, especially during times of severe fatigue or acute stress.

Another form of perceptual dysfunction is called an illusion. An *illusion* is a distortion or misinterpretation of an actual stimulus by the ego. For example, a patient in the intensive care unit may report that he has snakes crawling on his arm. He may distort the image of the intravenous tubing. In other words, an actual stimulus is sensed incorrectly. Illusions may be present in both organic brain syndrome and the functional psychoses (Solomon and Patch, 1974).

Two other forms of mental dysfunction are related to perception of one's self and the environment (Solomon and Patch, 1974):

1. *Depersonalization*
   A loss of sense of control over oneself, and a feeling of detachment from one's surroundings.

2. *Derealization*
   A sense of unreality about the environment or a distortion or frank loss of reality about the environment. This condition and depersonalization are signs of many types of psychiatric disorders. They also may be experienced by normal persons during times of acute stress or extreme fatigue.

Abstract Thinking and Judgment

Abstract Thinking

Abstract thinking is a person's ability to derive a conclusion from a logical reasoning process. *Concrete thinking* is a contrast to abstract thinking. When a person thinks concretely, he interprets what he sees and hears in a rigid way. He will perceive things exactly as they are sensed rather than applying an abstract judgment to decide the actual meaning. For example, a patient asked, "How did you happen to come to the clinic today?" may reply, "By bus," rather than by telling you the health problem that caused him to come to the clinic. Concrete thinking in a person of normal to high intelligence is often an indication of organic brain syndrome. Persons with a low level of intelligence may routinely think in a concrete manner. Concrete thinking may also be seen in schizophrenics (Langsley, 1979).

Judgment

Judgment is a person's ability to behave in a socially appropriate manner. In a formal mental status examination this can be determined by asking a person what he would do if he found a wallet containing a large sum of money lying in the street. Another question that could be asked is, "What would you do if you discovered a fire burning in a building?"

Informally, in the hospital setting, you can observe a patient's social judgment by the way he acts in his room or when he is with you or with other patients. For example, the patient discussed below was a major concern to the nurses on his unit:

Case Example

Joe is a 38-year-old married man. His father is a prominent lawyer (this causes you to expect that, under normal conditions, Joe should be aware of socially appropriate behavior). Joe's hospital room was located near the beginning of a busy surgical unit. Joe's normal attire was a loosely tied bathrobe. He declared that he did not like to wear underwear or pajamas; they were too constricting. On his head he wore a baseball hat that had wings protruding from each side. Joe refused to lie under the covers; his lack of modesty was an embarrassment to all.

Poor social judgment is frequently seen in patients with mental dysfunction caused by organic brain syndrome, schizophrenia, or severe depression (Langsley, 1979).

Assessment of Suicide Potential

If a patient is acutely or chronically depressed, another aspect of mental status evaluation is assessment of suicide potential. The mention of the word *suicide* results in an unpleasant feeling in most people. Because of this, the word is rarely mentioned. Instead, phrases such as "doing one-self in" or "ending it all" or other euphemisms are used. These are acceptable phrases for caregivers in the general hospital setting to use with physically ill patients who are acutely depressed. Although the concept of suicide may be unpleasant to caregivers, it does occur in the general hospital.

Many nurses in inpatient or outpatient settings come into contact with seriously depressed patients. The depression and hopelessness may be due to preexisting personality disorders or may be the result of living with chronic illness that has permanently disrupted quality of life. The hopelessness that results can eventually cause a person to want to die.

In Chapter 16: Nursing Intervention With the Emotionally Complex Patient, you will find specific recommendations to use in caring for depressed and potentially suicidal patients. Most persons who are not specifically trained in clinical psychiatric theory are afraid that if they ask a seriously depressed person if he has ever thought about committing suicide, they may introduce the idea into the person's head. It is also frightening for them to think that if they raise the idea, the patient may make it a reality.

Actually, when serious trouble occurs in the form of severe or prolonged physical or emotional pain, many normal persons can experience fleeting wishes to be dead so that they will no longer have to experience their distress. A person may wish that death would claim him, or he may think about killing himself in order to escape from his trouble. In either case, if such ideas are present, it can be a relief for the patient to acknowledge them. In fact, when patients have such thoughts, they are usually troubled by them but are afraid to share them with anyone.

The following dialogue can guide you in discussing this topic.

"Have you ever wished it would all be over?" If the answer is yes, continue on.

"What would you do so that it could all be over?" If the patient says "Nothing" or denies that he would do anything actively to kill himself, but would want the disease to kill him, then continue.

"What is it that keeps you from wanting to die?" Listen for him to tell you that his family needs him or one or more other specific reasons why he could not commit suicide. If he has no reason, then he is at greater risk. If he tells you that he wants to kill himself, it is important for you to find out how he would do it.

"How would you kill yourself?" If he has no suicide plan, his risk for suicide is less than that of a person who has one. *His intention to commit suicide must be taken seriously, however.* If he has a suicide plan, he is at strong risk for suicide.

Your assessment process may reveal that the patient has occasional or persistent thoughts of suicide. These thoughts are called *suicidal ideation.* He wants to die; his physical or emotional distress has caused him to give up hope. The only way that he sees out of his difficulty is to kill himself. If the patient has developed a *suicide plan* to use to kill himself, he is at greater risk for self-inflicted harm. Whether the patient has suicidal thinking or an active plan, the attending physician should be notified at once. If the patient has an active plan, you should strongly recommend psychiatric consultation in order to ensure the patient's well-being.

Another important consideration in making this recommendation is your legal responsibility as a caregiver to this patient. You could be held accountable if he harms himself while under your care. If you consider the patient to be a strong suicidal risk, then begin constant surveillance of the patient until the consultant arrives. The discussion of the care of the suicidal patient will appear in Chapter 16.

Conclusion

An evaluation of the mental status of all patients is strongly recommended. It only takes a few minutes to ask the questions recommended above. Your original assessment of a patient's mental status will be important if maladaptation to his illness should bring about changes in mental status. In addition, it is possible for *any* patient to develop an organic brain syndrome, since the physiological functioning of the brain is impaired by the toxic effects of illness or medications. When a baseline mental status evaluation is charted, and the *time* and *date* of the notation is present, later changes can be compared. It is important *always* to chart the time as well as the date of mental status observations.

Unlike functional psychiatric disorders, the psychiatric symptoms of organic brain syndrome can vary markedly within the hour (Dubin and Stolberg, 1981). With documentation of a changing mental status caused by maladaptation or organic dysfunction, medical intervention can often be initiated to diagnose and treat the underlying cause.

Organic brain syndrome (OBS) is frequently overlooked and underdiagnosed in the general hospital as a disease entity; it requires astute nursing and medical personnel to be aware of the multiple physical etiologies that can result in observable psychiatric symptoms. A simple definition of OBS is that it is a constellation of many psychiatric symptoms caused by a dysfunction of the physical structure or of the physiological functioning of the brain. (The specific psychiatric symptoms observed in a patient with organic brain syndrome will be presented later in this chapter.) This dysfunction results in emotional or intellectual changes in the patient's mental state. Another name for any type of organic brain dysfunction is *encephalopathy*.

Before you begin to believe that the nursing profession is negligent in not being more aware of the etiology and symptoms of OBS, read the following excerpts:

> Cerebral dysfunction and disease . . . have remained a no-man's land straddling the boundaries of psychiatry, neurology, and neuropsychology [Lipowski, 1975, p. 11].
>
> Mental disorders due to cerebral disease and dysfunction constitute an integral yet conspicuously neglected area of psychiatry. The currently used classification of these disorders is obsolete, their terminology is notoriously muddled, and data about their prevalence and incidence, pathogenesis, and pathophysiology are scanty [Lipowski, 1980, p. 674].

These are quotes from one of the most well-known U.S. experts on OBS. Although Lipowski is a psychiatrist, he states that psychiatry has done little to investigate the syndrome, and the diagnosis of OBS falls squarely on the shoulders of psychiatry (1980). This is because the psychiatric symptoms that result usually motivate puzzled attending physicians in other medical-surgical specialties to refer a patient for psychiatric consultation if his psychiatric symptoms become acute and psychosis occurs.

Importance of Nurses as Observers of Early Symptoms of Acute Organic Brain Syndrome

Nurses spend more time with patients than all other members of the health care team. Accord-

11

Organic Brain Syndrome

ingly, they are able to observe patients' mental status changes over several hours. The symptoms of acute OBS occur rapidly. For example, a nurse may give AM care to an alert patient who displays normal levels of energy, intellectual ability, and emotional stability. By 1 PM the patient may be lethargic, confused, and not able to remember seeing the nurse in the morning. Another possibility is that he may be restless, hyperalert, and suspicious of any treatment or medication you wish to give him. Within another hour he may tell you that the television set in the room is actually a camera that is spying on him. In other words, his mental state has changed markedly from what it was on admission, during the early days of his hospitalization, and as recently as a few hours earlier. It is essential that you note these specific changes and the exact time when you observed them.

When such a change in mental state is observed, it is important to watch closely for the variations and specific changes in functioning mentioned in the previous chapter. When slight differences in mental status occur, they can indicate the possibility of cerebral dysfunction due to physical causes. The patient's brain function may be deteriorating as the result of a new or worsening physical complication. Your early detection and call to the patient's physician may make a critical difference.

The Difference Between the Etiologies of Functional Psychiatric Disorder and Organic Brain Syndrome

One of the concepts that causes many nurses and physicians to miss the symptoms of early and acute OBS is the difference between functional and organically caused psychiatric disorders. A *functional psychiatric illness* is one with no known physical abnormality related to it (although researchers are continuing to look for relationships between catecholamine levels and such functional diseases as schizophrenia and depression). OBS is caused by specific deterioration in the physical structures or chemical functioning of the nervous system. An essential point to remember is that the psychiatric symptoms you observe in the patient with OBS may appear to be the same as the symptoms you observe in a hallucinating schizophrenic.

For this reason, one may hear a nurse remark, "Oh, Mr. Thomas is out of it again. Let's give him some more haloperidol (Haldol)." The nurse may not be aware that Mr. Thomas's hallucinations may actually be caused by a fluctuating mental state due to toxicity from an undiagnosed medical problem or even from the haloperidol itself. He or she may incorrectly believe that Mr. Thomas may be a former psychiatric patient who must be controlled with medication.

In observing the symptoms seen in patients with both organic *and* functional disorders, psychosis is present at the severe end of the continuum. How then, does one tell if the psychotic symptoms observed are more likely to be of organic origin and therefore medically treatable and potentially reversible? There are actually some basic differences between the two, and the chart on p. 121 will help to clarify them (Detre and Jarecki, 1971; Freedman and colleagues, 1976; Goldberg, 1980; Lishman, 1978; Murray, 1978; Thomas, 1973; Usdin and Lewis, 1979).

Types of Organic Brain Syndrome

Delirium

The most commonly observed acute form of OBS in general hospital patients is *delirium*. It can develop rapidly, in even a few hours. It is also called *toxic brain syndrome* (Kaplan and Sadock, 1981; Solomon and Patch, 1974). When delirium occurs, it frequently is associated with an already existing physical illness that may have precipitated the toxic brain reaction. The most important distinguishing characteristics of delirium are fairly rapid changes in the patient's wakefulness, alertness, attention span, and ability to perceive the environment accurately. If the organic process continues, symptoms will gradually increase to a psychotic state.

Visual hallucinations are common when the patient is delirious. This is in contrast to functional psychiatric disorders such as schizophrenia, in which auditory hallucinations are far more common than visual ones. When the delirious patient develops inaccurate ideas and thoughts, these delusional thoughts are usually paranoid. When the patient is stimulated to alertness, his intellect remains relatively unchanged.

A change in the patient's activity level usually occurs. Most often this is represented by a slowing

Differences Between OBS Psychosis and Functional Psychosis

Differentiating Factors	OBS Psychosis	Functional Psychosis
Etiology (the cause should be traceable to one of the categories noted)	Metabolic disorder Electrical (convulsive) disorder Neoplastic disease Degenerative brain disease Arterial (cerebrovascular) disease Mechanical (structural) disease Infectious disease Nutritional disorder Drug toxicity (Goldberg, 1980)	Schizophrenia Manic-depressive illness Psychotic depression
Past history	Evidence of recent infection, head trauma, metabolic disorder, or other incident related to categories above	Usually reveals past-psychiatric disturbances; recent history of an emotionally stressful precipitating event
Level of consciousness	Usually affected	Rarely affected
Orientation to time (usually first affected), place (less affected), person (least affected)	Usually one or more are affected	Rarely affected
Recent memory	Usually affected	Rarely affected
Distant memory	Less affected than recent memory	Rarely affected
Intellectual functioning (thinking and judgment)	Usually affected	Usually affected
Emotional functioning	Usually affected	Usually affected
Perception	Usually affected (hallucinations are more often visual)	Usually affected (hallucinations are more often auditory)
Neurological changes	Usually present	Rarely affected
Laboratory findings	Usually abnormal	Rarely affected

of movement, ranging to total stupor. Toxic OBS may cause psychomotor restlessness and overactivity. Another characteristic of both acute and chronic brain syndrome is a worsening of psychiatric symptoms at night (Kaplan and Sadock, 1981; Solomon and Patch, 1974). This syndrome is called *sun-downing.* (When this occurs, the use of a night light in the patient's room can be a help to him as he tries to orient himself.) If diagnosed promptly,

and the cause of the toxic brain reaction removed or treated properly, acute OBS reactions can frequently be reversed with no permanent effects.

Dementia

Dementia is a chronic form of OBS. It develops over an extended time, in contrast to acute OBS. When dementia occurs, the predominant characteristics are a gradual deterioration in a person's intellectual functioning; cognitive deficits slowly become evident. Most notable are decreases in ability to reason accurately, remember recent events, and use good social judgment. The patient remains fully oriented. Although delusions may occur, primarily of a paranoid nature, they are usually not as severe as those of the patient with the delirium form of acute OBS.

Other common symptom of dementia are changes in personality or an exaggeration of previously existing personality characteristics (Kaplan and Sadock, 1981; Solomon and Patch, 1974). For example, if the person had been thrifty in his buying habits he might become obsessed with finding the cheapest possible item or refuse to spend his money at all as the dementia progressed. Any type of new situation may be frightening to the patient because he is not able to process his observations accurately; he may feel overwhelmed by his helplessness. Marked anxiety ranging to panic levels may occur unless emotional support is available to relieve his fears. The term used for this type of overwhelming emotions is *catastrophic reaction* (Detre and Jarecki, 1971). Specific nursing interventions with both delirious and demented patients are presented in Chapter 16: Nursing Intervention With the Emotionally Complex Patient.

Causes of Organic Brain Sydrome

There are hundreds of possible causes of OBS. It would be impossible to try to remember each of these etiologies. Instead, a classification system devised by Richard Goldberg (1980) can help to simplify the list of conditions that may lead to brain dysfunction. He has made up a series of letters that can help you remember the possible causes of OBS. The mnemonic is MEND A MIND (*right*). The letters represent the etiologies listed. In this chapter each of these categories will be presented. Each category will include the most common conditions or disorders contained therein.

It is important to note that there are complex neurological changes as well as overt psychiatric symptoms present in OBS. You will find that *only* the psychiatric manifestations of each of the organic brain conditions are described in this chapter. The psychiatric changes are emphasized because the neurological changes are well described in most nursing and medical neurology

textbooks. The psychiatric symptoms are frequently not as well defined.

When a nurse knows what psychiatric changes to be aware of, his or her observations can make a critical difference in the data that the physician uses to make a diagnosis. Delay in determining the diagnosis results in extreme emotional discomfort and sharply increased physical risk to the patient. The increased physical risk has two causes. The first is the potential lethality of an undiagnosed underlying disease condition that is affecting the central nervous system. The second is the increased risk of injury to a delirious patient. He may either hurt himself by accidental injury or be injured as he is being restrained by caregivers.

Another consideration of the risks of OBS is the sequela of psychological discomfort related to the delirium episodes. Often, caregivers assume that the OBS patient will have no recollection of his terrors caused by hallucinations or delusions. In reality, many patients experience unpleasant aftereffects once the underlying cause is treated. Remember that, although these patients were delirious, an awareness of their thoughts, feelings, and surroundings during the delirious episodes is stored in their unconscious.

One of the emotional sequela that can occur is frightening nightmares related to the event(s). There also may be persisting fears. These puzzle the patient and his family because there is no conscious awareness of what caused them. These fears may include fear of the dark, fear of strangers, fear of hospitals, and so on. There also

---

Mend A Mind

M Metabolic disorder

E Electrical (convulsive) disorder

N Neoplastic disease

D Degenerative (chronic) brain disease

A Arterial (cerebrovascular) disease

M Mechanical disease (disease of the actual physical structures of the brain)

I Infectious disease

N Nutritional disease

D Drug toxicity

(Goldberg R: Psychiatry for the Primary Physician, 1st ed. Darien, CT, Patient Care Publications, 1980)

may be a vague awareness of an unpleasant event. This may have a mildly haunting quality to it.

One of the best ways to relieve these after-effects is to allow the patient to recall what happened after he has returned to his normal state. For example, you could say, "Mr. Smith, you've been very sick for the past few days. Do you remember anything that happened?" Because OBS is usually marked by a fluctuating mental status, there were periods when the patient was probably oriented. He will usually be able to remember some events. He may also recall some disturbing events. He may say, "I remember I saw bugs crawling all over my bed" or "I remember that I thought all of you were trying to capture me." If he remembers any disturbing thought or hallucination, ask him *how he felt at that time.* This is very important in releasing the unpleasant emotion that accompanied the event. Take your clues from what the patient is telling you and ask questions that allow him to express the negative feelings fully. You can then reassure him that his reactions (seeing bugs, having paranoid ideas, and so on) are very common when there is a physical crisis such as he had. It is the physical disease that caused his problems. This reassurance can bring tears of relief to the patient who has been silently suffering with fears that he may be crazy. The patient may also be afraid that it might happen again after he gets out of the hospital. You can tell him that unless all the conditions are duplicated (high fever, septic shock, or whatever his specific etiology was), it is highly unlikely. In addition, you can tell him that he may have dreams about what happened during his delirium or may remember aspects of it when he is awake. Unless they become more severe, they should go away in time. You can recommend that talking about feelings about these unpleasant events can help to relieve the unpleasant memories. If the memories are persistently troubling after discharge, suggest that the patient discuss them with his physician.

In the remainder of the chapter, many conditions will be described that are known to have the potential to change a person's mental status. The psychiatric symptoms that are presented with them, although sounding specific, can cover a broader range. Actually, the way in which a person responds to an organic change will vary depending on his premorbid personality style (Lishman, 1978). Accordingly, this guide should not be rigidly adhered to. It is written to introduce to you the many types of organic disease that can result in broad ranges of psychiatric dysfunctioning.

Categories of Organic Brain Syndrome

Metabolic

The metabolic etiology of OBS can include changes in endocrine gland functioning: the thyroid, parathyroid, adrenals, or Langerhans' islets (insulin-producing cells) in the pancreas and deficiencies in electrolyte blood levels (calcium, sodium, potassium, and base bicarbonate levels) (Lishman, 1978; Usdin and Lewis, 1979).

Endocrine Gland Disorders
The chart on p. 124 presents the most commonly occurring metabolic conditions caused by dysfunctions of the endocrine glands.

Electrolyte Imbalance
Another major metabolic cause of OBS is electrolyte imbalance. The chart on p. 125 includes a list of electrolytes, their normal laboratory values, and the psychiatric symptoms that occur when their level is either too high or too low (Freedman and colleagues, 1976; Kaplan and Sadock, 1981; Lishman, 1978; Solomon and Patch, 1974; Strub and Black, 1981).

It is important to be aware that sudden increases or decreases in these electrolytes are more likely to result in observable OBS symptoms than gradual, prolonged increases or decreases. Brain tissues are able to adapt gradually to slight changes that may eventually be surprisingly high or low after an extended period.

Electrical

The second major category of OBS etiologies is electrical disturbance, in which there is an excessive neuronal discharge within the brain (Brunner and Suddarth, 1975). The result is an epileptic seizure. Although there are four main classifications of seizures, only two are frequently accompanied by changes in psychiatric functioning: partial and generalized. In the partial seizure classification, there are two main types of seizure disorder. The categories, with their possible psychiatric effects, are presented in the chart on p. 126. Note that although mental status changes can and do occur in these conditions, their severity will depend on the patients' underlying personality

Mental Status Changes in Metabolic Conditions: Endocrine Gland Disorders

Name of Condition	Cause of Disorder	Changes in Mental Status*
Addison's disease (hypoadrenalism)	Deficiency in adrenocortical hormones of the adrenal cortex due to disturbed hypothalamic, pituitary, or adrenal functioning	Depression Negativism Suspiciousness Apathy
Cushing's syndrome (hyperadrenalism)	Excessive amounts of adrenocortical hormones of the adrenal cortex due to diseases of the hypothalamus or pituitary that produce excessive amounts of adrenocorticotropic hormone (ACTH) or to hyperplasia of the adrenal cortex; can also be caused by steroid drugs	Excitement Acute anxiety Emotional instability Depression (when disorder is result of internally caused elevated levels) Euphoria (when disorder is result of steroid drugs)
Hyperthyroidism	Excessive secretion of thyroid glands; basal metabolic rate is elevated	Nervousness Excitability Emotional instability Insomnia Psychosis (in acute stages)
Hypothyroidism (myxedema)	Deficiency of thyroid secretion; basal metabolic rate is decreased	Apathy Sluggishness Irritability Delusions and paranoid thinking (in acute stage) can sometimes persist for months afterward
Hyperparathyroidism	Excessive secretion of parathyroid glands results in increased levels of calcium and phosphorus	Mixed levels of anxiety and depression Weakness Irritability Psychosis
Hypoparathyroidism	Deficient parathyroid secretions	Apathy (if onset is rapid) Depression (if onset is slow) Psychosis
Hyperinsulinism	Adenoma of Langerhans' islets; excessive insulin in bloodsteam due to overdosage or undereating	Anxiety attacks Confusion Emotional lability
Pituitary problems of any kind, depending on etiology and course, can also cause psychiatric symptoms		Mixed, depending on etiology and course of the disease†

*Freedman and colleagues, 1976; Lishman, 1981; Kaplan and Sadock, 1981; Solomon and Patch, 1974.
†Pincus J: Personal communication, 1982.

style as well as on the severity of the electrical disturbance.

The majority of epileptics experience little or *no* emotional disturbance (Lishman, 1978). Epileptic disorder is a complex medical illness that requires the astute diagnostic ability of a neurologist. If emotional symptoms are present as well, the fine points of differential diagnosis should be evaluated by a psychiatrist. Psychiatric consultation will help to determine which aspects of the

Mental Status Changes of Metabolic Conditions: Electrolyte Imbalance

Name of Electrolyte	Normal Level	Abnormal Level	Cause	Changes in Mental Status
Calcium	8.5-10.5 mg/dl	+ Hyper- calcemia	Hyperparathyroidism	Loss of energy Depression Irritability
		− Hypo- calcemia	Hypoparathyroidism; deficiency of calcium or vitamin D in the diet	Psychosis in acute OBS caused by surgical removal of gland; nutritional deficiency results in less acute symptoms: ↓ concentration, ↓ intellectual functions, emotional lability, depression
Sodium	135-145 mEq/ liter	+ Hyper- natremia	Dehydration due to excessive water loss from body (vomiting, diarrhea) Diabetes insipidus Restricted fluid intake Excessive diuresis	Irritability Hyperactivity in intellectual ability Stupor
		− Hypo- natremia	Severe dietary restriction of sodium Addison's disease Excessive water consumption (polydipsia)	Depression Lethargy Withdrawal Anorexia
Phosphorus	2.6-4.5 mg/dl	− Hypophos- phatemia	Gram-negative septicemia Alcohol withdrawal Hyperalimentation Poor nutritional states	Apprehension Irritability Numbness Stupor
Potassium	3.5-5 mEq/ liter	+ Hyper- kalemia	Renal disease Potassium-sparing diuretics Level of potassium in intravenous fluids	Weakness Dysphasia
		− Hypo- kalemia	Renal disease Cushing's syndrome Loss of potassium due to diuretics Self-induced vomiting Gastroenteritis	Changes in mood and personality Tearfulness Hopelessness Helplessness

(continued)

Mental Status Changes of Metabolic Conditions: Electrolyte Imbalance (continued)

Name of Electrolyte	Normal Level	Abnormal Level	Cause	Changes in Mental Status
Base bicarbonate	Blood pH 7.38–7.42, bicarbonate level 24 mEq/liter	+Alkalosis	Prolonged vomiting Taking large amounts of sodium bicarbonate Hyperventilation	↓ Intellectual functioning Apathy Delirium Stupor
		− Acidosis	Severe respiratory illness: emphysema, status asthmaticus Renal failure Diabetes mellitus with ketosis	↓ Intellectual ability Drowsiness Confusion Delirium

psychiatric symptoms are due to the physiological dysfunction and which are caused by a separate but concurrent functional psychiatric disorder.

Neoplastic (Benign or Malignant Tumors)

Any neoplasm within the brain, benign or malignant, can produce psychiatric symptoms. At least half of all patients with primary sites of brain neoplasms demonstrate changes in psychological functioning. In addition to tumors that originate within the brain, the brain is also a common site of metastasis from other body sites. The tumors that most commonly metastasize are those from the lungs, breast, gastrointestinal tract, prostate, and pancreas. The most frequent type of metastasis to the brain originates from the lungs (Lishman,

Mental Status Changes in Different Types of Epilepsy

Type of Seizure	Change in Mental Status
Simple partial (no loss of consciousness)	Perceptual hallucinations Dizziness Nonsensical speech (Brunner and Suddarth, 1975)
Complex partial (temporary loss of consciousness)	Catatonia or Inappropriate movement Emotions of fear, anger, elation, or irritability No memory of seizure (Brunner and Suddarth, 1975)
Generalized seizures	↑ Irritability before seizure May be ↑ aggressive or emotional before seizure Confusion after seizure May demonstrate no confusion but may have transient episode of schizophrenialike symptoms of psychotic affect, disturbances in thinking, or perceptual distortion (Freedman and colleagues, 1976; Lishman, 1978; Solomon and Patch, 1974)

1978). In some instances, the psychiatric symptoms may appear before the existence of the primary cancer is known. Various psychiatric syndromes can occur. Depending on the location, size, and type of the tumor, dementia, delirium, or progressive changes in personality can be observed.* The major reason for the changes in psychiatric function is the increase in intracranial pressure, which applies pressure to all the brain structures.

Loss of ability to interpret sensory perceptions of vision, hearing, and so on (*agnosia*) and loss of ability to perform complex tasks or loss of motor control of all or specific parts of the body (*apraxia*) may occur.

In addition to intracranial tumors, psychiatric symptoms have been closely associated with another type of neoplasm, pheochromocytoma. *Pheochromocytoma* is a tumor of the adrenal medulla that, in most cases, is benign and can be treated (Thomas, 1973). The tumor releases increased levels of epinephrine. If you can recall your own mental status the last time you were *severely* stressed and adrenaline (epinephrine) was flowing in sharply increased levels in your bloodstream, you can understand the potential effects of this illness. The most predominant symptom of this patient is a high level of anxiety, with episodic anxiety or "panic" attacks (Usdin and Lewis, 1979).

Another neoplastic illness with a high incidence of associated psychiatric symptoms is pancreatic carcinoma. Patients with this illness frequently become despondent and apathetic. Their mental state is that of a very depressed person (Usdin and Lewis, 1979).

Degenerative

The next category of organic brain syndrome includes diseases that lead to deterioration of the tissues of the brain. The diseases included in this category and the type of neurological deterioration that occurs are as follows (Strub and Black, 1981):

Multiple sclerosis	Widespread destruction of myelin in the sheath of nerve fibers
Systemic lupus erythematosus	Antibodies attack neurons; cerebral vasculitis
Alzheimer's disease	Premature degeneration of neurons

*DeBell P: Personal communication, 1982.

Huntington's chorea	Frontal lobe atrophy
Creutzfeldt-Jakob disease	Motor neuron involvement; cerebellar, pyramidal tract damage

These diseases are accompanied by marked changes in neurological status and, depending on the illness, gradual to marked changes in psychological functioning. Creutzfeldt-Jakob disease is suspected to be transmittable (Lishman, 1978).

For a full description of the pathological process, as well as accompanying neurological symptoms of each of these conditions, refer to any standard neurology textbook. The chart on p. 128 presents the psychiatric symptoms that are commonly seen as these illnesses progress.

Arterial

The type of mental status symptoms that develop as the result of failure of blood supply to the brain depend on the disease process that causes the normal blood supply to be changed. For example, depending on the location and extent of the disease process, there can be a continuum of mental status changes ranging from no changes in mental functioning to unconsciousness.

Cerebrovascular Accident

Cerebrovascular accidents (CVAs) are the third most common cause of death in the Western hemisphere (Lishman, 1978). CVAs are caused by atherosclerosis or hypertension that ultimately results in either infarction or hemorrhage. Infarction outnumbers hemorrhage 3:1.

Thrombosis, caused by the atherosclerotic process, is the most common cause of obstruction to the cerebral arteries that eventually results in CVA. In a CVA there is a loss of blood supply to particular regions of the brain. It is usually the specific region affected and the functions it performs that determine the range of psychiatric symptoms observed. The mental status symptoms that accompany the profound neurological symptoms fall within both the delirium and dementia categories. There can be fluctuating mental confusion and visual hallucinations or mental slowing, permanent personality changes, and other symptoms of dementia caused by permanent changes in the structures of the brain. Characteristics common in some stroke patients are emotional lability and hostility. Such patients can demonstrate mild paranoia, as well as aggressiveness in the face of

Mental Status Changes of Degenerative Brain Diseases

Multiple Sclerosis

Age of onset: 20-40 years

Incidence: 50:100,000 (more common in women)

Prognosis: long course; early symptoms may cause diagnostic confusion

Changes in Mental Status

Changes in mental status occur in 50% of patients; personality changes include lability, euphoria, ↓ intellectual ability progressive to gross mental deterioration (Kaplan and Sadock, 1981)

Systemic Lupus Erythematosus

Age of onset: 20-40 years

Incidence: women 8:1

Prognosis: long course; early symptoms may cause diagnostic confusion

Changes in Mental Status

Changes in mental status occur in 15% to 50% of patients; varied changes possible; thought disorder, depression, confusion (Kaplan and Sadock, 1981)

Alzheimer's Disease

Age of onset: 40-60 years

Incidence: 2 or 3:1 (women:men)

Prognosis: death within 2-5 years

Changes in Mental Status

First phase (lasts 2-3 years): ↓memory, ↓general functioning, ↓emotional stability

Second phase (lasts approximately 1 year): ↓intellectual ability, personality deterioration, dysphasia, apraxia, agnosia, acalculia, symptoms of Parkinson's disease (gait and muscular changes)

Third phase (lasts approximately 6 months): profound dementia, grand mal seizures, delusions and hallucinations (Kaplan and Sadock, 1981; Lishman, 1978)

Huntington's Chorea

Age of onset: 25-50 years

Incidence: 6:100,000

Prognosis: death within 10-20 years

Changes in Mental Status

Initial phase: involuntary movements, changes in personality: quarrelsome or apathetic, paranoid, anxious, depressed

Later phase: dementia, ↓intellectual ability (memory may be impaired), psychotic episodes (Kaplan and Sadock, 1981; Lishman, 1978)

Creutzfeldt–Jakob Disease

Age of onset: 40-50 years

Incidence: 1:1 (women:men)

Prognosis: death within 9 months-2 years

Changes in Mental Status

Early phase: fatigue, insomnia, anxiety, depression, mental slowness, unpredictable behavior, slowly developing ↓memory and ↓concentration

Later phase: ↓intellectual ability, uncontrollable laughing or crying, clouding of consciousness or delirium, auditory hallucinations or delusions, eventual profound dementia (Kaplan and Sadock, 1981; Lishman, 1978)

new experiences, new medical regimens, and so on. Approximately half the patients with sub-arachnoid hemorrhage show mental status changes, including mental confusion, loss of drive, irritability, and anxiety (Storey, 1970).

Degenerative Changes of Cerebral Arteries

A second category is the chronic, gradual changing of mental functioning caused by degenerative changes of cerebral arteries. This category includes those persons with cerebral arteriosclerosis or "hardening of the arteries." They have no history of CVA but demonstrate chronic changes in mental functioning, typically during the seventh and eighth decades of life but sometimes as early as the sixth decade. The changes in mental status are those of a senile dementia, including increasing loss of memory regarding recent events, poor social judgment, decreases in general intellectual ability, and anxiety in new social situations.

Multiple Infarct Dementia

The third category, multiple infarct dementia, is usually caused by hypertension. The mental status changes are similar to those of degenerative cerebral arteriosclerosis described above.*

Mechanical

Head trauma, subdural hematoma, and normal-pressure hydrocephalus fall within the mechanical OBS category. In these conditions, a force or pressure exerted on the brain results in changes in the patient's psychiatric functioning.

Head Injury

The most common aftereffect of moderate to severe head injuries is loss of consciousness and amnesia about the accidental event. The cause of these two phenomena is possibly related to the rapidly accelerating or decelerating brain tissue that impacts on the inside of the cranium during the accident (Russell and Schiller, 1949; Lishman, 1978).

A head injury results in structural changes as well as major changes in neurological functioning caused by differences in the circulatory, electrical, and biochemical functions of the brain. It has been suggested that the shock of the injury produces a sudden and very great neuronal discharge at the moment of injury, resulting in the release of large

amounts of acetylcholine into the cerebrospinal fluid (CSF). The CSF normally does not contain acetylcholine. It may continue to be present for days or weeks. It usually is present in proportion to the changes in brain electrical status as measured by electroencephalograph (EEG). This neuro-transmitter is also found in proportion to the degree of change in level of consciousness. As the level of acetylcholine in the patient's CSF decreases, his overall mental and physical status usually improves (Lishman, 1978).

Following head injury, the patient may be unconscious for several hours yet recover spontaneously with no ill effect. Generally speaking, prolonged coma of 1 or several days is the result of more serious injury to brain tissues. (See Chap. 10 for ways to identify the level of consciousness of the patient with an acute head injury.) Mild to severe cognitive, behavioral, or physical deficits may be permanent when unconsciousness lasts more than a month (Lishman, 1978). Cases do occur, however, in which people regain consciousness after a prolonged period and progressively return to their previous level of functioning.

No matter what part of the brain receives a direct blow or what causes the injury, the life-threatening aspect of head injury is caused by the resulting stress on the brain stem. The brain stem contains the life-supportive centers of respiration, cardiac rate, and blood pressure regulation as well as the reflexes of swallowing and of the iris. (It is the iris that contracts in response to light and regulates the size of the pupil.)

The acute psychiatric effects of head injury are loss of consciousness and amnesia about the accident as well as loss of memory about events following the accident. In mild to moderate head injury, the cognitive functions of the ego, such as reasoning, problem solving and judgment, are affected. It is not unusual for perceptual disturbances to occur in the form of decreased spatial relationship perception in milder forms. Another outcome of this sudden change in ego functioning is a decrease in the ability of the ego to control emotion. Increases in the range of emotion normally experienced are due, I believe, to a decrease in ego defensive capability. As a result of these changes, the patient may experience mild to severe episodes of anxiety. Panic episodes may also occur.

These changes in psychiatric functioning may last anywhere from 4 weeks to 6 months or longer, depending on the severity of the blow to the head. Exaggeration of preinjury personality characteristics can also occur. Recent memory is frequently

*DeBell P: Personal communication, 1982.

impaired. Confabulation to cover up the memory deficits is another potential outcome. In severe head injury, mental status changes can include coma, delusions, hallucinations, and marked disorientation to time, person, and place. These changes are caused by physical stresses on the brain structures from the accident. This type of OBS can be further complicated by biochemical, circulatory, infectious, or other sequelae of the injury.

In addition to the acute effects of head injury, patients with complex head injuries may experience chronic psychiatric dysfunction after they are discharged from the hospital. If the psychiatric dysfunction is specifically related to the accident, rather than a preexisting personality disorder, the patient may be depressed, experience high levels of anxiety, or become phobic. Some patients also demonstrate mild to marked permanent changes in personality or in cognitive functions (Lishman, 1978). There is a low tolerance for effects of alcohol consumption for a few weeks to many months.

Subdural Hematoma

Subdural hematoma may or may not be present in the patient admitted for acute head trauma. If it is an acute phenomenon accompanying a head injury, then the psychiatric changes viewed in the patient will be similar to those in the previous section on head injury. The discussion of subdural hematoma in this section will be limited to the psychiatric effects of subdural hematomas that are undiagnosed at the time of injury and develop slowly and are not diagnosed for weeks or months. This type of chronic subdural hematoma is most commonly seen in the elderly patient who does not remember the precipitating fall or head injury.

The symptoms of chronic subdural hematoma usually begin with a vague headache. There may be mental slowness characterized by poor concentration and lethargy. This gradually progresses to fluctuating levels of consciousness, that is, changes from wakefulness to drowsiness that may occur as often as every 1 or 2 hours. Without medical attention the patient will eventually lapse into a coma. Because of chronic and slow progression, the patient with subdural hematoma may be mistakenly diagnosed as having senile dementia (Lishman, 1978). Brain scan examination is an important diagnostic aid in differentiating between the two conditions.

Normal-Pressure Hydrocephalus

Normal-pressure hydrocephalus (NPH) is a condition that has been recognized only during the last two decades. The complex and sophisticated diagnostic screening advances developed during that time have helped to diagnose and treat this brain condition, which can sometimes be reversed if an early diagnosis is made. Hydrocephalus is a condition in which the ventricles of the brain enlarge because of increased amounts of CSF. It differs from other forms of hydrocephalus because there is no increase in spinal fluid pressure (Thomas, 1973).

The symptoms of NPH can be confused with those of senile dementia. Again, brain scanning will help to differentiate the two conditions. The specific symptoms of NPH are ataxia (abnormal gait), urinary incontinence, and dementia. The dementia associated with NPH includes symptoms of depression, agitation, changes in organization of thoughts, and forgetfulness (Gilroy and Meyer, 1975; Lishman, 1978; Murray, 1978). With early diagnosis and surgical treatment, the prognosis for the patient with NPH is excellent (Gilroy and Meyer, 1975).

Infections

Several infectious diseases of the brain can result in psychiatric changes. They are encephalitis, meningitis, cerebral abscess, and the late stage of syphilis.

Encephalitis

Encephalitis means inflammation of the brain. It can occur as a complication of viral diseases such as mumps, infectious hepatitis, herpes zoster and simplex, and rabies. It can also develop as a result of a further inflammatory reaction to brain abscess or meningitis. In addition to the physical symptoms of central nervous system (CNS) disease, the psychiatric symptoms include changes in level of consciousness. Seizures or delirium or both may also occur, depending on the type of encephalitis. The delirium symptoms can include general confusion and disorientation, hallucinations, or delusions.

After the acute phase is over, there usually is a prolonged recovery period of several months. If the patient is a child, it is not uncommon, especially in boys, for there to be personality changes and behavioral problems (Greenbaum and Lurie, 1948). Studies of children after recovery from infectious brain disease have shown that there usually is no change in intellect, but there are problems of impulsiveness, restlessness, poor concentration, and antisocial behavior (Greenbaum and Lurie, 1948). These symptoms are similar to the personality changes noted with electrical disturbances in the brain (Kaplan and Sadock, 1981).

Meningitis

Meningitis is an infectious disease of the meninges, the three layers of membranes that surround the brain and the spinal cord. There are three different etiologies of meningitis: pyogenic, with meningococcal and pneumococcal causative organisms predominating; aseptic, which is usually caused by a virus; and tubercular, which is caused by the tubercle bacillus.

Pyogenic meningitis has a rapid onset with high temperature, severe stiffness of the neck, and CNS symptoms. In addition, the psychiatric disturbance is that of an acute delirious brain reaction. There is a change in consciousness, and coma may occur. Disorientation, excitability, and hallucinations may also be present. Following treatment, psychiatric sequelae such as depression and low energy level may last for several months in adults. Permanent changes in intellectual functioning or in personality are rare. Usually people recover with no complications (Lishman, 1978).

Aseptic meningitis is the mildest form of meningitis. The patient displays symptoms similar to those of pyogenic meningitis. The course of the illness is usually rapid, and there are no negative psychiatric effects.

Tuberculous meningitis is the most severe form of meningitis. Its symptoms differ from those of the other two forms of meningitis; accordingly, the diagnosis may be delayed. The physical symptoms may develop over a 2- to 3-week period. There is vague malaise and a low-grade temperature. There may be no neck stiffness at the onset, and then it may develop slightly. Mild psychiatric symptoms are usually present at the beginning of the illness. These include poor attention and minor memory deficits. Gradually, changes in consciousness occur and drowsiness becomes prominent. Disorientation may proceed into frank organic psychosis. With delirium, the patient may be terror stricken by hallucinations or delusions.

Once the acute phase is over and the disease is treated, there are usually no consistent personality changes other than amnesia, which may improve slowly over several months (Lishman, 1978).

Cerebral Abscess

The most common presenting symptom of a brain abscess is a change in mental status (Gates and Kernohan, 1950). It is rare for a brain abscess to develop as a primary lesion. Usually it is preceded by infection elsewhere in the body; frequently this infection is in the ears or the facial sinuses. Another cause is a penetrating head injury. The onset of symptoms may occur immediately or may be delayed if the abscess is dormant.

An abscess in the frontal lobe will produce more pronounced psychiatric symptoms than one in the temporal or occipital lobe. Frontal lobe symptoms include a decrease in concentration and memory as well as obvious changes in personality. If the development of the abscess is slow, regardless of the site of infection, mild delirium may be present. There also can be general changes in neurovegetative functioning. These include low energy level and loss of appetite. Depression and irritability may also be included in the clinical findings.

The prognosis regarding psychiatric complications after the acute stage depends on the extent of the infectious process and the time before diagnosis occurred as well as the duration of the acute stage.

Syphilis

Because of public information programs and the availability of penicillin, cases of syphilis in the Western world rarely advance to the later stages. Psychiatric complications can be severe during the third and last stages of syphilis. There are three different ways that syphilitic CNS involvement can occur: meningitic disease, tabes dorsalis, and general paresis. The meningitic form takes approximately 1 to 5 years to develop. The psychiatric symptoms begin in a mild form and gradually worsen. They are intellectual slowness, poor concentration, failing memory, dementia, and occasional psychotic episodes.

General paresis is a form of syphilis in which the syphilis spirochetes actually invade the brain tissue. With general paresis the mental status changes of meningitic syphilis are present. In addition, marked changes in temperament and personality occur. Poor social judgment, mania, depression, or schizophrenialike symptoms may dominate the personality. If treatment is begun early in the clinical course, it is possible to reverse the disease process and restore the person to a more acceptable level of physical and mental health (Lishman, 1978).

Tabes dorsalis is another form of syphilitic disease that occurs in approximately 20% of cases of general paresis. It may not occur until 8 to 12 years after the primary infection. It results in severe neurological disease but rarely causes mental status changes. Severe depression has been reported in some cases of tabes dorsalis.

The depression could also be the result of the severe physical disabilities that the syphilitic victim experiences.

Nutritional

Under the heading of nutrition are included many types of vitamin deficiencies. The vitamins that are most important in promoting psychological well-being are those of the B complex. These vitamins are essential to adequate brain metabolism and are also involved in the brain neurotransmitter process. The mental effects of B vitamin deficiencies will appear before physical manifestations of malnutrition. The symptoms include fatigue, weakness, and emotional disturbances.

Vitamin B$_{12}$

The vitamin implicated in pernicious anemia is B$_{12}$. People with pernicious anemia cannot absorb vitamin B$_{12}$ into the stomach. Such patients are known to have an increased incidence of mental disorder in as high as 64% of the cases (Geaga and Amanth, 1975). Included in the mental status changes are depression and lethargy progressing to confusion, paranoid delusions, and schizophrenialike psychotic symptoms. (It is noteworthy that gastrectomy patients are at risk for pernicious anemia.)

Folic Acid

A common result of malnutrition is folate deficiency due to inadequate intake of folic acid. The psychiatric manifestations of this B vitamin deficiency are depression, progressive dementia, or epilepsy. It is noteworthy that studies of patients in homes for the elderly and in psychiatric institutions frequently find that the folic acid levels of the elderly patients are subnormal (Carney, 1967; Carney and Sheffield, 1970; Reynolds and associates, 1970). When the folic acid level returns to normal after treatment, it may take several months for the patient's mental status to return to normal (Lishman, 1978).

Nicotinic Acid

A deficiency in nicotinic acid is the cause of pellegra. The initial mental changes of pellegra are weakness, nervousness, and memory disorder. There are swings in mood, and emotional instability is common. Serious depression usually accompanies the illness. As the deficiency progresses, dementia occurs; confabulation to cover the mental deficits is common. In the later untreated stages organic psychosis and delirium of a hallucinatory or delusional type occurs. Nicotinic acid restores the patient to normal functioning very rapidly (Lishman, 1978).

Thiamine

Thiamine deficiency results in Wernicke's encephalopathy. It is commonly seen in patients with chronic alcoholism but may occur in those with carcinomas of the digestive tract, toxemia, or tuberculosis. The mental effects of this syndrome are general disorientation and confusion. Replacement of thiamine in these patients may improve their mental status but does not change the often terminal underlying illness.

Beriberi is another disease caused by thiamine deficiency. Patients present with psychiatric symptoms similar to those of Wernicke's encephalopathy. The condition can be reversed with thiamine replacement.

Drugs

This category includes toxic reactions to drugs or substances that cause changes in normal brain functioning. These include alcohol, hallucinogens, heavy metals, and prescribed medications such as CNS depressants, digitalis, quinidine, and steroids. Actually, any drug can be suspected of causing an OBS. Drugs and substances are metabolized differently by each person (Pincus and Tucker, 1974).

Alcohol

Alcohol can cause OBS in several ways. The most commonly recognized is the immediate effect of excessive alcohol intake, in which the drunk person may develop poor social judgment, excitability, and mild disorientation. When alcohol abuse is chronic and addiction occurs, the withdrawal from alcohol results in the hallucinations and seizures of delirium tremens. The specific symptoms of alcohol withdrawal are presented in Chapter 16: Nursing Intervention With the Emotionally Complex Patient in the section about the alcoholic patient. When alcoholism is chronic, there are nutritional deficiencies that result in Wernicke's encephalopathy (see section on thiamine deficiency earlier in this chapter). Korsakoff's syndrome is another alcohol-related OBS, and patients with it display prominent psychiatric symptoms of delirium. They include disorientation, insomnia, hallucinations, delusions, and incoherent muttering (Thomas, 1973). Liver disease is a physiological sequela of alcoholism and contributes toward the development of OBS because of the progressive inability of the liver to metabolize toxins. In addition, there can be brain degeneration because of the excessive exposure of brain cells to alcohol.

Hallucinogens

Many hallucinogenic drugs are available for illegal sale in the United States. Generally speaking, the population has become more wary of these substances because of massive information campaigns warning of long-term ill effects from using them. One of the most commonly used hallucinogenic drugs during the last decade was lysergic acid diethylamide (LSD-25).

LSD causes a wide variety of mental status changes. Large doses produce vivid hallucinatory experiences and marked changes in perception and body image. There is an accompanying strong sense of unreality. Unlike other OBS conditions, there usually is no change in intellectual functioning. This allows the person to maintain an awareness of the marked unreality. This awareness can lead to strong anxiety and panic in people who are unprepared for the severe perceptual distortions that can occur (Lishman, 1978). After the acute reaction is over, there can be unexpected psychiatric aftereffects of the drug. These include acute depressive reactions, hallucinations, overwhelming nightmares, and a schizophrenialike mental state.

Heavy Metals

In the Western world, the most common cause of OBS caused by heavy metals is related to occupational exposure. The metals that may cause problems are lead, mercury, manganese, and arsenic. People employed in chemical plants, the photoengraving industry, ore refining, steel or battery manufacture, electrowelding, insecticide production, the glass-making industry, and lawn care products factories are at risk for heavy metal poisoning (Lishman, 1978). Children, especially those in surroundings where there is old furniture painted with a lead-based paint (no longer manufactured), are also at risk for lead poisoning by ingestion from chewing.

Prescribed Medications

A detailed description of the types of psychiatric symptoms that can be drug induced could fill a volume. Most prescription and over-the-counter drugs can have psychiatric side-effects. As discussed above, people metabolize drugs in different ways. Psychiatric side-effects are surprisingly common with many drugs. It is very important for nurses to be aware of the possible negative psychiatric effects of drugs because of their liability in administering them to patients as well as the need to observe for negative side-effects.

The most notable changes in mental status are found with steroids, belladona derivatives, bromides, digitalis preparations, and all CNS depressants. In addition, there are hundreds of reports of negative psychiatric effects of commonly prescribed drugs used for medical, surgical, and obstetrical conditions. Table 11-1 lists commonly prescribed medications and the mental status changes they can cause.

Another medication-related phenomenon that can cause toxic side-effects is called *synergism*. Synergism is the action of two or more drugs that, when taken together, produce a total effect that is stronger than if either was taken alone. The synergistic effects of even low doses of medication can produce either a delirium or dementia type of OBS. Nurses who work with patients with chronic illness or the elderly are likely to see patients with this type of encephalopathy.

Prevalent Types of Organic Brain Syndrome

Postoperative

A phenomenon that has not been well described in the medical literature but has been reported nonempirically by many people after all types of general surgery is a *subtle* but changed mental status that can last up to 6 weeks. The cause of this changed mental functioning can possibly be attributed to the medications and drugs administered during the immediate preoperative and postoperative periods as well as during the intraoperative period itself.

Most people who undergo surgery are not accustomed to medications that have psychotropic alteration potential. The surgical patient's pharmacological regimen usually includes preoperative and intraoperative tranquilizing agents, curarelike paralyzing medications, general anesthetic, around-the-clock postoperative narcotics, and sedation at bedtime. Although the time of exposure to these drugs may only last a few days, it is important to remember that they are not normally present in the brain. Accordingly, brain tissues respond to a change in their normal homeostasis.

(Text continues on p. 137.)

Table 11-1.
Some Drugs That Cause Psychiatric Symptoms

Drug	Reaction	Comments*
Amantadine (Symmetrel)	Visual hallucinations, nightmares	Occasional; more frequent in elderly[1]
Aminocaproic acid (Amicar)	Acute delirium, with auditory, visual and kinesthetic hallucinations	Immediately following bolus injection[2]
Amitriptyline (Elavil; others)	Anticholinergic psychosis	See Atropine
Amphetamines	See Dextroamphetamine	
Amphotericin B (Fungizone)	Delirium	IV and intrathecal use[3]
Anticonvulsants	Tactile, visual and auditory hallucinations, delirium, agitation, depression, paranoia, confusion, aggression	Usually with high doses or high plasma concentrations[4]
Antihistamines	Anxiety, hallucinations, delirium	Especially with overdosage
Asparaginase (Elspar)	Confusion, depression, paranoia, bizarre behavior	Occur frequently in some studies[5,6]
Atropine and anticholinergics	Confusion, memory loss, disorientation, depersonalization, delirium, auditory and visual hallucinations, fear, paranoia	More frequent in elderly and children and with high doses[7]
	Sudden incoherent speech, delirium with high fever, flushed, dry skin, visual and tactile hallucinations	From eye drops, with high or repeated doses, and particularly when confusion with nose drops leads to overdosage[7]
Baclofen (Lioresal)	Visual and auditory hallucinations, paranoia, insomnia, nightmares, mania, depression, anxiety, confusion	Sometimes with treatment, but usually after sudden withdrawal[8]
Barbiturates	See Phenobarbital	
Belladonna alkaloids	See Atropine	
Benztropine (Cogentin)	See Atropine	
Bromocriptine (Parlodel)	Mania, delusions, visual hallucinations, paranoia, aggressive behavior	Occasional, not dose-related;[9] symptoms may persist 6 weeks after stopping the drug[10]
Chlordiazepoxide (Librium)	Probably same as diazepam	
Chloroquine (Aralen)	Confusion, agitation, violence, personality change, delusions, hallucinations	Several cases, one within 2 hours of single 1-g dose[11]
Cimetidine (Tagamet)	Visual and auditory hallucinations, paranoia, bizarre speech, confusion, delirium, disorientation, depression	Many reports; usually with high dosage, more frequent in elderly and with renal dysfunction[12]
Clonazepam (Clonopin)	Probably same as diazepam	
Clorazepate (Azene; Tranxene)	Probably same as diazepam	
Contraceptives, oral	Depression	15% in one study[13]
Corticosteroids (prednisone, cortisone, ACTH; others)	Mania, depression, confusion, paranoia, visual and auditory hallucinations, catatonia	More common with high dosage or rapid increase but can also occur with low doses for short periods[14]
Cyclopentolate (Cyclogyl)	See Atropine	Eye drops
Cycloserine (Seromycin)	Anxiety, depression, confusion, disorientation, hallucinations, paranoia	Common
Dapsone (Avlosulfon)	Insomnia, irritability, uncoordinated speech, agitation, acute psychosis	Occasional, even with low doses[15]
Desipramine (Pertofrane)	Anticholinergic psychosis	See Atropine
Dextroamphetamine	Bizarre behavior, hallucinations, paranoia	Usually with overdose or abuse[16] but can occur with lower doses
	Depression	On withdrawal
Diazepam (Valium)	Rage, excitement, hallucinations, depression, suicidal thoughts	Can occur with usual doses; depression and hallucinations can occur on withdrawal[17]

*Frequency is unknown with many drugs; adverse effects are usually underreported.

Table 11-1.
Some Drugs That Cause Psychiatric Symptoms *(continued)*

Drug	Reaction	Comments*
Diethylpropion (Tenuate)	See Dextroamphetamine	
Digitalis glycosides	Nightmares, euphoria, confusion, delusions, amnesia, belligerence, visual hallucinations, paranoia	Usually with excessive dosage or high plasma concentrations; more frequent in elderly.[18]
Disopyramide (Norpace)	Agitation, depression, paranoia, auditory and visual hallucinations, panic	3 patients, within 24-48 hours after starting treatment[19]
Disulfiram (Antabuse)	Delirium, depression, paranoia, auditory hallucinations	Not related to alcohol reactions[20]
Doxepin (Adapin; Sinequan)	Anticholinergic psychosis	See Atropine
Ephedrine	Hallucinations, paranoia	Excessive dosage[21]
Ethchlorvynol (Placidyl)	Agitation, confusion, disorientation, hallucinations, paranoia	Continued use or on withdrawal[22]
Ethosuximide (Zarontin)	See Anticonvulsants	
Fenfluramine (Pondimin)	See Dextroamphetamine	
Halothane (Fluothane)	Depression	Postoperative period[23]
Imipramine (Tofranil; others)	Anticholinergic psychosis	See Atropine
Indomethacin (Indocin)	Depression, confusion, hallucinations, anxiety, hostility, paranoia, depersonalization	Especially in elderly[24]
Isoniazid (INH; others)	Depression, agitation, auditory and visual hallucinations, paranoia	Several reports[25]
Ketamine (Ketalar; Ketaject)	Nightmares, hallucinations, crying, delirium, changes in body image	Frequent with usual doses[26]
Levodopa (Dopar; others)	Delirium, depression, agitation, hypomania, nightmares, night terrors, visual and auditory hallucinations, paranoia	More frequent in elderly; risk increases with prolonged use[27]
Lidocaine (Xylocaine)	Disorientation	
Methamphetamine	See Dextroamphetamine	
Methyldopa (Aldomet)	Depression, hallucinations, paranoia, amnesia	Several reports[28]
Methylphenidate (Ritalin)	Hallucinations	In children[29]
Methysergide (Sansert)	Depersonalization, hallucinations	Occasional[30]
Metrizamide (Amipaque)	Confusion, disorientation, hallucinations, depression	Can occur frequently[31]
Nalidixic acid (NegGram)	Confusion, depression, excitement, visual hallucinations	Rare
Niridazolle (Ambilhar)	Confusion, hallucinations, mania, suicide	More likely with higher doses[32]
Nortriptyline (Aventyl)	Anticholinergic psychosis	See Atropine
Pentazocine (Talwin)	Nightmares, hallucinations, disorientation, panic, paranoia, depersonalization, depression	During treatment[33]
Phenelzine (Nardil)	Paranoia, delusions, fear, mania, rage, aggressive behavior	Symptoms may resolve quickly after drug is stopped[34]
Phenmetrazine (Preludin)	See Dextroamphetamine	
Phenobarbital	Excitement, hyperactivity, visual hallucinations, depression, delirium-tremens-like syndrome	On withdrawal, or with usual doses in some children and the elderly, or with overdosage in epilepsy
Phentermine (Fastin; others)	See Dextroamphetamine	

*Frequency is unknown with many drugs; adverse effects are usually underreported.
(continued)

Table 11-1.
Some Drugs That Cause Psychiatric Symptoms *(continued)*

Drug	Reaction	Comments*
Phenylephrine (Neo-Synephrine)	Depression, visual and tactile hallucinations, paranoia	Overuse of nasal spray[35]
Phenytoin (Dilantin; others)	See Anticonvulsants	
Primidone (Mysoline)	See Anticonvulsants	
Procainamide (Pronestyl)	Paranoia, hallucinations	Uncommon[36]
Procaine Penicillin G	Terror, hallucinations, disorientation, agitation, bizarre behavior	Probably due to procaine; occurs occasionally; 33 patients in 1 report[37]
Propoxyphene (Darvon)	Auditory hallucinations, confusion	Usually with high doses[38]
Propranolol (Inderal)	Depression, confusion, nightmares, visual and auditory hallucinations, paranoia	Several reports, with usual doses and after dosage increase[39]
Protriptyline (Vivactil)	Anticholinergic psychosis	See Atropine
Quinacrine (Atabrine)	Bizarre dreams, anxiety, hallucinations, delirium	Can occur with usual doses but more common with high doses[40]
Rauwolfia alkaloids (reserpine—Serpasil, others; rauwolfia—Raudixin, others)	Depression	Occurs commonly with doses higher than 0.5 mg daily; may continue for months after drug is stopped[41]
Scopolamine (Hyoscine)	See Atropine	
Sulindac (Clinoril)	Paranoia, rage, personality change	Reported in 5 patients[42]
Thiabendazole (Mintezol)	Hallucinations	Occasional
Tricyclic antidepressants	Anticholinergic psychosis	See Atropine
Trihexyphenidyl (Artane)	See Atropine	
Trimipramine (Surmontil)	Anticholinergic psychosis	See Atropine
Vinblastine (Velban)	Depression	Occasionally
Vincristine (Oncovin)	Hallucinations	Less than 5% of patients; high doses[43]

*Frequency is unknown with many drugs; adverse effects are usually underreported.

1. Borison RL. Am J Psychiatry 136:111, 1979: Harper RW, Knothe BUC. Med J Austr 1:444, 1973
2. Wysenbeek AJ et al. Clin Toxicol 14:93, 1979
3. Winn RE et al. Arch Intern Med 139:706, 1979
4. Franks RD, Richter AJ. Am J Psychiatry 136:973, 1979; Tollefson G. J Clin Psychiatry 41:295, 1980; Woodbury DM et al (eds): Antiepileptic Drugs, pp 219, 377, 449, New York, Raven Press, 1972; Stores G. Dev Med Child Neurol 17:647, 1975
5. Carbone PP et al. Recent Results Cancer Res 33:236, 1970
6. Moure JMB et al. Arch Neurol 23:365, 1970
7. Greenblatt DJ, Shader RI. N Engl J Med 288:1215, 1973; Adcock EW III. J Pediatr 79:127, 1971
8. Skausig OB, Korsgaard S. Lancet 1:1258, 1977; Lees AJ et al. Lancet 1:858, 1977; Jones RF, Lance JW, Med J Austr 1:654, 1976; Arnold ES et al. Am J Psychiatry 137:1466, 1980
9. Vlissides DN et al. Br Med J 1:510, 1978; Parkes D. N Engl J Med 302:1479, 1980
10. Caine DB et al. Lancet 1:735, 1978
11. Torrey EF. JAMA 204:867, 1968; Bomb BS, et al. Trans R Soc Trop Med Hyg 69:523, 1975
12. Adler LE et al. Am J Psychiatry 137:1112, 1980; Barnhart CC, Bowden CL. Am J Psychiatry 136:725, 1979: Arneson GA. Am J Psychiatry 136:1348, 1979; Flind AC, Rowley-Jones D. Lancet 1:379, 1979; Agarwal SK, JAMA 240:214, 1978; Nouel O et al. Gastroenterology 79:780, 1980; Jefferson JW. Am J Psychiatry 136:346, 1979; Basavaraju NG et al. NY State J Med 80:1287, 1980; Beraud J-J et al. Nouv Presse Med 7:2570, 1978
13. Leeton J. Aust NZ J Obstet Gynaecol 13:115, 1973
14. Sullivan BJ, Dickerman JD. Pediatrics 63:677, 1979; Baloch N. Br J Psychiatry 124:545, 1974; Clark LD et al. N Engl J Med 246:205, 1952
15. Sahu DM. Indian J Dermatol 17:47, 1972
16. Petursson H. Aust NZ J Psychiatry 13:67, 1979
17. Floyd JB Jr, Murphy CM. J Ky Med Assoc 74:549, 1976; Ryan HF, et al. JAMA 203:1137, 1968; Karch FE. Ann Intern Med 91:61, 1979
18. Shear MK, Sacks MH. Am J Psychiatry 135:109, 1978; Sodeman WA. N Engl J Med 273:35, 1965; Volpe BT, Soave R. Ann Intern Med 91:865, 1979; Riesman D. Am J Med Sci 161:6, 1921
19. Falk RH et al. Lancet 1:858, 1977; Padfield PL et al. Lancet 1:1152, 1977; Ahmad S et al. Chest 76:712, 1979
20. Rainey JM Jr. Am J Psychiatry 134:371, 1977; Quail M, Karelse RH. S Afr Med J 57:551, 1980
21. Herridge CF, Brook MFA. Br Med J 2:160, 1968
22. Garza-Perez J et al. Med Serv J Can 23:775, 1967; Heston LL, Hastings D. Am J Psychiatry 137:249, 1980; Flemenbaum A, Gunby B. Dis Nerv Syst 32:188, 1971
23. Davison LA et al. Anesthesiology 43:313, 1975
24. Gotz V. Br Med J 1:49, 1978
25. Kiersch TA. US Armed Forces Med J 5:1353, 1954
26. Hawks WN Jr. et al. J Pediatr Ophthalmol 8:171, 1971: Dundee JW et al. Lancet, 1:1370, 1970
27. Shader RI (ed): Psychiatric Complications of Medical Drugs, p. 149. New York, Raven Press, 1972; Presthus J, Holmsen R. Acta Neurol Scand 50:774, 1974; Moskovitz C et al. Am J Psychiatry 135:669, 1978; Birkmayer W. J Neural Transam (Suppl) 14:163, 1978

Table 11-1.
Some Drugs That Cause Psychiatric Symptoms (*continued*)

28. Kellaway GSM. Drugs (Suppl) 11:91, 1976; Hawkins DJ. Miss Med 73:476, 1976; Riddiough MA. Am J Hosp Pharm 34:465, 1977; Endo M et al. Psychoneuroendocrinology 3:211, 1978
29. Lucas AR, Weiss M. JAMA 217:1079, 1971
30. Persyko I. J Nerv Ment Dis 154:299, 1972
31. Richert S et al. Neuroradiology 18:177, 1979; Schmidt RC. Neuroradiology 19:153, 1980
32. Calloway SP. Med J Zambia 10:70, 1976
33. Kane FJ Jr, Pokorny A. South Med J 68:808, 1975; Wood AJJ et al. Br Med J 1:305, 1974; Miller RR. J Clin Pharmacol 15:198, 1975; Hamilton RC et al. Br J Anaesth 39:647, 1967
34. Sheehy LM, Maxmen JS. Am J Psychiatry 135:1422, 1978
35. Snow SS et al. Br J Psychiatry 136:297, 1980
36. McCrum ID, Guidry JR. JAMA 240:1265, 1978
37. Bjornberg A, Selstam J. Acta Psychiatr Neurol Scand 35:129 1960; Green RL et al. N Engl J Med 291:223, 1974; Eggleston DJ. Br Dent J 148:73, 1980

38. Fraser HF, Isbell H. Bull Narc 12:9, 1960
39. Fleminger R. Br Med J 1:1182, 1978; Steinert J, Pugh CR. Br Med J 1:790, 1979; Gershon ES et al. Ann Intern Med 90:938, 1979; Greenblatt DJ, Koch-Weser J. Am Heart J 86:478, 1973; Hinshelwood RD. Br Med J 2:445, 1969; Voltolina EJ et al. Clin Toxicol 4:357, 1971
40. Engel GL JAMA 197:515, 1966
41. Goodwin FK, Bunney WE Jr. Semin Psychiatry 3:435, 1971; Freis ED. Am Fam Physician 11:120, 1975
42. Thornton TL. JAMA 243:1630, 1980; Kruis R, Barger R. JAMA 243:1420, 1980
43. Holland JF et al. Cancer Res 33:1258, 1973 (Abramowicz M [ed]: Some drugs that cause psychiatric symptoms. Med Lett Drugs Ther 23:9, 1981)

It appears to take some people several weeks to return to their normal preoperative mental status. The following changes in functioning have been reported:

Changes in cognitive functioning
Decreased problem-solving ability
Tendency toward more concrete than abstract reasoning
Distractability
Decrease in recent memory retention
Egocentrism; less aware of needs of others (ego is protecting the self during the recuperation period)

Changes in mood
Increased emotionality
Unexpected mood swings

Changes in neurovegetative functioning
Changes in sleep patterns
Difficulty falling asleep

As noted, these changes are mild and usually disappear 4 to 6 weeks after surgery. They appear to be part of the normal response to the acute surgical period.

Another factor that can contribute to the mental status changes of postoperative patients is that surgery is a threatening event. It requires a major coping effort of the ego. One of the results of this major effort may be the temporary egocentrism identified above. It causes the person to focus on himself and his rehabilitation at a time when he lacks the physical energy to support the well-being of others.

Because of the possibility of these slight changes in mental functioning, it is advisable that patients follow their physician's recommendations on the length of their recuperation period before returning to work, even though they may feel physically well enough to return to work earlier.

Common Examples

The following case examples of OBS are presented in order to increase your awareness of its potential and prevalence.

Case Examples

While dieting, and just before *mealtimes*, Ann notices that she is tremulous, anxious, and dizzy. She is irritable with her roommates. She finds her thinking "fuzzy" rather than clear. Ann's low blood sugar (hypoglycemia) has resulted in inadequate glucose availability to her brain cells (Kaplan and Sadock, 1981).

Jerry is normally a shy, unconfident person who does not enjoy being with people. After having two drinks at a party, he notices that he has no trouble finding things to talk about and feels comfortable being with people. He finds almost every conversation amusing. The effects of alcohol have relaxed Jerry's normal ego and superego functioning.

Stephanie experiences depression, irritability, and poor emotional control during the few days before her menstrual period each month. She believes it must be "all in my head."

Actually, Stephanie is partially correct, except that she is not imagining these emotional changes. They are due to temporary premenstrual changes in physiology, which are caused by retention of fluid (resulting in slight swelling of all body tissues, including the brain) and rapid electrolyte and hormonal changes. Once her period begins, Stephanie's hormone and electrolyte levels return to normal and her symptoms disappear (Kaplan and Sadock, 1981).

Andy had a wisdom tooth removed before a final examination. He took analgesic tablets that contained codeine before he entered the examination room. Within half an hour, he was surprised at his drowsiness and inability to quickly remember facts that he had been actively studying during the week before the examination.

Conclusion

This chapter was written to raise your awareness of the incidence of OBS in patients in the general hospital. It occurs far more commonly than is normally recognized. When OBS results in a delirious episode, patients, families, and caregivers are frightened by the event. By being alert for subtle changes in mental status, it is possible to reverse or reduce progression to delirium by rapid nursing and medical intervention. Knowledge of the complex symptoms of OBS can help you in your nursing assessment and ongoing evaluation of patients. Another important point to remember in determining the nursing diagnoses of your patients is that OBS is a potential etiological consideration in *each* of the nursing diagnosis categories (Barry, 1982).

12

Counseling Techniques for Nurses

Nurses usually have a good sense of "where" their patients are emotionally. This ability, as mentioned earlier in the book, is thought of by many as intuition. Actually, it develops because nurses are well skilled in observing and assessing patients' nonverbal communication: the barely perceptible cues given by their eyes, voices, moods, and body posture. When nurses' exposure to patients is combined with good judgment and assessment skills, they frequently are the primary forces in identifying patients who need extra emotional support in adjusting to their illnesses or new life situations.

Many times, patients with physical illness respond within normal limits when their adaptive response is delayed. At other times, their coping abilities are severely taxed when sudden catastrophic illness occurs. In addition, there are people with immature personalities who need additional support during their hospitalizations, although their illness itself is not considered life threatening by hospital personnel. Entering a hospital, for whatever reason, is a severely threatening experience for many people.

At times, the families of patients need extra attention from hospital caregivers. If their family member is dying, chronically ill, lying in an intensive care unit, or waiting for a possibly frightening diagnosis, they frequently look to nurses for understanding and for the opportunity to talk about their concerns. The interpersonal relationship established by a nurse with patients and family members can promote the adaptation and mature coping of all these people.

This chapter presents theoretical material and practical suggestions that can improve your ability to alleviate some of the anxiety that you have previously observed in patients but perhaps have felt inadequately prepared to relieve. Dartington and co-workers (1977) have written that these skills are not intended "to prepare nurses to be counselors but to enhance their counseling skills within the professional role" (p. 54). With a basic knowledge of counseling theory and a warm, caring approach to patients, you are in an excellent position to help your patients. It is possible that you may prevent more serious emotional and physical complications from occurring during patients' hospitalizations by relieving some of the emotional stress caused by their illnesses.

Which Patients Are Appropriate for Nursing Intervention?

Any patient in the general hospital or outpatient setting who demonstrates minimal to moderate levels of anxiety, depression, or any of the psychosocial diagnostic categories (see Chap. 13: Psychosocial Nursing Assessment and Diagnosis) is a suitable candidate for nursing intervention. These skills may be especially helpful with patients who have chronic conditions, such as cancer, respiratory disease, burns, orthopaedic problems, and so on. They also can be well used by nurses in outpatient departments or visiting nurse agencies who work with clients and families.

It is essential that nurses be able to recognize whether the patient is appropriate for nursing intervention or whether psychiatric consultation is indicated. If you have any question, or if the patient's problem is moderate to severe, discuss it with a clinical supervisor. A decision can then be made about whether to approach the medical team about ordering a psychiatric consultation.

When nurses identify patients who need psychiatric referral, there usually are strong indications present that the patient is maladapting to his illness or hospitalization. He needs support in order to cope more adaptively with these stresses. Other reasons for psychiatric referral in the hospital and outpatient settings are a marked change in the previously observed mental status of the patient or a mental status of a patient that appears abnormal from the beginning (see Chap. 10: The Mental Status Examination). If a consultation is ordered, talk to the consultant to obtain recommendations about the best therapeutic approach you should use with the patient.

Caution is recommended to nurses about using newly acquired counseling skills. Family members and friends of nurses often perceive them to be good listeners and advisors. Nurses should be wary of filling the advising or counseling role with them when they have complex emotional problems. Objectivity is difficult to maintain when people are emotionally tied to one another. Bias can sway a person from being empathetic and helpful to being too involved and intrusive.

Empathy vs. Sympathy

It is important to clarify the meaning of empathy, an essential quality in a helping relationship.

Kalisch (1975) differentiates *empathy* from *sympathy* as follows:

> In empathy the helper *borrows* his patient's feelings in order to fully understand them, but he is always aware of his own separateness. He realizes that the feelings of his patient are not his own.
>
> Sympathetic understanding, on the other hand, involves a process in which the helper loses his own separate identity and *takes on* the patient's feelings and circumstances as if he were in his place [p. 275].

Many nurses are required to memorize the meanings of empathy and sympathy during their nursing preparation. Frequently, however, the terms are confusing. The following examples may make the differences more understandable.

If a person is walking near a frozen lake and sees a person who has fallen through the ice, he can either (1) carefully walk on the ice and throw him a rope or pull him to safety with a piece of wood or (2) walk on the ice and, in his desire to help, get so close to the edge that the ice breaks and he falls in; then two people need help. A similar example is if someone were caught in quicksand. The helper can (1) find a board to slide under his feet or hold the board out to him so that the trapped person can help himself or (2) get into the quicksand to help the victim out, is of no help, and then needs help himself. In the two examples described above, the first course of action chosen is similar to empathy in a caring relationship. The second action is comparable to a sympathetic one, in which the desire to help a person in difficulty ultimately may cause both people to need help. *A common mistake of beginning-level counselors is assuming that the person needing help is helpless.*

The process of relieving another person's psychological distress involves an empathic caring; the caring is much like the rope or board mentioned above. The person being helped is not passive. He *is* able to help himself. Remember that the patient, in the great majority of cases, was emotionally stable on admission. His normal coping ability has been temporarily disrupted by the multiple stressors involved in hospitalization. The objective caring of another person can lend him the strength to help himself. A caregiver is at risk for sympathetic overinvolvement if he or she needs to "jump in" to make the other person feel better.

Richards (1975) described the differences between "caring for" and "caring about" in his definition of the term *caring*. In "caring for," the caregiver expresses his concern by taking charge of another's life. This type of caregiver enjoys his work when he has an invalid or passive person to care for. The other person is reduced to an object and therefore becomes predictable and controllable. "Caring about," on the other hand, is described as the caregiver meeting the other as a complete person and respecting his abilities and decision-making capacities. In order to promote a patient's normal coping abilities, it is necessary to care *about* him.

Brammer and Shostrom (1968), Rogers (1976), and May and colleagues (1976) state that the person being helped is responsible for his own life and has forces locked inside that will help him to achieve optimal development. The helper may turn the key, but the client must ultimately solve his own problem.

The Difference Between Informal and Formal Counseling Relationships

Staff nurses will usually engage in less structured types of counseling relationships with their patients because of time constraints. In a hospital, it is usually difficult for them to set aside specific times in which to talk with patients. What happens instead is that they frequently combine physical care with an informal counseling approach. Once the physical care has been administered, they may continue to stay and talk with the patient about his concerns. Despite being called *informal counseling*, this type of relationship should not be underrated. It has the potential to be the most therapeutic emotional experience the patient has in the hospital.

When it is not possible to find a private place on the unit and the patient has a roommate, respect your patient's need for privacy if you are engaging in a sensitive discussion about his background or current illness. Always close the curtain between the two beds. One of the best ways to promote privacy under these less than ideal conditions is to place a chair on the side of the patient's bed that is not adjacent to the roommate's bed. The chair should be placed close to the head of the bed. This way, the patient's conversation will be directed away from his roommate.

Formal counseling can be differentiated because it is prearranged and contacts are made on a scheduled basis (Litwack and associates, 1980). For nurses involved in a formal counseling rela-

tionship, an important component is the provision for lack of interruptions; for example, a clinician's beeper should ideally be left elsewhere. Sometimes an empty room on the nursing unit can be used if privacy cannot be guaranteed elsewhere. This should be prearranged with the head nurse.

Whether talking with patients formally or informally, one of the most important things that nurses can do to signify their interest in patients is to *sit down*. The importance of this gesture to the patient cannot be overemphasized. How many times do caregivers ask patients, "How are things going for you?" as they stand with their hands on the door knobs? The "hand on the door knob" approach is the quickest way to tell patients that we really do not have the time to find out.

The Patient's Readiness for Help

The most important aspect of any counseling relationship is that the patient recognizes his need for help. If the patient is not receptive to counseling, he will derive little, if any, value from it. Additionally, he usually will become more resistant to future assistance. An important motivator for any patient in a counseling relationship is his feeling of emotional discomfort and *his* desire to relieve it.

Important Personal Qualities of a Counselor

The most important characteristics in a helping person are listed below:

1. A genuine feeling of warmth for the person being helped. Rogers (1976) has termed this *unconditional positive regard*. The helper must care about the other person and be free of his own judgments of what he thinks or feels. He accepts him *as he is*.

2. A capacity for empathic understanding of the patient's *internal frame of reference* (Rogers, 1976). This means *really* understanding how the patient feels. It does not mean how the helper thinks the patient feels after a quick conversation. Unbiased understanding is essential and takes time to develop. It is important to remember that total understanding of the patient's situation is never constant. The listener must always be open to changes in the patient's thoughts and feelings and able to revise his awareness of the patient's problems.

3. The ability to be human and real in the relationship. These qualities have also been called *authenticity* (Jouard, 1971), *transparency* (Brammer and Shostrom, 1968), and *genuineness* (Cormier and Cormier, 1979). This does not mean sharing one's own opinions or personal history with the patient. It is instead a sharing of one's *self*. This concept has also been called "encounter . . . not merely as a self but also a being-together with another" (May and colleagues, 1976, p. 433).

A Counseling Deterrent: "Professional Distancing"

Because of their constant exposure to illness and death, nurses may unconsciously defend themselves psychologically in the stressful hospital environment. They may cope by pulling back their awareness of what is actually occurring emotionally in their patients and themselves. Nurses are rarely aware when this happens to themselves because it is an unconscious defensive tactic of the ego. This is the cause of "*professional distancing*" from patients (Barry, 1978); the result is a cool, detached demeanor. Nurses, accordingly, give technical care and have intimate physical contact with their patients; however, they tune out their awareness of patients' emotional states. Nurses who are professionally distanced are not capable of giving good-quality supportive emotional care. Because of distancing and avoidance, they lack the three important personal characteristics of a counselor mentioned above. Flaskerud and co-authors (1979) have identified five strategies that many nurses use to avoid closeness with patients:

1. Concentrating on impersonal and regimented aspects of care
2. Presenting self as impotent to change the system
3. Complaining of inadequate staffing
4. Being involved in indirect care
5. Seeking promotion and advancement (p. 165)

Stewart (1975) describes nurses as professionals who are taught that they should not show their feelings. They are also taught to make decisions *for* patients rather than *with* them. These behaviors are the opposite of those required in an open interpersonal relationship.

The Nurse's Attitude Toward Counseling

Nurses must be able to analyze *honestly* their normal way of relating with patients if they plan to be effective in a counseling situation. If they have been socialized into giving opinions and advice before the patient has a chance to say what *he* needs, their potential for therapeutic work is diminished.

Probably one of the most important characteristics of helpers in a helping relationship is that they must have attained healthy levels of personal growth (Brammer and Shostrom, 1968; Rogers, 1976). If they are immature, guarded, or professionally distanced, they will lack the ability to know themselves and be honest about their own reactions in the relationship. The following guidelines, extracted from Litwack and colleagues (1980), may help nurses who are ready to move into a more active role in helping their patients cope with their new or chronic health conditions:

1. There is no *right* way to counsel (p. 25). (By following the guidelines you can potentially avoid the wrong ways.)
2. Individuals have inner resources to help themselves (p. 25).
3. Start where counselees are and accept them where they are (p. 26).
4. Each human being must be respected and potentialities for growth recognized (p. 27).
5. Our role as counselors is not to preach or impose our values (p. 27).
6. The key to successful counseling is nonevaluative listening (p. 28).

The Meaning of Support

One of the most beneficial aspects of a good therapeutic relationship is the emotional support given to the patient (Litwack and colleagues, 1980). In many nursing circles, support means reassurances and words of positive encouragement; *this is different from the support demonstrated in the counseling setting*. In a counseling relationship, the support comes from the counselor's ability to convey total understanding, acceptance, and caring about the client and his problems. *Open listening* is the hallmark of the supportive counselor. No matter what the client says or feels, the counselor totally accepts the client as he is. If, for example, a diabetic man is told that his foot must be amputated, the nurse will allow him to express his feelings freely. He should not be "shut off" or encouraged to feel that "everything will be all right." If nurses feel compelled to hold back patients' emotions, it may be due to their *own* anxiety.

This anxiety in a nurse seems to have two main sources: the nurse feels helpless in the situation and is not able to tolerate this feeling of helplessness; or he or she has experienced similar feelings and was never able to resolve them. The patient's distress is a reminder of his or her own similar problem. In either case, quick reassurances to the patient usually cut off the anxious feeling for the caregiver but *not* for the patient. His anxiety usually increases with this approach. He feels even more alone and abandoned. Instead of "shutting off" patients' emotions and expressions, nurses can allow patients more therapeutic ventilation of feelings and fears using techniques outlined in the remainder of the chapter.

Is There Such a Thing as Too Much Support?

It is also important to understand the consequences of too much support (Litwack and colleagues, 1980). Most nurses have a strong need to nurture and make things better for people. It is important for nurses to be aware of this tendency in themselves. Support can cause problems in a relationship if overused. If the helper helps too much, the resulting feeling in the other, if he is a mature person, is frequently resentment or guilt. This occurs because the helper is fostering the other's dependence on him or her. A dependent, immature person may enjoy the excessive support, but it further encourages his dependency and discourages his personal growth.

Too much warmth from the caregiver is threatening to many people, especially those for whom a close experience with another is difficult; it is viewed as intrusive. Too much support by the nurse also may be interpreted by the patient as shallowness or a "Pollyanna" attitude about a medical condition that may have potential inherent complications. This may sour the patient's attitude toward the caregiver. He may doubt the helper's honesty and pull back from the relationship. For the dependent person, too much warmth is construed as an effort on the caregiver's part to establish a relationship that will be maintained after

the patient's discharge. In conclusion, too much support by a helper also risks a sympathetic rather than an empathic relationship (remember the consequences of "falling in"?).

The Importance of Assessment

When nurses begin an informal or formal type of counseling relationship with a patient, their first responsibility is to assess what is happening with the patient emotionally. The theory presented in the previous chapters should be used in assessing the patient's emotional status. The question that a nurse should be able to answer after assessment is, "*What* treatment, by *whom*, is most effective for *this* person with *this* specific problem, under *which* set of circumstances?" This will provide the framework on which to base the intervention. As with any problem-solving process, assessment should be ongoing during the nursing process.

The Structured vs. the "Tree" Assessment Approach

Two main types of approaches can be used in the psychosocial assessment process. One is rigidly structured and formal; the helper has a set format of questions and a set time in which they must be answered. The approach allows little flexibility and spontaneity. It is like an agenda that must be closely followed. If a patient presents interesting sidelights to the problem, the helper usually delays exploration of them until the established list of questions has been answered. Often they are never returned to.

The second approach is one that is informally called the "tree" approach. It is the preferred method to use in the assessment process. Using this approach, the helper uses a loosely structured format and takes his or her clues about the types of questions to ask from the patient. It consists of an open-ended questioning approach. The nurse asks a specific question, and as the client gives the answer and begins to explain a problem, the nurse tries to understand every aspect of it. The problem is explored in the same manner that a squirrel explores a tree. The squirrel usually climbs up from the trunk to a large limb, then on to the branches, then on to the twigs. He does not jump from large limb to large limb. The use of too structured an assessment process can be compared to the squirrel jumping from large limb to large limb. If the patient is asked specific questions and is told that you will "get back" to the details, the details never evolve in a natural way. You may miss valuable information.

Content and Process

Content and *process* are important concepts to understand. They describe what is occurring in a helping relationship (Brammer and Shostrom, 1968). *Content* is the actual accounting of what occurred during the interview period; it is the factual recording of the conversation between the nurse and the patient. *Process* is how and why the conversation occurred. For example, a patient may say, "I am worried." The nurse may respond by saying, "What are you worried about?" or "You are worried. Here, let me take you for a walk to take your mind off things" or "I noticed that your wife was in earlier. Does it have something to do with her visit?" In the above examples, the content would include all the discussion in the interchange. The process includes all the underlying dynamics of what happened and why. The dynamics of the nurse's personality respond in particular ways to the dynamics of the patient's personality and can prompt several types of responses. Similarly, the nurse's response to the patient prompts different reactions in him. To understand the latter point, what effect did the three different nurse responses have on you as you read them? Did one of them make you feel that you could talk freely? Did one of the responses tell you that the nurse was not "open" to your feelings?

Specific Characteristics of the Relationship

Rogers (1976) has written, "The counseling relationship is one in which warmth of acceptance and absence of any coercion or personal pressure on the part of the counselor permits the maximum expression of feelings, attitudes, and problems by the patient" (p. 407). Brammer and Shostrom (1968) explain that there are various levels of the helper's impact on the one being helped:

1. *Friendship level.* The helper likes certain qualities in the patient, and the relationship is pleasurable.

2. *Encounter level.* The helper disregards qualities he may like or dislike in the patient.
3. *Altruistic level.* The helper loves the patient because he is a fellow human being.
4. *Erotic level.* The helper responds sexually to the patient, but may or may not be consciously aware of it. His effectiveness with the patient can be impaired, and his objectivity can be distorted.

The ideal levels in a counseling relationship are numbers 2 and 3 above.

Underlying Dynamics of the Relationship

There are three important dynamics present in any helping relationship that are not generally known to most hospital caregivers. These phenomena were originally described by Freud (1933). They are called *transference*, *countertransference*, and *resistance*. The awareness of these dynamics may be helpful whenever the nurse is puzzled by events occurring in the relationship.

It is important to understand that these phenomena arise in the unconscious of the nurse and the patient. They are not part of one's normal awareness. Whenever nurses do not understand why they or their patients are reacting in particular ways, the answer may be that one or more of these dynamics are operating.

Transference

Freedman and colleagues (1976) describe transference as "an unconscious phenomenon in which the feelings, attitudes, and wishes originally linked with important figures in one's early life are projected onto others" (p. 1334). For example, if a normally mature person, after hospitalization, begins to be very demanding and needy with a particular nurse, it is possible that there is a maternal transference. The female nurse, because of physical or personality qualities, reminds the patient of his mother. Feelings that he had long forgotten come to the surface when, because of his illness, he regresses and reverts to immature defense mechanisms or a childlike dependency.

Countertransference

Countertransference is the "conscious or unconscious emotional response of the therapist to the patient. It is determined by the therapist's inner needs, rather than by the patient's needs" (Freedman and colleagues, p. 1293). If, in the hospital setting, a nurse finds himself or herself inexplicably drawn to, or repelled by, a particular patient, it is possible that the dynamic of countertransference is occurring; the patient reminds the caregiver of a well-loved (or perhaps a disowned) family member.

Take, for example, a student nurse who became heavily involved in the care of a 50-year-old man dying of cancer. She requested that he be her patient every day. When she was transferred to another unit, she continued to visit him daily. Her nursing instructor was concerned about her overinvolvement. Eventually it became known that the student's father had died of cancer, and she had never adequately resolved the loss.

When transference or countertransference issues occur in a relationship, the most important thing for nurses to do about them is just to be *aware* of them. It is important to remember that a patient's transference to a particular nurse and the possibly concurrent reduction in optimal emotional functioning may have two important precipitants. The first is a reduced coping level because of the stress of hospitalization. The second is an altered mental state due to organic causes such as residual effects of anesthesia or narcotics, elevated temperature, dehydration, and so on. Trying to confront such a patient with the fact that he is treating you like his mother would not have any beneficial effect. Likewise, telling a patient that he reminds you of your dead father is information he could probably do without.

Resistance

Resistance is the "conscious or unconscious opposition to the uncovering of the unconscious. Resistance is linked to underlying defense mechanisms" (Freedman and colleagues, p. 1326). Sometimes nurses find it difficult to believe that patients will defy physicians' orders and engage in behaviors that have been sternly prohibited. The physician has usually warned the patient that death or serious consequences will occur if the orders are not obeyed. Examples of patients who fall into this category are the diabetic who eats anything he wants or the patient with cardiac or respiratory disease who smokes or exercises excessively. Another patient who demonstrates the same "inability to hear" is the patient recently diagnosed with terminal illness.

For each of these patients, the threat to their self-image, in addition to their fear of death, causes the ego to use defense mechanisms to defend itself.

These defense mechanisms cause the patient to be resistant. It seems as if he cannot hear. This is the result of the need of the ego to shut out full awareness of reality.

The most pronounced of these defense mechanisms is denial. Others are distortion, repression, avoidance, rationalization, and suppression (see Chap. 4). For people with strong egos, it may take only a day or two until the ego is able to tolerate reality; then the defense disappears and the patient is ready to accept the physician's words. For others, reality remains too threatening, and they continue to block out the physician's diagnosis and recommendations for much longer periods. No matter how maladaptive this resistance seems to be, it is important to remember that it protects the patient's emotional equilibrium. Without the protection of these defense mechanisms, his ego might be overwhelmed. When resistance is present, we may "test" it with gentle questions to determine its strength. The following case example may clarify this approach:

Case Example

Ed is a 50-year-old middle-level executive. For the past year he has become increasingly forgetful, and his working ability has deteriorated. He has poor social judgment and poor emotional control. His primary physician admitted him to the general hospital for a neurological workup and psychiatric evaluation. Diagnostic tests indicated that he was experiencing presenile dementia as a result of Alzheimer's disease. Immediately after he was told the diagnosis and prognosis, Ed continued to be very cheerful. Three days later he was very positive about the future and talked about returning to work as soon as possible. He confided to his nurse that he was hoping for a promotion to the home office in another city.

This patient is behaving contrary to our normal expectations of a recently diagnosed and ultimately terminal patient with a frightening illness. This should tell us that the patient's emotional status would be very threatened if he were fully aware of the awful reality of his situation.

In working with this patient, one can ask gentle probing questions such as, "How long do you think you will be in the hospital?" or "How do you think things will go for you when you get home?" or "How does your wife feel about your illness?" The responses to these questions will be good indicators of the level of his denial. He may respond that he expects to be fine when he goes home and hopes to return to work very soon. If he should also tell you that his wife is hopeful and not concerned, then his level of defense is very strong.

Any attempt to force reality and break through his denial may result in some type of emotional decompensation or further strengthening of his denial. If, for example, you were frightened and alone in a room and someone began to threaten you on the other side of a closed door, would you open it or *would you further reinforce it with a chair and anything else available?* Remember that the ultimate task of the ego is to defend itself. It will do exactly what *you* would do in that room if you were frightened.

If this type of extreme resistance occurs and is of concern, it is advisable to request psychiatric consultation. Frequently, however, the questioning approach described above will gradually help the patient to become aware of the situation. As he responds to the questions, the reality will slowly become apparent to him. His ego will become less defended as it becomes able to cope more adaptively and tolerate his new life circumstances.

Under no condition should a newly diagnosed and highly resistant patient be blatantly confronted with a statement such as, "Now, Ed, you know you have cancer. The doctor told you you have only a year to live. Why do you keep ignoring his words?" There are far more therapeutic ways in which patients can be helped to accept their prognoses.

Different Types of Relationships

The many types of relationships in which health caregivers engage with their patients include interviewing, advising, supporting, guiding, teaching, and counseling (Litwack and colleagues, 1980). The following descriptions of these relationships should help to differentiate the various roles in which nurses meet their patients' needs.

Interviewing

The *interview* is primarily a question and answer situation in which the caregiver seeks historical data. The interviewer is usually not seeking opinions from the interviewee. *Example:* obtaining a past medical history from a newly admitted patient.

Advising

Advising is a helping process in which the advisor works with an advisee who is trying to make a decision. The advisor knows about the various options open to the advisee. Using this knowledge and the knowledge of the advisee's situation, the advisor makes a strong recommendation about the option *he* thinks is best for the advisee. He essentially takes away the advisee's ability to make a decision.

Health care consumers are frequently in this position. In all fairness to their caregivers, the limitations of time may contribute to the frequency with which this approach is used. The information about *all* the options open to the advisee is frequently withheld by well-intentioned caregivers. *Example:* a nurse in an outpatient gynecology clinic suggests that a welfare patient use a particular type of birth control without fully explaining all the options open to the patient and learning the advisee's opinions about each of the options.

Supporting

Litwack describes a *supporting relationship* as one in which the supporter approves of the actions of the person being supported. The value system of the supporter enters strongly into the relationship. (Note that there is a difference between approval support and the acceptance support discussed earlier in the chapter, which is essential to a counseling relationship.) In *acceptance support* the listener supports the *person.* In *approval support* the listener supports the person's actions and experiences. *Example:* A Reach to Recovery Cancer Society volunteer visits a mastectomy patient in the hospital. She compares the patient's experiences with her own and assures the patient that everything is fine.

Guiding

In a *guiding relationship,* the caregiver is similar to the advisor discussed above. The difference is that he knows the options open to the health care consumer and presents all of them so that the patient can make his own decision about the best choice for his particular circumstances. *Example:* a 66-year-old man is experiencing urinary frequency. The physician diagnoses benign prostatic hypertrophy. The patient has been planning on a trip to visit his daughter when she has a baby in 1 month. The physician tells the patient that he can be admitted before or after the trip for cystoscopy and a diagnostic workup. He explains the consequences if a malignancy is found if surgery is delayed until after the trip is over. The patient ultimately makes his own decision after he has all the necessary information to do so.

Teaching

In a *teaching relationship,* the teacher presents information about a subject that the teacher believes the students need to know. It is a strongly dominant-subordinate relationship. The teacher is in control of the relationship, and two-way communication is minimal. *Example:* A diabetic class on use of insulin and self-administration by syringe.

Counseling

In a *counseling relationship,* the counselor serves as a catalyst for self-exploration by the counselee as he strives to resolve conflicts, make decisions, and solve problems. Some readers may question the difference between counseling as described here and psychotherapy. A psychotherapy relationship contains the same elements as counseling. In addition, it includes the use of interpretation of unconscious elements by the therapist. (Interpretation is explained later in this chapter.) *Example:* A cardiac rehabilitation nurse sits with a recent myocardial infarction (MI) patient as he talks about the changes he must make in his life and his feelings about his new status. As he talks, he uncovers concerns and begins to examine ways that he can learn to adjust his life style.

Attending Behaviors in the Nurse Counselor

Another very important aspect of a helping relationship is the way the nurse acts during the time he or she is with the patient. This is called *attending behavior.* Attending behavior is the manner in which a listener responds to someone. It can either encourage or discourage clients from wanting to confide in them (Brammer, 1973; Brooke Army Medical Center, 1973). These behaviors, also called *kinesics,* include eye contact, posture, gesture, and verbal behavior.

Eye Contact

If the helper is an open, unthreatened person and genuinely cares for the patient, consistent eye contact communicates this to him.

Posture

As discussed above, in counseling situations the nurse should be sitting whenever possible. The helper should demonstrate a relaxed and attentive attitude. An erect but casual posture, rather than one in which the helper either looks ready to fall asleep or bolt out of the chair, encourages the patient as he is relating his problem.

Gesture

The way the nurse moves his or her head, hands, arms, and legs and shows facial expression indicates interest in the patient's problem. A slight nod of the head will signify understanding to him. Some negative gestures are frequent movements of the arms and legs, arms folded across the chest, a hand held in front of the mouth, or a blank stare. They may indicate anxiety or an unwillingness to openly participate in the helping process.

In the three attending behaviors presented above, the emphasis is on the nonverbal messages the nurse gives to the patient. In developing helping relationships, nurses should also be attentive to the nonverbal messages their patients give to them. If a patient demonstrates poor eye contact, posture, or gestures with negative implications, it is possible that the client is not motivated to be in a counseling situation. Another possibility is that anxiety, depression, or other personality conflicts may be preventing him from being free and open in the counseling situation. A neutral or negative response by a patient to a nurse's counseling intervention can also cause the nurse to feel unfullfilled or unwanted as a caregiver.

Verbal Behavior

The last of the attending behaviors includes the ways in which nurses usually respond to patients. These responses, if positive, will promote the relationship rather than end it prematurely. They include the three listening skills of *paraphrasing, clarifying,* and *perception checking* (Brammer, 1973).

In *paraphrasing,* the helper "feeds back only the helpee's message and avoids adding his own ideas" (Brammer, 1973, p. 84). In other words, the helper listens to what the patient says and repeats or rephrases it in his own words; he "mirrors it back." Paraphrasing concentrates on the cognitive components of the client's problem. This is also known as *reflection of content* (Brooke Army Medical Center, 1973). After paraphrasing, watch for a nod or some other sign that you have accurately understood the patient's message.

Clarifying differs from paraphrasing in that it does more than rephrase what the patient has said. Instead, the listener takes a guess about what the patient means. The listener asks, "Are you saying that—?" He then asks the patient if his statement is correct (Cormier and Cormier, 1979). It is advisable not to do this too soon (Brammer, 1973). Otherwise, you may misinterpret what the patient is saying, and he may feel even more alone and misunderstood. It is also possible that the patient may feel compelled to agree with a clarifying statement you make if he is intimidated by persons who represent authority.

A more perceptive paraphrasing and clarifying approach is for you to listen for and observe the affective or feeling component of what your patient is saying and to share your observations with the patient. If you accurately reflect the true feelings of the patient, it can cause the interview to shift to a deeper and more meaningful level (Brooke Army Medical Center, 1973). It helps the patient to feel, "Finally, someone understands."

A colostomy patient, for example, may frequently repeat that her colostomy is messy, smelly, and so on. In an informal hospital situation the nurse may respond, "Oh, Mrs. Decker, it may seem smelly to you, but I really can't smell it." Or a chair can be pulled up to the patient's bed and the nurse can sit down and say, "Mrs. Decker, you seem worried about this colostomy."

The last of the three responding skills is *perception checking.* It occurs after the patient has made several statements (Brammer, 1973). You then reflect back your perceptions of the general theme of what the patient has been saying to you. Then, follow this statement with a request for the client's response to your statement. For example, you might say, "Mr. Paige, it sounds as if you're depressed because you don't think you'll be able to go back to work because of your respiratory disease and you wonder how you will be able to make your house payments. Is that your biggest concern at this time?"

Leading Skills

The next important set of skills are the *leading skills.* Particularly important in establishing a helping relationship, they include indirect leading, direct leading, focusing, questioning, confronting, interpreting, and advice giving (Brammer, 1973). As you read about the leading skills described below, take the time to picture yourself in a discussion with a patient you have actually cared for. Imagine the way you would carry out each of the leading skills described in this section. If you are a student, it can be very helpful to role play these leading skills in a group of fellow students. One student should be the "patient" and should be assigned a specific diagnosis and accompanying set of psychosocial problems.

Leading types of statements invite the patient to respond. The *indirect leading* statement is deliberately vague and general, such as, "Tell me about your father." The *direct lead* asks for more specific responses, for example, "You said your father was an alcoholic?"

Focusing is best used after the client has had the chance to discuss various topics, usually with indirect leading. The helper would then "zero in" on a specific aspect of the client's explorations. "You mentioned earlier that it was hard for you having an alcoholic father. What was it like?" The helper's focusing techniques should help to uncover feelings.

Questioning is a very important leading skill when *open-ended questions* are used. An open-ended question is a question that is structured to avoid a single answer from the person being questioned. It should bring forth a response from the patient that requires him to formulate a more detailed answer. For example, a nurse may ask a patient, "How did you feel when your father was in a sanatorium?"

A *close-ended question* is one that requires only a one-word answer. A one-word answer can bring the flow of questions to an abrupt halt. When asked "Did you ever feel angry toward your father when he was in the hospital?" The person who replies "no" may make the interviewer uncertain about how to proceed with questioning. Instead, the counselor can say, "What kind of feelings did you have when your father was in the sanatorium?" When you are in a counseling situation with a patient, a good rule to keep in mind is that the most therapeutic outcome usually occurs when feelings are discussed. Patients, when asked about their illnesses, often will reply with cognitive statements. For example, if a patient is asked how he feels about the leg amputation scheduled for next week, he may reply, "Oh, I think it will be rough" or "I hope it will be O.K." Maintain your focus on his feelings rather than on his thoughts or opinions. You can follow up with the question "How does it make you feel when you think about your amputation next week?" or "When you go home after surgery how do you think you will feel about things?"

Often, a patient will describe how he feels physically when he is asked how he feels. Remember, that is the aspect of him that most caregivers are concerned with. If this happens, clarify for him that you want to know how he feels emotionally. It is often a very special relief for him to be able to talk about his fears and concerns. It is highly therapeutic for him to release the anxiety that these fears generate in him.

The examples above should clarify how the process of the interview can be partially blocked or halted completely if the question is phrased poorly. The patient's intellectual and affective response to open-ended vs. close-ended questions is that with an open-ended questioning approach, he usually feels freer in the interview and has fewer constraints imposed on him. Close-ended questions, similar to the one above, sometimes introduce the helper's judgment and bias into the interview. Another advantage of the open-ended question is that it may bring forth feelings and attitudes not previously mentioned; these responses may suggest other important and unexplored areas (Brooke Army Medical Center, 1973).

Summarizing is an important skill in a helping relationship. Using this ability, the helper is able to extract the essence of what a patient has intellectually and affectively experienced during their time together. It is a statement made at the close of a discussion that summarizes the content and the process of the interview time. Skillfully and accurately done, it leaves the client with a feeling of knowing what he feels and gives him a sense of having accomplished something during the interview.

Confronting is a skill that should be used cautiously at this level of counseling. Confrontation is a direct statement made by the nurse that challenges the patient with realistic information that opposes his own beliefs. It can be harmful if used before adequate assessment has occurred. If, for example, a patient or family member is under exceptional stress because of hospitalization and is

using denial as a way of coping with it, caregivers frequently think that the person should be confronted. The following case is an example of how stresses other than hospitalization can be having a profound effect on the patient and contribute to his need to deny the situation. In many cases, a sudden illness or hospitalization can be "the straw that breaks the camel's back."

Case Example

John was a 38-year-old executive recently transferred to the midwest from the West coast. At age 35 he experienced an MI. Two months after the move he had a second massive MI and was not expected to live. His caregivers were concerned and angry that his wife did not understand the seriousness of his illness and, instead, was more concerned about finding a job in the new community.

In talking with her, the psychiatric liaison nurse discovered that her father had died 6 months earlier of a heart attack and that her two teenage sons had been doing poorly in school since the move. In addition, she had been strongly opposed to, and was very unhappy about, the move away from her family and friends on the West coast.

His wife needed a chance to talk about the anger and grief she was experiencing because of the overwhelming events that had occurred in the previous 6 months. After only 2 half-hour discussions, her denial about her husband's terminal status disappeared. Without understanding the serious underlying issues, a confronting caregiver could have prodded her into a severe crisis situation. An important guideline to use when strong and *apparently* inappropriate denial is observed is as follows: *what* is the denial defending the patient from knowing, and *why* can't he tolerate knowing it? This involves taking the time to know what else is occurring in the patient's life.

The type of confrontation discussed in the case example above is different than that used in a true counseling situation. In a counseling setting, confrontation is used to give the patient information and feedback about his behavior. Confrontation can aid the client in developing insight by making him aware of information about himself that he had not been aware of. Generally speaking, direct confrontation by a nurse in any situation is not recommended. Instead, a less threatening indirect approach such as, "Is it possible that there is a connection between the severe arguments you told me that you have with your husband and the beginning of your asthma symptoms?" could be stated. This approach, which still would be threatening to many people, at least gives the client the opportunity to deny it.

When the statement is phrased as a question preceded by the words "Is it possible that—?" the patient may initially respond by saying "no." Remember, however, that your comment has registered in his unconscious. Later, when the reality is less threatening (sometimes days or weeks later), your question may reenter his conscious awareness, and, in the process of answering it by himself, he will gain insight.

"*Interpreting* is an active helper process of explaining the meaning of events to helpees so that they are able to see their problems in new ways" (Brammer, 1973, p. 102). Interpreting is a high-level skill that requires much training and expertise. It is described as "a psychotherapeutic technique used in psychoanalysis, both individual and group. The therapist conveys to the patient the significance and meaning of his behavior constructing into a more meaningful form the patient's resistances, defenses, transferences, and symbols (dreams)" (Freedman and colleagues, 1976, p. 1310). It should be used only in a psychotherapy setting. Nurses should not attempt to interpret in this manner because the effects of an interpretation are never predictable and the patient may be unnecessarily upset. If the earlier skills of paraphrasing, clarifying, perception checking, open-ended questions, and accurate reflection of content and affect are mastered, the patient usually finds his own answers in the counseling setting.

Advice giving is the last category to be discussed under this heading. In almost every counseling situation, and many hospital circumstances, advice is contraindicated. Many of the events that occur during hospitalization have an unexpected or crisis component to them, however (Brammer, 1973). As a coping aid to patients and families in these situations, it is possible that some advice may be appropriate. For example, an adolescent may be diagnosed as diabetic and react maladaptively by ignoring his diet, doing poorly in school, and engaging in antisocial behavior. The diabetes nurse specialist can, in addition to letting him talk about how he feels about the illness, give him information about how others have dealt with the problem. This may give him some alternatives to consider, raise his level of hope, and reverse his maladaptive pattern.

Because advice may seem to be "the easy way out" in many situations, it is important to be aware of the negative effects of inappropriate adivce giving. Frequently, dependent types of persons will ask nurses what they should do about a particular problem. Solving "all" problems for patients in this way further encourages their dependence on the caregiving system. Frequently, clients do not follow the advice of caregivers but may blame them if their situations continue to deteriorate. The caregiver(s) then may feel angry and used. Another negative effect of advice giving is that the caregiver may react to the patient's resulting dependence by feeling pressured to continually come up with solutions to seemingly impossible problems. Eventually, the burdened caregiver "distances" from the demanding, dependent patient. The result is that the patient feels abandoned and rejected without understanding why.

Other Characteristics of the Relationship

Contracts

An important aspect of any relationship is that the two people involved have an understanding of what their responsibilities are and what the relationship means to each. In formal counseling settings, this is known as a *contract*. The two types of contracts in which nurses engage with their patients are *formal* and *informal* contracts. Formal contracts occur whenever nurses tell patients they will take care of them and patients agree verbally or nonverbally to receive their care. These are verbal contracts and appear informal, but they are taken seriously by the patient. A primary nurse, for example, is someone who makes a formal contract with a patient.

As described in Chapter 6: Major Psychosocial Issues of Patients With Physical Illness, one of the first issues confronting a newly hospitalized patient is trusting an alien environment. For many of these patients, their nurses are the second most trusted people in the hospital (their physicians are usually first). If nurses do not value themselves properly, they may overlook their importance to patients (Barry, 1979). Accordingly, they may neglect to tell a patient that they will be off for 2 days. When told this by the head nurse or nurse's substitute, their confidence in the nurse *and* the environment erodes.

If a clinical specialist promises a patient that he or she will be in to see the patient *every other day,* the patient should be told in advance if this schedule will change. If it is necessary to cancel the visit for a particular day, a call should be made to the nursing unit. A message should be relayed to the patient by a staff member about the cancellation and another time given when he can plan on a visit.

Incidents that actually are informal types of contracts with patients are requests for pain medication, and nurses' promises that they will be back in 5 minutes, or a promise to a patient in the operating room that the nurse will stay with him until the anesthesia is given. Although these may seem incidental, they form the foundation of trust for the hospital patient.

Termination

Termination is the psychological term for saying goodbye. Most people have been negatively socialized about saying goodbye. As a result, they may, figuratively speaking, bury their heads in the sand, try to avoid unpleasant feelings, and assume that there will be no consequences if they do not say goodbye. Accordingly, although nurses are aware that patients will be discharged from the hospital on a specific day, they may avoid discussing their feelings about the patient's leaving until the day the person is being discharged; a quick "good luck" may be the only goodbye the nurse expresses. The patient may be someone to whom the nurse has become attached during a long hospitalization, or there may have been a close primary nurse-patient relationship.

In these instances, what do you think happens to both the patient's and the nurse's feelings? These feelings of loss, although they are not the same as the loss of death, are feelings of loss nonetheless. If not expressed, they are repressed or avoided. The more adaptive behavior is to acknowledge them and allow them to be felt.

When the nurse avoids discussing feelings about a special patient's discharge, he or she may be blocking the patient from expressing similar feelings. A special time of validation of both the patient's worth to the nurse and the nurse's worth to the patient is also lost. This openness in a relationship is an example of the intimacy that Erikson (1963) has described as essential to mature and adult relationships. An important responsibility nurses have to their patients is to say goodbye before the actual moment when the patient is being wheeled out the door. This allows the patient to express his feelings about the nurse and the care he received. He may also express

some anxiety about going home and leaving the protective hospital environment that otherwise has not been explored. All this is a healthy and normal conclusion to the nurse-patient relationship. If a formal type of counseling relationship has been established with a patient, the discussion of termination should be brought up in a session before the final one. This gives the patient a chance to work through some of his feelings about leaving the relationship, and it will also promote a more mature way of handling losses in the future.

Referral

In the course of working with a patient, the nurse may become aware that the patient's mental state is deteriorating or is more impaired than originally evident. These symptoms of changed mental status (see Chapter 10: The Mental Status Examination) should be discussed with the head nurse and physician. The staff nurse in the inpatient or outpatient setting is usually the first caregiver to notice the changes. If warranted, a recommendation for psychiatric consultation can be made to the head nurse. In a primary nursing setting, make the recommendation directly to the physician, taking care to be articulate about the various aspects of the patient's mental status or psychosocial functioning that concern you.

The most important reason for referring a patient to another caregiver is that the helper does not possess the skills the client requires. The decision and rationale for referral should be discussed with the patient so that he does not feel abandoned or hopeless about his outcome (Farr, 1979). If the nurse knows some positive information about the consultant, a low-keyed statement to that effect could help allay some of the patient's anxiety about the referral. Overselling the consultant's abilities could be detrimental, however.

If referral occurs and time permits, do not withdraw from the patient. Remember that an unexpressed fear of most patients is abandonment. You may have become an important person to him. If you do not maintain your relationship with him, it could undermine his confidence and trust in the environment. Remember to ask the consultant what types of approaches and interventions with the patient could be most helpful to him.

Support Groups

A new role for nurses in many settings is serving as a leader or co-leader of a support group for inpatients or outpatients who have similar types of problems in dealing with a chronic health problem. Some examples of these are groups for parents of infants in a neonatal intensive care unit, groups for cancer patients and their family members, and groups for patients who have had an MI. It is important for nurses to understand the difference between support groups and therapy groups. The purpose of a *support group* is to provide people with a setting in which they can discuss their illness-related problems with other people who have the same illness. By sharing their feelings, they receive mutual support and caring from others who can fully understand the problem. The recommended training for a nurse group leader is that he or she have attended a group dynamics course in the university setting. The course should have theoretical and group membership components. The new leader also should have served as an assistant or coleader with another, more experienced support group leader before attempting to lead a group on his or her own.

It is essential that support group leaders realize that their clinical preparation has not prepared them to conduct a therapy group. The leader of a therapy group has had graduate-level training in psychiatric and counseling skills.

In order to understand the difference between a support group and a therapy group, the purpose of a *therapy group* is to examine all areas and aspects of a person's intrapsychic and interpersonal functioning. The leader is an active force in the dynamics of the group. He may use interpretation (see above) as an aid to group process. The purpose of the support group leader is very different; the leader's role is to *reflect back* the statements of the various members. The function of the leader is to *assist* the group members as *they* support one another. A common mistake of inexperienced support group leaders is to become *actively* involved in the group members' process. It is more difficult to maintain an empathic objective stance in a group than in a one-to-one relationship because of the cumulative effect of the activity and emotional level of the group. It is easy to be swept up in the feelings of the group.

In a support group, a person may raise intrapsychic and interpersonal issues not relating to the illness. He may also raise intrapsychic and interpersonal issues that relate to the illness but are very emotionally complex. In either case, tell him, in the presence of the other group members, that discussing these types of issues is not a function of the group and that you will talk with him after the session about other sources of assistance

available to him. This will prevent the further complication for you of having other members raise subjects that are inappropriate and not within your background and capabilities to manage therapeutically. After the support group session is over, the leader can discuss referral possibilities if any clients want them. Patients should be encouraged to remain in the group even if they become involved in individual counseling.

When support groups fail, the leaders usually are very disappointed. They wonder why patients do not return after the first few sessions. Frequently, it is because of the leader's overinvolvement in the process and lack of experience in keeping the group members focused on the *original* purpose of the group.

Formation

The number of people in the group should range from 8 to 12. With fewer than eight people in the beginning stage, the possibility of losing a few members during ensuing weeks may be detrimental to good group dynamics. More than 12 people results in a group with multiple dynamics, which could prove too complex for an inexperienced leader. It also results in incomplete participation from all members because of the large number. Group cohesiveness thus may not occur.

Before beginning the group, it is essential to establish admission criteria. An interview with each prospective member should be conducted. If members are automatically allowed to enter, the possibility of having inappropriate members in the group, with resulting failure of the group, is greatly increased. The purpose of the interview is to rule out persons with moderate to severe psychopathology. The best clue to a potential problem is that the prospective leader feels anxious in the interview. In a group setting, this person could arouse high anxiety in the other group members as well as in the leader.

Potential leaders, in their eagerness to start a group, frequently dislike having pregroup screening interviews, but they are strongly recommended. Some of the questions that could be asked are as follows: "Why do you think the group would be helpful to you?" "What do you think you'll gain from the other group members?" and "Tell me how things have been going for you following your heart attack?" The answers to these questions should give the leader a general idea of how the person relates with others. If the client seems inappropriate for the group, then a referral to a private therapist or public mental health clinic should be given.

When the Group Begins

At the start of the first session, the leader should explain the rules of the group. He or she should say, "The function of this group is to talk about the feelings we have about cancer and the changes that cancer has caused in our lives." *It is very important to keep the group focused on this goal.* Because feelings are difficult to talk about, group members often will try to divert to "thinking" types of statements. If the group leader does not gently pull them back into the feeling area, the group usually is not as effective and the group members may gradually drop out. The most successful support groups are ones in which feelings about the effects the illness has caused are discussed. The discovery of mutuality in a group is very comforting to members and is one of the most important outcomes. They begin to realize that the feelings that they thought were too intense or extreme and their response to this unexpected life change are normal when compared with those of the other group members.

Most support groups are of limited duration, usually 6 weeks. The duration of the group and the length of each meeting should be announced before the first session. Ninety minutes is usually the most effective time period. It should be *strictly* adhered to.

Stages of Group Development

It is important to be aware that all time-limited groups have set stages of development. If the group is of 6 weeks' or 1 year's duration, each of the three stages will take approximately one third the time. The middle stage in the year-long group may take up somewhat more than one third the time. The stages, adapted from Yalom (1975), are as follows:

1. *Opening stage.* Search for goals and structure takes place.
2. *Middle or working stage:*
   a. Various members vie for positions within the group
   b. A cohesive group forms; teamwork is dominant
3. *Last or termination stage.* Characterized by increased self-disclosure; group may become

more subdued; discussions of death may occur.

In this type of support group, the last stage frequently also involves a strong sense of mutual understanding, caring, and support. An intimacy may develop between members that is carried into relationships that endure beyond the group. Because of the similar problems members share, they find the support they may have lacked from other people.

The stages described above will develop only in a group that has a specific starting and end point. This is called a *time-limited group.* It usually occurs only in an outpatient setting. As a contrast, support groups in the general hospital usually have open membership, with members attending for a few sessions and dropping out when discharged. This type of group, which has no definite beginning and completion time, is called an *ongoing group.*

All the counseling theory presented in this chapter can be adapted to the group setting. The concept of process is even more dynamic in the group setting than in the individual setting (Litwack and colleagues, 1980). The transference and resistance issues of several members interacting with each other *and* with the countertransference and possibly resistance issues of one or two co-leaders results in numerous effects. All are beyond the full awareness of any group leader. For this reason, it is strongly recommended to record the entire session so that the leader(s) can listen to it after the session. Usually the recording introduces many new awarenesses that the leader(s) missed during the actual session. The request to record the group session should be introduced just before the first session begins. If the leader explains that it will be confidential and he is doing it only so he can help the participants, members usually have no objection.

Another recommendation is for the group leader to negotiate one hour of supervision time after each group session from a psychiatrist, psychologist, psychiatric nurse specialist, or psychiatric social worker who works in the same hospital and has had experience leading groups. It is important to remember that support groups relating to illness usually involve discussion of life's deepest issues: dying, hopelessness, conflict within the family, anger, and so on. An inexperienced group leader can begin to feel overwhelmed if he or she does not have an experienced consultant available to review the group's progress and issues. Usually someone is willing to spare an hour of time to listen to the tapes, supervise the leader's work, and answer questions.

Conclusion

This chapter has presented many concepts that are part of the counseling process. If you are new to the caregiving role, remember that it can take a long time to develop these skills. A psychiatrist acquaintance once remarked that it took him at least 10 years of training to learn psychiatric theory and be able to use it comfortably in his work with patients.

It is important to be aware of these concepts so that you can recognize that "talking with patients" is actually a very complex and potentially highly therapeutic clinical skill. If you work in nursing for 10 years and read and apply this chapter every year, you will discover that each year you can acquire higher levels of skill in your assessment of patients' psychosocial status. In addition, you may be able to conduct therapeutic interventions that more strongly support patients' adaptation to illness. Without knowing appropriate psychosocial theory and counseling skills, nurses may stand by helplessly as their patients maladapt because they do not know what to do. Knowing *what* to do for a patient in emotional distress and *how* to do it can be one of the most challenging and rewarding aspects of being a nurse.

This section of the book is the "how to" part. Nursing textbooks often urge nurses to intervene with patients who are at risk for psychosocial maladaptation. Nurses often feel uncertain about what they should or should not do with these patients. Traditionally, recommendations for intervention have included the following: encourage verbalizing, support coping, promote ventilation, and so on. This section is written to give you more definite guidelines on which to base your nursing intervention process. The recommendations are derived from the fields of nursing, medicine, and social work and from my own experience in working with physically ill patients and their families who are struggling to cope with the effects of illness. The process of assessing patients' and family members' responses to illness can be carried out effectively using the structure of the nursing process.

The nursing process is a flexible approach to patient care that can be used in any type of setting. It is not intended to be a rigid process or one that imposes restrictions on a nurse's creativity in designing care. Rather, it is intended to give the nurse a structure on which to develop his or her nursing care plan. It allows for the uniqueness of patients and nurses and is intended to meet the needs of both.

The steps of the nursing process are briefly reviewed below.

The Nursing Process

1. *Assessing.* Assessing involves collecting information about the patient and his family to compile a nursing history and diagnosis. The information includes data about physical, intra-psychic, and social functioning. The nursing diagnosis should be based on the approved list of nursing diagnosis categories presented at the end of Chapter 13: Psychosocial Nursing Assessment and Diagnosis. Further information on the etiology and defining characteristics of each diagnostic category can be found in the appendix.
2. *Planning.* The planning phase uses the nursing diagnosis(es) as its base. The information obtained in the assessment phase is used in your initial problem-solving process. When a general plan is being formulated, include the patient in the process whenever possible. You can review appropriate aspects of your plan with him and seek his opinions and recommendations. When the alternatives have been

Part Two

Application of Psychosocial Nursing Theory to the Nursing Process

worked through, the nursing care plan is complete.

3. *Implementing.* Implementing is the action phase of the nursing care plan. An important aspect of the nursing care plan is that it be used by *all* nursing team members so that the caregiving system approaches the patient in the same or similar ways. This phase is strongly interactive. The patient, family members, caregivers from other disciplines, and nurses all contribute in their own way to the patient's psychosocial response to the stress of illness.

Another very important contribution to this response is the patient's intrapsychic functioning: his normal personality style, his mental status (which may be temporarily altered because of the effects of illness or drugs on the brain), and his normal response to stress. The implementation phase includes ongoing assessment of the interactions described above and the flexibility of the nurse in modifying the original care plan.

4. *Evaluating.* Evaluating involves assessing the patient's response to your nursing intervention. Has the problem identified in your nursing diagnosis been resolved? Is it still present? Is it worse? Depending on your assessment, your care plan will be subject to modification and new approaches may be necessary. In reality, the evaluation phase can actually be the first phase in a circular nursing process that is continually responding to patients' needs.

13

Psychosocial Nursing Assessment and Diagnosis

Nursing assessment has been defined by Marriner (1978) as

> the first phase of the nursing process. Before the nurse can plan the patient's care, she must identify and define the patient's problems. Consequently, this phase includes collection of data about the health status of the patient and ends with the nursing diagnosis, a statement of the patient's problem [p. 1].

The term *data collection* may seem somewhat technical to nurses. It seems to be a computer-age concept. Actually, data collection is what nurses have always done since Florence Nightingale's time. Data collection is the assembling of all information about the patient's physiological, psychological, and social functioning. The sources of information used are many: the patient, physician, laboratory and other test findings, family, social worker, and so on. As part of the nursing process, you will be the data processor who pulls together all these bits of information. As part of the assessment process, you will integrate all these bits of information and apply the multiple theories you know about normal and abnormal physiological, psychological, and social functioning to formulate a list of the patient's problems. As you integrate all these concepts (something that many experienced nurses have been doing all along, before all these high-sounding terms were applied to the steps involved), you will actually be using a systems approach.

In many institutions the basic nursing approach to patient assessment is to emulate the medical model of patient assessment, which is based on evaluating physical pathology. Rarely obtained is the history of social stressors that the patient has experienced, especially those experienced during the year preceding the development of physical illness. Similarly, no history of the patient's normal way of coping with stress is obtained. Little attention is paid to the effects of illness on the psychological processes and family dynamics until the patient or a member of the family develops psychiatric symptoms. If psychosocial assessment and ongoing patient evaluation is carried out by nurses, it can and *does* result in fewer psychological emergencies for patients and families both in the hospital and after discharge.

Justification for Importance of Psychosocial Nursing Assessment

The importance of nursing assessment of psychosocial status can be understood when you consider that the National Conferences on Nursing Diagnosis (1974, 1976, 1978, 1980, and 1982) have identified that two thirds of the disorders that nurses are capable of independently diagnosing and treating are in the psychosocial categories (Kim and Moritz, 1982). Clearly, our priority setting in delivering professional patient care may be shifted as the nursing diagnosis movement becomes more widely accepted.

As nurses, you have the potential to identify patients who are beginning the process of emotional maladaptation to physical illness. If intervention does not occur and the process continues, two responses are probable:

The patient may experience an in-hospital crisis and the problem may continue after his discharge.

The patient and his family will experience a decrease in the quality of their lives because of his ongoing postdischarge maladaptation. The effects will eventually be experienced by all members of the family system.

With astute nursing assessment, the precrisis types of maladaptive processes such as depression, anxiety, and other signs of inadequate coping can be reversed.

The maladaptive process can be identified only if an adequate psychosocial assessment is part of the admission and ongoing evaluation data base. Some hospitals require that nurses obtain little or no psychosocial history from the patient. I strongly recommend including in all nursing histories questions that will give the nurses who care for the patient a good personality and coping profile of the patient. Nursing has unfortunately taken many of its clues about what data to include on an admission assessment from the medical model and frequently performs minimal psychosocial assessment. It is important to remember that nursing and medicine are different caregiving disciplines with different objectives in their care delivery to patients. Nursing is the only primary caregiving discipline prepared to monitor the psychosocial as well as the physical response of the patient and his family to illness.

The Psychosocial Nursing Assessment Interview

The psychosocial assessment interview presented here takes approximately one half hour to complete. It can be modified to a shorter form, but none of the major categories should be deleted. Before beginning the interview, take the time to explain to the patient that one of your responsibilities as a nurse is to understand how he is feeling about and reacting to his illness in order to help him during his recovery. This introduction during the admission process helps the patient to feel understood. It can give him a sense of security at a time when he usually is feeling apprehensive and alone (but frequently has no one in whom he can confide). Remember that he often will hesitate to tell his family his fears because he may need to be "strong" for them. In addition, this introduction will give a professional stamp to your questions, some of which are very personal.

Ideally, the interview should take place in a setting that affords privacy for you and the patient. Realistically, most hospitals have no provisions for quiet discussion with patients because space is limited.*

In the actual interview, use the techniques recommended in Chapter 12 to promote trust and openness. Your approach to the patient should primarily be that of a nonjudgmental listener. If the patient begins to ask your opinion about the various information he is presenting to you, return the question to him by asking, "What do you think?" This often happens during the admission process. The patient is essentially looking for your *acceptance*, not your opinion. Regardless of what you say, his level of anxiety will often prevent him from fully hearing your response. The patient may tell you, for example, how his family usually responds to trouble or that he has difficulty falling asleep at night and ask you what you think it might mean. By returning the question to him, you are saying, "Your own opinion about this situation is important. Tell me more about it." You are validating *him* with this approach. Sometimes,

---

*The best you can do to insure privacy is to pull the curtain between him and his roommate. Do not pull it completely around the bed, however. In an interview a completely closed curtain often leaves the patient with an uncomfortable feeling of being closed in. In addition, if he cannot see the door he may wonder if someone other than his roommate has entered the room. By sitting on a chair close to the head of the bed, you should be able to maintain a fairly reasonable level of privacy.

nurses will respond to this type of patient question with the response, "I don't know. Why don't you ask your physician?" Put yourself in the patient's place. Imagine yourself as a patient in the hospital. What would be your own response to this nurse? Would you feel accepted by him or her? Would you feel a developing level of trust? Or, would you feel avoided and put off?

Whether a family member can be present during this interview is left to your own discretion. If the patient is a child or is not a reliable informant, a family member should give the information. It can be a valuable part of your assessment to have a family member (usually a spouse) present. His or her presence can ensure a far more realistic impression of the response of both the patient and his family to the stress of illness. It is understandable, however, that family members' visits and nurse's available time often do not coincide. Accordingly, an interview with the patient alone can provide adequate information.

Psychosocial Nursing Assessment Process

Several areas are included in a psychosocial nursing history, and they will be outlined and described in this section. The rationale for including each of these categories will be explained. The categories included in the assessment process are as follows:

1. Social history
2. Level of stress during year before admission
3. Normal coping ability
4. Neurovegetative changes
5. Patient's understanding of illness
6. Mental status
7. Personality style
8. Major psychosocial issue(s) of illness
9. Psychosocial nursing diagnosis and potential for maladaptation

In the process of obtaining information from the patient about the first five categories listed above, you should consider using the psychosocial assessment rating form that begins on page 160. Before you begin the interview, explain to the patient that your job as his nurse is to oversee his overall response, both physically and emotionally, to his illness. In addition, the information can ensure that his family receives the support it needs. In this way, he can better understand the nature of the questions. He may inquire why you need to

know specific bits of information because they do not seem relevant to nursing or his illness. You will find that in the section following the rating scale I have described the reasons why this information is important in your assessment of the patient's potential for adaptation. If the patient should inquire, it can offer a fine opportunity to you to teach him about the effects of stress and life stressors on human beings.

In order to complete the last four categories on the assessment rating scale, you can return to the nurses' station and review the patient's interaction with you. It is helpful during the interview to keep in mind the various objective assessments that you will be completing after the session. For example, if, during the interview, you see indications of a mildly abnormal mental status, you will want to ask your questions in such a way that you can better observe the patient's style of thinking, memory, judgment, and so on.

The same is true regarding the patient's response to his illness. If you ask him how he feels about his illness, how he thinks it will affect him in the future, and so on, you may observe a strong potential for maladaptation. If so, obtain more data so that you have the information you need to implement the nursing process properly.

The psychosocial assessment rating scale appears in the following chart. After the psychosocial assessment rating scale, you will find a justification for including each category as well as a more detailed explanation of the evaluation process of each category.

Rationale for Psychosocial Assessment Categories

Social History

The social history includes basic data about the patient, such as name, age, date of admission, religion, and marital status. Use the demographic data on the patient's chart for this information.

Religion
The patient's religious affiliation is a routine piece of demographic information in most hospitals. It becomes more important data, however, if the patient's ability to cope is weakened by the threat of illness. When this occurs, any available persons

(Text continues on p. 163.)

Psychosocial Assessment Rating Scale

Social History

Name ———————————————— Age ———— Date of admission ——————

Religion —————————— Is pastor a supportive person? ————

Date of assessment ————

Marital status S —— M —— W —— D —— How long ——————

Occupation ————————————————

Admitting diagnosis ———————————————

With whom do you live? ————————————

Members of immediate family (names not necessary). Relationships should be listed. Include deceased members and dates of death.

Position of patient in relation to brothers and sisters (e.g., second oldest, youngest) ——————

How often do you see your parents and brothers and sisters? ——————————

Is there someone you confide in when you have a problem?

Yes ——— No ——— Who?———————

What goes on in your family when something bad happens? What do most of the members do?

Smoking history

Do you smoke? ———— How long have you been smoking? ————

How many packs per day? ————

Alcohol use history

Do you drink? ———— How often? ———— How much? ————

History of alcoholism in family? ———— Who? ————

Level of Stress During Year Before Admission

How long have you been out of work with this illness? ——————

Changes in family during the last 2 years. Which family members are involved? Include dates.

Death ———— Was this someone you were close to? ————

Divorce ————

Child leaving home ———— Cause? ————

New baby ————

Illness in other family member ————

Change in residence Yes ———— No ————

Cause? ————

Changes in relationships within the immediate and extended family ————

If so, to what do you attribute the cause? ————

Has there been any unusual stress during the last year that is still affecting the family? ———— Describe it.

Psychosocial Assessment Rating Scale (continued)

Change in job or school (if student) _____

(Delete remaining questions if student)

Unusual job stress during the past year _____
What was the cause? _____ Do you expect it will still be present when you return to work? _____

Retirement _____

Fired _____

Same job but new boss or working relationship _____

Promotion or demotion _____

Normal Coping Ability

When you go through a very difficult time, how do you normally handle it?

Talk it out with someone _____

Ignore it _____

Get angry and yell _____

Get angry and hit or throw something _____

Drink _____

Become anxious _____

Become depressed _____

Other (Explain) _____

What is the most difficult time you have experienced in your life? _____
How long did it take you to get over it? _____

What did you do to cope with it? _____

Neurovegetative Functioning

Normal sleeping pattern

How many hours per night? _____

What hour to what hour? _____ to _____

Changes in normal sleeping pattern

Difficulty falling asleep _____

Middle of night awakening _____

Early morning awakening _____

Sleeping more or fewer hours than normal _____ How many? _____

Change in appetite?   Increase _____ Decrease _____

Change in energy level? Increase _____ Decrease _____

Change in sexual functioning? _____

How? _____

For how long? _____

Have you associated your change in sexual functioning with some other event? _____

Do you think that this illness could change your normal pattern of sexual functioning? _____

How? _____

Patient's Understanding of Illness

What was the original problem that caused you to come to the hospital? _____

(continued)

Psychosocial Assessment Rating Scale (continued)

On what date did you first become ill? ————————

How are things going for you here in the hospital?

How do you feel about being in the hospital?

How can the physicians and nurses help you most?

How will this illness affect you when you are out of the hospital?

Do you think it will cause any changes in your life?

How will it affect your family?

This is the end of the formal interview process (the subjective part of the assessment). The remainder of the psychosocial assessment will be based on your objective assessment of the patient.

Mental Status

In this section state whether the patient's mental status was within normal limits. If not, briefly describe the presenting problem.

Time and date of mental status evaluation ————————

Orientation and level of awareness ————————

Appearance and behavior ————————

Speech and communication ————————

Mood ————————

Thinking process ————————

Perception ————————

Abstract thinking ————————

Social judgment ————————

Personality Style*

Write brief sentence explaining choice.

Dependent ————————

Controlled ————————

Dramatizing ————————

Suspicious ————————

Self-sacrificing ————————

Superior ————————

Uninvolved ————————

*If limited data are available, this category can be completed within 48 hours after admission.

Psychosocial Assessment Rating Scale (continued)

Mixed (usually two styles predominate) _____

No predominate personality style _____

Response to interviewer: Guarded? _____ Open? _____

Able to maintain good eye contact? _____

Major Psychological Issue(s) of Illness

What are the major issues of *this* illness for *this* patient? Explain why.

Trust _____

Self-esteem _____

Body image _____

Control _____

Loss _____

Guilt _____

Intimacy _____

Psychosocial nursing diagnosis and potential for psychosocial maladaptation? Use one or more of the approved nursing diagnoses. Justify briefly your reasoning for each category.

Nursing diagnosis

(This rating scale was developed by Patricia D. Barry.)

whom the patient or family view as support persons should be called on. If the patient identifies his pastor as someone whom he trusts and has confidence in, he can be a valuable ally in the midst of a psychosocial crisis response to illness.

Marital Status

Whatever the patient's marital status, it is important to ask him how long he has been married, widowed, or divorced. Any one of these categories, if it occurred during the previous year, is a major stressor. Research has demonstrated that the rates of physical and mental illness and death are sharply increased in the recently bereaved (Maddison, 1968; Parkes and associates, 1969). Holmes and Rahe (1967) also found that marital separation, as well as the process of being married, were significant stressors in the lives of their research participants.

Occupation

The patient's occupation, as mentioned in an earlier chapter, can give you many clues, such as how this illness is likely to affect his working status. For example, someone who works as an auto body repairman and has suffered a myocardial infarction (MI) will not be able to return to work as easily

as an accountant; in addition, an accountant may be more inclined to be a type A personality for whom control is important. This need could be potentially identified early in his admission, rather than after several days when his anxiety level requires sedation. Occupation can also give you a general idea of the patient's social and intellectual status. This is a less threatening question than asking a patient how much he earns a year or how many years of schooling he has completed. Remember that some illnesses can leave a patient impaired so that return to his normal role is not possible. This increases the risk of maladaptation for both the patient and his family.

The next part of the social history gives you important information about the patient's support system. The answers to these questions will give you very good data about the strength of his support system and his ability to relate to others. Based on his responses to these questions, you can begin the deductive process of listening for clues about personality style.

Family Relationships

It is not necessary to obtain the names of family members. Instead, you are seeking the types of relationships that exist in the family: for example, mother, father dead, two sisters, and a brother. Ask the patient about deceased members of his immediate family and the dates they died. This will give you information about his family's experience with major object losses.

The position of the patient in relation to siblings, although not entirely predictable, can give you an idea of the patient's personality style. In general, oldest children tend to be more highly motivated and have more need for control than youngest children, who tend to be more dependent and passive (because many people met their needs in their original families). Middle children, on the other hand, tend to be more flexible and adaptable (Toman, 1976).

How often the patient sees his parents and siblings and whether he has someone in whom he can confide are very important pieces of information. They will tell you how able this person is to relate to others. If he develops any type of complication in the hospital, will he be able to receive support from someone close to him? Persons with suspicious or aloof personality styles are unlikely to have a close relationship with anyone. In many cases, the controlled person may also have difficulty with openness in a relationship. Watch for the patient's emotional response to the following relationship-related questions. Does he demonstrate pleasure, sadness, anger, and so on? "What goes on in your family when a very bad event happens? What do most of the members do?" This will tell you the normal family coping style, an important clue to how the family system will respond if the patient faces a crisis. Remember, too, that in some families, a member entering a hospital for any type of illness is a strong enough stress to begin family maladaptation.

Smoking History

If the patient is a heavy smoker and is admitted for an illness, such as cardiac illness, that will require him to give up smoking, his anxiety level will be increased.

Alcohol Use History

It has been reported that from 27% to 60% of all hospital admissions are alcohol related (Barcha and colleagues, 1968; Gomberg, 1975; Kearney, 1968). Such questions as "Do you drink? How often? How much? Is there a history of alcoholism in your family? Who?" may elicit an answer.*

*If the patient does have a drinking problem, he may not acknowledge it. By observing for body language and evasive eye contact at the time of the question, you will have a better indication about the reliability of his answer.

Without obtaining information about the patient's drinking history, it is possible that the patient will receive full medical treatment, be discharged in good condition, and return to the hospital in 3 months because his drinking has precipitated another disease process. This is an expensive omission caused by lack of adequate assessment of caregivers.

Many hospitals have alcohol counselors who work with patients and promote Alcoholics Anonymous concepts with alcoholic patients. The question about history of alcoholism in the family is important because the child of an alcoholic parent is five times more likely to be an alcoholic (Estes and colleagues, 1980).

Level of Stress During Year Before Admission

As Chapter 9 suggested, research has demonstrated a high correlation between high levels of stress and the development of illness. Newly admitted patients frequently report a high level of change in their lives during the year or so before admission. *If questions about stress are asked on admission, the patient will frequently attribute the development of his illness to one or more of these stressors.*

Realistically, the physician, using a medical model, is not likely to obtain a good history of the patient's stress because the patient's psychosocial sphere is not his or her major interest. (Remember, the nursing diagnosis movement *has* identified the psychosocial sphere as the major interest of the nurse because nearly 70% of its diagnostic categories are in the psychosocial realm.)

If this information is not routinely obtained, we may miss one of the original precipitants of the patient's illness. We can patch him and heal him only to let him be discharged at the same inadequate coping level into the same social system that may have caused the stress that helped bring on his illness. If we are aware of these problems, there are interventions that can promote more adaptive patient responses.

Changes in Family

Changes in the family, such as death, divorce, a child leaving home, a new baby, an illness in another family member, a change in residence, and a change in job or financial state can all be stressful. Remember that Holmes and Rahe (1967) found that positive changes could be as stressful as negative changes because of the necessary adjustment process.

Changes in Work or School

How long the patient has been out of work with his current illness will tell you the level of stress the patient and family may be experiencing because of economic hardship. If a breadwinner is out of work for several weeks or more, there are usually major strains in the relationships between all family members.

Normal Coping Ability

In this part of the history you will learn how the patient normally copes. By asking the few questions below, you will find out what *conscious* coping strategies the patient uses when he is severely stressed. The word *conscious* tells you that these are actual strategies that he is aware of using. Coping strategies are different from unconscious defense mechanisms, which the patient is not aware of. This is very important information as you plan your nursing intervention. Your care plan should support the patient's normal coping style.

Most patients know what coping method works best for them in reducing stress. You may have to ask a few questions to discover what it is. When you find out, you can assess whether it may help during the current illness. The following case examples clarify this point.

Case Examples

Jim is 28 years old and a garage mechanic. One day, while he was working in the garage, a car fell onto him. His neck was broken, and he was permanently paralyzed from the neck down. Jim's wife said that his normal way of handling stress was to pound his fist against the wall. Given this information, what would you expect Jim's ability to cope adequately to be?

Diane is a 32-year-old schoolteacher. She and her husband were happily expecting their first child. During her fifth month of pregnancy the fetus was unexpectedly aborted. Diane says that when she is under stress, she normally shares everything with her husband, who is very understanding and caring. Given this information, what would you expect Diane's ability to cope adequately will be?

Can you see how obtaining this type of information can help you to anticipate coping problems and potential for patient maladaptation? As a further point, how would you evaluate Diane's coping potential if she told you that her husband was working in the Middle East for 6 months as a management consultant and would be given only a 2-week leave of absence?

The questions to ask your patient are as follows: "When you have stress in your everyday life, what do you do to decrease it?" or "When you go through a very difficult time, how do you normally handle it?" Many patients are able to immediately tell you what they do. Others may need more help in finding their answer. If they should ask, "What do you mean?" you can inquire, "What is the worst thing that ever happened to you? How did you get over it?"

Remember that hospitalizations can be a major crisis for the patient and family. Their normal, everyday stress responses may not work for them. It is important to keep in mind that the way that people respond to stress usually does not change significantly over a lifetime. If, for example, the patient experienced a major crisis in his 20s and responded with serious depression, there is an increased possibility that depression can occur as the result of this current crisis.

Usually patients are able to identify their normal response specifically if you describe some possibilities:

Talk it out with someone

Ignore it (actually, defense mechanisms of repression, denial, or avoidance are being unconsciously used)

Get angry and yell

Get angry and hit or throw something

Drink

Become agitated

Become depressed

Anything that I have not mentioned?

Another important question to elicit the patient's previous response to crisis is, "How long did it take you to get over it?" The patient's answer will tell you about his adaptive ability. Remember, however, that major losses of significant persons usually take a year to resolve. Be realistic in your evaluation of whether the patient's crisis resolution time was within normal limits.

Neurovegetative Functioning

Some of these neurovegetative functions may already be included in the nursing or medical assessment histories in your institutions and agencies. *All* the functions should be assessed for an accurate data base. If abnormal, they may indicate unresolved emotional conflict in patients.

These conflicts are usually manifested as depression or anxiety. It is possible that your patient has been depressed or anxious for several months or longer. These difficulties often progress to the physical symptoms in this category. They occur as the result of changes in the autonomic nervous system, which are caused by intrapsychic stress.

Frequently, mystified physicians admit their patients for diagnostic workups based on these chronically occurring physical symptoms. Too often, they fail to ask the patients if they are experiencing any emotional difficulty or unusual stress in their lives. If, in your assessment of neurovegetative functioning, you learn that many of these physical problems are present, be alert to the possibility that the patient may have underlying emotional conflict. Questions about the patient's sleeping pattern (see chart) may provide some insight into his neurovegetative functioning. Likewise, questions about sexual functioning are significant because sexual functioning is an important indication of a person's ability to enjoy life. When people become chronically depressed or anxious, are involved in a conflicted relationship, or have underlying personality disorders, diminished capacity for sexual enjoyment is often one of the first indicators of a problem. In addition, many illnesses and different types of medications cause physiological changes that alter sexual functioning. The patient may associate his changed capacity for enjoyment to his MI of 3 years ago, the birth of his first child, or the beginning of his treatment for hypertension. Many of these causes can be potentially reversed with appropriate intervention. A section on sexual dysfunctioning in Chapter 16: Nursing Intervention With the Emotionally Complex Patient, discusses many of these issues. In addition, information about the threat to intimacy caused by many diseases or conditions is presented in Chapter 17: Psychosocial Aspects of Specific Physical Conditions, and Chapter 18: The Coping Challenge of Chronic Illness.

Patient's Understanding of Illness

During this part of the psychosocial assessment, you will be asking the patient questions that will give you information about how he perceives his illness and the potential threat that it holds for him. Based on your careful observation of him as he answers these questions, you will be able to form your impressions of his mental status, personality style, and potential risk for psycho-

social maladaptation. These questions are more complex than those asked in previous sections. These questions involve not only memory but require the nurse to use more complex thought processes such as problem analysis and problem solving, as well as anticipatory reasoning and judgment.

"What was the original problem that caused you to come to the hospital?" or any similar question that is appropriate for your patient that tells you his reason for being in the hospital provides important information because it tells you how long the patient has had to prepare for the changes that this illness is causing in his life. For example, in Chapter 1 you read about a young man who faced a leg amputation with very little warning. Generally, the shorter the warning, combined with the seriousness of the illness, results in more strain on a patient's and family's ability to cope with major illness.

Your observations of the patient and your memory of the assessment interview should be used to complete the last three sections of the psychosocial assessment.

Mental Status

The responses to these questions will give you information about the patient's cognitive, perceptual (reality testing), and emotional functioning:

> How are things going for you here in the hospital?
>
> How do you feel about being in the hospital?
>
> How can the physicians and nurses help you most?
>
> How will this illness affect you when you are out of the hospital?
>
> Do you think it will cause any changes in your life?
>
> How will it affect your family?

In addition, they will enable you to evaluate his judgment, abstract thinking, and memory.*

Orientation and Level of Awareness

If, during your discussion with the patient, you detect any evidence of confusion, it is recommended that you specifically question if he knows who and where he is as well as the day of the week, month, and year. Many times patients who appear

---

*If the patient's functioning in each of these categories appears to be within an acceptable range, the letters WNL (within normal limits) can be used.

oriented are actually masking mild to moderate confusion.

Appearance and Behavior

What was the patient's general appearance? Was he neat or disheveled? Was there anything remarkable about his posture and overall behavior? Remember, in all these categories, if you observe a normal range, make sure you state it. Otherwise, if there is any change later on, there will be no comparative data.

Speech and Communication

Was the speech garbled, slurred, distinct, rapid, slow, accented? Was there anything remarkable about the patient's nonverbal communication with you?

Mood

What was his emotional state? Did you see a normal range of emotions as the patient discussed various issues with you, or was the range of emotions very constricted? Was he depressed or anxious? Were there wide swings in his emotions when you were with him? Was his mood appropriate for the content of his discussion? Did his emotions match the topic of his discussion?

Thinking Process

Did the patient's statements make sense and proceed to logical conclusions? If so, they reflect a well-ordered thinking process. There are many abnormalities in this category, especially for patients with organic brain syndrome (OBS) of either the dementia or delirium type. Refer to the cognitive section of Chapter 10 for specific references if you observed any abnormalities. These abnormalities in thinking are subject to marked change in the patient with delirium over even a few hours. It is important that you be as specific as possible and note the time of your observations.

Perception

You will not be able to assess fully the patient's perception unless you ask him specific questions about whether he ever sees or hears things that are not really there. Usually this is an inappropriate question for a nurse to ask the majority of general hospital patients, who function well perceptually. Unless you see a patient who appears to be experiencing an organic or functional emotional disorder, you need not ask the question.

Abstract Thinking and Social Judgment

The responses to these categories are based on the manner in which the patient responded to your questions. As the patient presents his thoughts to you, listen for examples of concrete thinking (see Chapter 10: The Mental Status Examination). If the patient is thinking concretely, this will be apparent at various points during the interview. Impairment in judgment may be seen in association with a concrete thinking style. Again, the patient's answers to your questions will indicate his social judgment.

Personality Style

You will be able to evaluate the patient's normal personality style by reflecting on the way he interacted with you. One of the clues will be his eye contact with you. Was he able to maintain eye contact consistently or not? Dependent persons, for example, tend to maintain strong eye contact; they seem to be waiting for your response, looking for approval, or wanting something from you. On the other hand, the suspicious patient, the aloof patient, and sometimes the controlled patient will avoid eye contact with you.

Descriptions of feelings can be another strong indicator of personality style. At any time during the interview, the suspicious or aloof patient will avoid discussing feelings. Feelings may seem strangely missing or absent in the controlled patient. (Remember that one of his strong defense mechanisms is to overintellectualize. He is able to describe his intellectual reaction to something in detail and, at the same time, to repress his feelings about the situation.) His emotions are constricted and lack a normal range. Patients who may demonstrate normal to abnormal levels of feelings are those with dependent personalities, dramatizing, emotionally involved personalities, and long-suffering, self-sacrificing personalities (guilt is a dominant feeling in these patients). The personality styles in which feelings seem dispensed with and in which the patients seem "above" having feelings are the antisocial and the superior personality types.

Descriptions of relationships with other persons are also strong indicators of the patient's normal personality style and the way that he interacts with others. Watch for signs of emotions as the patient describes his family's reaction to his illness or as he tells you about his original family. You can observe the following clues in the different personality types:

Dependent	Needy, clingy, demanding, overly trusting
Orderly, controlled	Neat, intellectual, impatient; asks many questions; may be slightly anxious because of lack of control in the hospital
Dramatizing	Increased level of emotions; captivating; quickly engaged with caretaker but at a more mature level than dependent patient; dramatic
Suspicious, guarded	Low level of trust, poor eye contact, fault-finding about caregivers, food, hospital
Self-sacrificing	Seems unusually tolerant of sick role; refuses pain or sleep medications; illness may have been brought on by patient's exhaustion due to trying to meet others' needs; when discharge planning, states that family's needs are more important than own
Superior	Judges level of care, hospital policies, food to be inferior; requests special services; talks about important people he knows; tries to impress others
Uninvolved, aloof	Generally avoids others; poor eye contact; difficulty talking with others (not to be confused with the shy person, who wants to talk with others but is embarrassed; the aloof patient is completely uninterested); hermit type

Reaction of Patient to Nurse-Interviewer

The way that a patient responds to a nurse-interviewer is usually similar to the way that he reacts to others in his life. Was he comfortable and at ease, or was he anxious and tense? Could he maintain eye contact with you? Or did his eyes consistently look around or at the floor?

Major Psychosocial Issues of Illness

Your evaluation of the degree of risk that the patient's illness presents is based on the uniqueness of your patient. Remember, *all* the major developmental issues of patients are threatened by illness. Your assessment of the threat of *this* illness to *this* patient will be based on the information you obtain in all the categories above. In this section you are asked to evaluate which psychosocial issues will most likely bring about maladaptation.

Identifying the potentially most threatening issues will help you to be more aware of the stress the patient will experience in coping. You may check one or all of the categories. After checking it off, briefly justify the reasoning you used. It can be helpful to begin to identify the potential major issues of the patient's specific condition before you begin the assessment process. For example, a 38-year-old patient who is undergoing a mastectomy will probably experience a challenge adapting to the issues of self-esteem, changed body image, loss, and intimacy. During your assessment process of the patient, you can test your hypothesis based on her coping style, personality style, and so on.

Remember, too, that although you will not be formally assessing the patient's family members, you should be aware of their potential for maladaptation with each of the following major issues. These overall guidelines in assessment of risk should be integrated with the threats of the specific illness. For example, the major issues of a patient following mastectomy, laminectomy, or herniorrhaphy can all be different.

Trust

Persons who are most at risk for problems with trust:

Dependent patients because of overly trusting and dependent behavior

Controlled patients because of need to control all situations

Suspicious patients because their ability to trust is minimal and yet they must follow caregivers' recommendation and accept their care

Uninvolved patients because of desire to be separate and independent of others

Self-esteem

Persons who are most at risk for problems with decrease in self-esteem:

Controlled patients because part of their need for control is related to self-esteem

Persons with a type A personality because there is often a great need to achieve; if the illness results in a change in their ability to work, it will present a greater threat

Superior patients because their behavior is motivated by a need to bolster their self-esteem

Body image change is actually a subheading under self-esteem. A highly significant factor in the risk of the illness is the degree of perceived threat of body change. The following two examples may help to clarify this point: a 24-year-old newly married woman must undergo a hysterectomy due to diethylstilbesterol (DES)-induced cancer, and a 48-year-old menopausal woman must undergo a hysterectomy because of frequent menorrhagia due to benign fibrosis.

Control

Persons who are at risk for problems of control:

Controlled patients because of lack of control in hospital setting

Suspicious patients because of inability to trust caregivers' control of his care

Self-sacrificing patients because their actions, behavior, and motivation seem to be largely controlled by others' needs or by their own exaggerated perception of others' needs; these patients frequently overexert themselves physically after discharge because their own well-being and convalescence are sacrificed on behalf of others

Superior patients because one of the ways that they maintain control over others is frequently by impressing them with their possessions, clothes, and so on; with hospitalization, the patient loses his reliance on these status symbols because he is socially "leveled"

Uninvolved, aloof patients because of their normally very independent state, which is threatened by hospitalization

Loss

Persons who are at risk for problems with loss:

All patients because this category is similar to body image changes; the degree of threat will depend on the level of emotional investment in the lost person, body part, or function

Guilt

Persons who are most at risk for problems with guilt:

Dependent patients whose normal way of interacting with others is passive; frequently, the person is motivated by guilt; if guilt is a major dynamic, then the level of dependency may increase

Controlled patients because their superegos (consciences) are already critical of themselves; extra guilt is a difficult burden

Self-sacrificing patients because their behavior is often motivated by feelings of guilt and unworthiness

Intimacy

Persons who are most at risk for problems with intimacy:

Suspicious patients because closeness is threatening to them

Uninvolved patients for the same reason

All patients, to some extent, because of fear of self-disclosure related to impersonal hospital policies; need for intimate types of information; loss of modesty and privacy; violation of body boundaries; different tubing, catheters, endotracheal apparatus, and so on imposed upon them

All patients are also affected by the change in interpersonal relationships that hospital admission inflicts on them. They are removed from their normal social system; opportunities for privacy and closeness with loved ones are limited in the impersonal hospital environment

Psychosocial Nursing Diagnosis and Potential for Maladaptation

In this final subsection you are asked to review the material you learned in the patient's psychosocial history and to formulate a nursing diagnosis based on one or more of the approved nursing diagnoses from the list presented by the National Conferences on Nursing Diagnosis (Kim and Moritz, 1982; Kim and colleagues, 1984). If the patient does not have any presenting signs of psychosocial maladaptation, but based on his history you believe that there is a potential for maladaptation, the diagnostic categories should be preceded by the words *potential for psychosocial maladaptation*. For example, this final subsection on psychosocial assessment can read:

Nursing diagnosis:
Grieving anticipatory

Potential for maladaptation:
Coping, ineffective individual
Coping, ineffective family: compromised
Home maintenance management, impaired

Nursing Diagnosis of Psychosocial Maladaptation

One of the accepted beliefs about a profession is that its members use a specific body of knowledge in their practice. During the 1970s, a group of nurse clinicians and educators began to identify specific patient states that nurses were qualified to diagnose and treat within the scope of their practice. The right to practice nursing within this framework has been stated as the keystone of the American Nurses' Association *Social Policy Statement* published in 1981. In it, nursing is defined as "the diagnosis and treatment of human responses to actual or potential health problems." Several state legislatures have incorporated this definition in their nurse practice acts.

There have been five National Conferences on Nursing Diagnosis, held approximately every 2 years since 1973. The group has been chaired by Marjory Gordon (1982) of Boston College. Its function has been to identify, develop, and classify the categories of nursing diagnosis. During the Fourth National Conference on Classification of Nursing Diagnosis, held in 1980, the following categories of nursing diagnosis were identified:

List of Nursing Diagnoses Accepted at the Fourth National Conference (1980)

Airway clearance, ineffective

Bowel elimination, alteration in: constipation

Bowel elimination, alteration in: diarrhea

Bowel elimination, alteration in: incontinence

Breathing pattern, ineffective

Cardiac output, alteration in: decreased

Comfort, alteration in: pain

Communication, impaired verbal

Coping, ineffective individual

Coping, ineffective family: compromised

Coping, ineffective family: disabling

Coping, family potential for growth

Diversional activity, deficit

Fear

Fluid volume deficit, actual*

Fluid volume deficit, potential

Gas exchange, impaired

Grieving, anticipatory

Grieving, dysfunctional

Home maintenance management, impaired

Injury, potential for; poisoning, potential for; suffocation, potential for; trauma, potential for

Knowledge deficit (specify)

Mobility, impaired physical

Noncompliance (specify)

Nutrition, alteration in: less than body requirements

Nutrition, alteration in: more than body requirements

Nutrition, alteration in: potential for more than body requirements

Parenting, alteration in: actual

Parenting, alteration in: potential

Rape-trauma syndrome: rape trauma, compound reaction, silent reaction

Self-care deficit (specify level): feeding, bathing/hygiene, dressing/grooming, toileting

Self-concepts, disturbance in: body image, self-esteem, role performance, personal identity

Sensory perceptual alteration: visual, auditory, kinesthetic, gustatory, tactile, and olfactory perceptions

Sexual dysfunction

Skin integrity, impairment of: actual

Skin integrity, impairment of: potential

Sleep pattern disturbance

Spiritual distress (distress of the human spirit)

Thought processes, alteration in

Tissue perfusion, alteration in: cerebral, cardiopulmonary, renal, gastrointestinal, peripheral

Urinary elimination, alteration in patterns

Violence, potential for

---

*Two sets of defining characteristics with two etiologies for the same nursing diagnosis. (Kim M, Moritz D [eds]: Classification of Nursing Diagnoses: Proceedings of the Third and Fourth National Conferences, pp. 281-282. New York, McGraw-Hill, 1982. By permission of North American Nursing Diagnosis Association)

It was decided that the list developed by the Fourth National Conference in 1980 would not be altered at the Fifth National Conference in 1982. Instead, the entire list was retained and the conference participants approved of eight new categories, which were accepted for clinical testing. They include the following:

List of Nursing Diagnoses Added at the Fifth National Conference (1982)

Activity intolerance

Anxiety

Family processes, alteration in

Fluid volume, alteration in: excess

Health maintenance alteration

Oral mucus membrane, alterations in

Powerlessness

Social isolation

(Kim M, McFarland G, McLane A [eds]: Classification of Nursing Diagnoses: Proceedings of the Fifth National Conference. St. Louis, CV Mosby [in press]. By permission of North American Nursing Diagnosis Association)

In order to dramatize the importance of psychosocial nursing care, the list of nursing categories is repeated in the chart below. All categories with predominately psychosocial dynamics in their etiology are preceded by one asterisk. Other categories are customarily viewed as having physiological etiologies. Actually, they may have one or more psychosocial dynamics in their developmental course. These dynamics may also contribute to the ongoing problem and are preceded by two asterisks.

Nursing Diagnosis Categories (1980)

**Airway clearance, ineffective

**Bowel elimination, alteration in: constipation

**Bowel elimination, alteration in: diarrhea

**Bowel elimination, alteration in: incontinence

**Breathing pattern, ineffective

**Cardiac output, alteration in: decreased

*Comfort, alteration in: pain

*Communication, impaired verbal

*Coping, ineffective individual

*Coping, ineffective family: compromised

*Coping, ineffective family: disabling

*Coping, family: potential for growth

*Diversional activity, deficit

*Fear

**Fluid volume deficit, actual

**Fluid volume deficit, potential

**Gas exchange, impaired

*Grieving, anticipatory

*Grieving, dysfunctional

**Home maintenance management, impaired

*Injury, potential for; poisoning, potential for; suffocation, potential for; trauma, potential for

*Knowledge deficit (specify)

**Mobility, impaired physical

*Noncompliance (specify)

*Nutrition, alteration in: less than body requirements

*Nutrition, alteration in: more than body requirements

*Nutrition, alteration in: potential for more than body requirements

*Parenting, alteration in: actual

*Parenting, alteration in: potential

*Rape-trauma syndrome: rape trauma, compound reaction, silent reaction

**Self-care deficit (specify level): feeding, bathing-hygiene, dressing-grooming, toileting

*Self-concepts, disturbance in: body image, self-esteem, role performance, personal identity

*Sensory perceptual alteration; visual, auditory, kinesthetic, gustatory, tactile, and olfactory perceptions

*Sexual dysfunction

**Skin integrity, impairment of: actual

**Skin integrity, impairment of: potential

*Sleep pattern disturbance

*Spiritual distress (distress of the human spirit)

*Thought processes, alteration in

**Tissue perfusion, alteration in: cerebral, cardiopulmonary, renal, gastrointestinal, peripheral

**Urinary elimination, alteration in patterns

*Violence, potential for

*The causes of these conditions contain primarily psychosocial dynamics.

**The causes of these conditions contain primarily physiological dynamics but may include one or more psychosocial dynamics.

*Nursing diagnosis categories accepted
for clinical testing (1982)*

**Activity intolerance

*Anxiety

*Family processes, alteration in

**Fluid volume, alteration in: excess

**Health maintenance alteration

**Oral mucus membrane, alterations in

*Powerlessness

*Social isolation

*The causes of these conditions contain primarily psychosocial
dynamics.
**The causes of these conditions contain primarily physio-
logical dynamics but may include one or more psychosocial
dynamics.
(Kim M, Moritz D [eds]: Classification of Nursing Diagnoses:
Proceedings of the Third and Fourth National Conferences, pp.
281-282. New York, McGraw-Hill, 1982; and Kim M, McFarland
G, McLane A [eds]: Classification of Nursing Diagnoses:
Proceedings of the Fifth National Conference. St. Louis, CV
Mosby [in press]. By permission of North American Nursing
Diagnosis Association)

In order to familiarize you with the etiologies
and defining characteristics that have been identified for each of the diagnostic categories, refer to
the complete listing of the categories, which were
approved in 1980 and 1982. They appear in the
Appendix.

Documentation of
the Psychosocial
Nursing Process

Many nurses carry out psychosocial assessment
and diagnosis, formulate a plan, intervene, and
evaluate the results of their psychosocial interventions with the patient. They concurrently carry out
the nursing process in promoting physiological
homeostasis. Notes about the patient's physical
status are routinely written. Documentation of the
psychosocial nursing process, however, is frequently omitted, although there may be sporadic
notes about the patient's appearing depressed or
anxious. Although nurses may be aware of the
underlying stresses and conflicts that are causing
these responses and may be actively intervening
with their patients to promote adaptation, they
may omit describing their findings and efforts.
    Why is this so? One of the reasons may be the
past emphasis on and use of the medical model by
nursing to document patient care. Because of

the primary emphasis of medical caregivers on the
physiological processes (which *is* their identified
caregiving role), nursing has used a similar approach in documenting its assessment of the
patient. The value system that nurses developed
between 1900 and 1950 seems to have been based
on becoming physicians' assistants in the hospital
setting. However, in the last decade or so, nursing
has moved to establish a more autonomous role in
patient care.
    It is time that the nurses' charting reflected
their awareness of the patient's psychosocial
response to illness and their interventions to
promote adaptation. Many nurses lament the fact
that physicians rarely take the time to read their
notes. Could part of the reason for physicians' lack
of interest in nurses' notes be that the nurses'
observation of the patients' status is so much like
their own—based on physical assessment? They
can read the notes of fellow attending physicians
and house officers if they want to know the
patients' physical status during the previous 24
hours. They usually are not able to determine the
patient's psychosocial responses to illness from
physicians' notes, however. Unless the patient is in
emotional crisis, there may be no documentation
of his emotional status.
    The patient's psychosocial response to illness
is highly important. Remember that 3 months after
discharge, the patient's physical condition has
usually returned to normal. If psychosocial maladaptation occurred in the patient or his family
during his hospitalization, however, the quality of
their life can be permanently disrupted. Nursing is
the caregiving discipline that is trained to perform
an initial assessment and care plan for the patient
with a maladaptive response to illness. Accordingly, do you think that documenting your observations of these responses can help physicians
to develop more of an awareness of this essential
aspect of the effects of illness? Many physicians
who initially discounted the patient's psychological
reaction to illness or the family's response to the
illness of their loved one are changing their
opinions. Articulate nursing documentation of the
coping responses of patients and families introduces them to a side of illness that they had
previously overlooked. They will increasingly respect this knowledge base of nursing.

Conclusion

When a nursing plan is formulated using the
assessment guidelines presented in this chapter, it

can help a nurse to review many aspects of the nursing care plan that previously may have been overlooked. Once a psychosocial nursing diagnosis is established, it is important to provide daily documentation of the ongoing nursing process. This is necessary to ensure that nursing peers know how to proceed with the patient in your absence. It helps to establish continuity and an overall systems approach. This promotes the patient's sense of security and trust in his nursing caregivers. Psychosocial nursing care provides the patient with essential support, which can avert a crisis and contribute toward optimal coping for all concerned.

Psychosocial nursing can be one of the most challenging aspects of caring for patients. The reason is that much of the assessment is based on deductive rather than on the concrete reasoning used in physical assessment based on specifically measurable data. Perhaps it is because of the abstract nature of working with a patient's feelings and thoughts that makes some nurses feel uneasy and uncertain about whether their own perceptions are accurate.

At one time I worked as a psychiatric-mental health clinical instructor in an upper division baccalaureate nursing program. The students were registered nurses who ranged in age from 23 to 50 years. As part of their basic nursing educations they all had spent 3 months working in psychiatric institutions. Most of them reported that they had felt uncomfortable talking with psychiatric patients. They were not sure what to say to the patients or how the patients would respond. Many of them said they were frightened of the patients but did not acknowledge it to anyone. Because they were not sure what to say or do, they often played cards with the patients and engaged in superficial conversation.

The clinical setting used by the university for its mental health clinical experience was an inpatient drug and alcohol treatment hospital. The patients were coherent and rational. They were generally eager to share their thoughts and feelings with the nurses. Although the nurses were not in an acute psychiatric setting and the patients were not likely to have any psychotic episodes or to harm them, they reported feeling very uneasy. On reflection, the nurses discovered that they were not afraid of the patients but of encounter between themselves and the patients. Perhaps, also, they feared what they did not know about themselves. One nurse said, "Usually when I'm with a general hospital patient there's something I have to do for him. I'm taking his blood pressure or checking a dressing or something; I may talk to him as I'm doing it, but at least I have something to *do*."

Sitting and talking with a patient about his major life issues was something most of them had never done before. Gradually, as they relaxed, they discovered that the patients were eager for someone to listen and care, not to utter magical words that would change the course of their lives. The students learned that it was their listening and the skill of their questions, not their talking, that was most therapeutic.

In Chapter 12: Counseling Techniques for Nurses you learned many techniques that are essential for therapeutic intervention with patients.

14

A Model for Psychosocial Nursing Process

You can make a difference for patients and families. The following factors are important in determining the outcome of psychosocial nursing interventions.

1. Your openness and warmth with a patient
2. Your ability to withhold judgment until you have an understanding of the patient's perceptions of himself, his illness, and his social system
3. Your assessment skill
4. Your willingness to become involved when you see maladaptation or the potential for maladaptation

In encountering a patient who is hurting emotionally, many nurses unfortunately have believed that they should be able to actively *do* something about his emotional pain, that they should be able to come up with a sentence or idea that could eliminate his distress. Would you believe this to be a fair expectation for a nurse to have of himself or herself? It is not. Remember that a patient's emotional pain is usually the result of the combined effects of an inadequately coping ego *and* a social system that may also be inadequate. These dynamics have been operating for years and possibly for a lifetime. Is it reasonable to think you can effect a major change in a patient's thinking or feeling state with just a few words.

Is It Realistic to Teach a Patient New Coping Skills?

It is not unusual to see written on a patient's care plan *teach patient new coping skills.* Let me explain why this expectation, which many nurses impose on themselves, is not realistic. First of all, patients enter the hospital with a repertoire of defense or coping mechanisms that they have been using since childhood. They use most of them unconsciously. They also have a series of conscious coping skills. When the stress of hospitalization occurs and gradually becomes more threatening, the patient's normal ability to cope regresses. His unconscious defense mechanisms progressively become more immature and are increasingly used by the ego in its effort to adapt. Remember that the patient is usually unaware of his use of defense mechanisms. They are *automatic* as the ego works to protect the person.

If a patient is astute psychologically and has a high level of differentiation between his thinking and emotions (see Chapter 8: The Family as a System) it is possible that he is able to use conscious stress management in his response to the stress of day-to-day life. Hospitalization for serious illness, however, usually removes the potential for these conscious stress reduction techniques such as jogging, meditation, exercising, and so on. The reasons for his decrease in coping ability are that it may be impossible for him physically to carry them out; most important, the threatening nature of the illness will decrease his normal ability to cope consciously. Unconscious defenses will be used by the ego to protect the unpleasant awarenesses of the environment as well as the patient's internal anxiety level.

The nurse may be conversant with many types of defense mechanisms and coping skills. He or she may be an excellent teacher. Is it possible, however, to teach someone who is under psychological stress a new way to use defense mechanisms? Or is it possible to tell the patient to stop using unconscious maladaptive denial or repression and, instead, to use a more adaptive defense against the threats he is experiencing? I don't think so. Remember, he has been using them unconsciously for most of his life.

Instead, there are ways that the nurse can help to decrease the patient's level of anxiety by allowing him to talk about his fears, by providing reality testing, and by encouraging support from family members and other caregivers. These approaches can allow the patients' ego to obtain a gradual awareness of reality. A more adaptive use of defense mechanisms can then occur. Gradually, the patient may be able to apply his normal coping skills in order to reduce his level of anxiety and conflict.

Now that we have clarified what is reasonable for nurses to expect of themselves, let us talk about intervention.

Psychosocial Intervention With General Hospital Patients

As described in the beginning of the chapter, the process of helping a patient to adapt to the stress of hospitalization and the effects of illness can be one of the most challenging aspects of nursing care. If maladaptation occurs, it can have a profound and lasting effect on the patient's and family's quality of life. You *can* have an effect with a maladapting patient. It is important, however, not to expect too much of yourself in this process. You are a change agent, but you cannot make changes happen. Adaptation and the changes required for it to occur greatly depend on the patient's ego functioning. You can be a catalyst in the process, but it is ultimately the *patient* who must change and adapt.

An essential aspect of being a change agent is providing ego support to the patient whose coping ability is weakened. The major causes of a weakened ego are as follows:

1. *High levels of stress.* Stress due to hospitalization, fear of death, changes within family due to illness, and so on can alter coping ability.
2. *Normally weak personality style.* For example, dependent and inadequate personality styles have trouble coping with hospitalization and illness.
3. *Organic brain syndrome (OBS).* When brain tissue is affected by an organic dysfunction, it alters normal cognitive and perceptual abilities, and mood. All these are ego functions.

In most cases, the ego is weakened only temporarily. When the nurse provides extra ego support by encouraging the patient to release emotion through talking, providing reality testing, and so on, this can help the patient to work through and resolve a potential crisis. This type of ego support can be compared to the use of sandbags as an extra support to the walls of a dike that are under strain of breaking because of a flood.

The Nurse as a Change Agent

When you assist patients in adapting to illness or to longlasting or permanent changes in body image, there is a very important change process that must occur in you *before* you can actually be a change agent: *letting go.* Letting go can be compared to what the parents of teenagers must do if their children are to develop as autonomous adults. It can also be compared to what bicycle riding and swimming instructors must do when their young charges are feeling insecure about their own abilities.

The emotional and intellectual ability of the nurse to "let go" in the counseling process has perhaps never been emphasized enough. Nurses sometimes feel a heavy responsibility that they must "do it all"; accordingly, the idea of taking on such a challenge may be frightening.

It is the rare nurse who is not conscientious and cautious when talking with an emotionally overwhelmed patient. If you are mindful of the theory that has been presented in this text and are genuinely concerned for your patient, the next step is to pull up a chair and be *with* the patient. I am aware that this can feel risky for a young nurse who feels inexperienced. This is understandable.

The process of engaging in such a relationship can seem more threatening for the nurse than it is for the patient. Be aware of your own feelings, thoughts, and reactions; just allow yourself to be aware of them rather than judging them unacceptable and repressing them or avoiding the patient altogether. Above all, the involvement should be one that feels right for you and the patient. If it is uncomfortable for you, there *are* other nurses available to the patient. If you are the patient's primary nurse, however, consider discussing your hesitation with a peer on your unit, an impartial supervisor (with whom you can be honest with no fear of a negative evaluation), or a psychiatric liaison nurse whose clinical background can help you to understand your response. It is important for you to examine your reaction to the situation so that you do not consistently avoid such situations in the future. You and your future patients would perhaps miss some very valuable and special experiences.

A Model for Promotion of Psychosocial Adaptation

In keeping with traditional clinical nursing theory, it is important to have a formal conceptual model on which to base your psychosocial interventions. The model that I have developed is designed to promote the patient's adaptation to a change in his health status. The emphasis in this model is to increase the nurse's awareness of the multiple subsystems and their forces that affect the patient's psychosocial response to the stress of illness.

The nurse can promote the patient's psychosocial adaptation by constantly monitoring and assessing the response of the patient and his social system to his illness. When you are aware of factors in the patient's environment that have the potential to undermine his adaptation, these factors can be subject to alteration and change. The nurse can also change his or her approach with the patient and temporarily give the patient the extra ego support he needs. When the patient's adaptation is at risk because of weakened intrapsychic defenses, organic failure, or temporary or chronic personal or family stress, there are intervention choices available to the nurse that can promote change and reverse a maladaptive process.

Conceptual Approach to Psychosocial Nursing Intervention

The words *conceptual model* often seem to frighten many readers. Actually, in order to clarify the term and make it seem less awesome, think of it by contrasting it to the word *idea*. When you think of an idea, it actually is an incomplete form of a concept. An idea is like a wall of brick that has no mortar or "glue" to keep it together. A conceptual model, on the other hand, is like a brick wall that has mortar to connect all the bricks. An idea, when analyzed, may actually be unworkable because it is missing connectedness. A conceptual model has a framework or structure on which theory is built. Concepts are presented that build on each other and become the actual model. My intention in presenting this model is that it be used as a guide. I encourage you to use flexibility rather than rigidity in applying it to the unique circumstances of your patients.

This section includes the basic concepts of my proposed approach to psychosocial nursing care. The important concepts in this approach to psychosocial nursing intervention are as follows:

1. All people are constantly subject to stress from many subsystems and systems:
   a. Physical
   b. Intrapsychic
   c. Family
   d. Other social relationships in the environment
2. The constancy of stress produces ever-changing dynamics in these subsystems and systems
3. The person's responses to stress partially depend on the strengths and weaknesses in these same subsystems and systems; they continually feed into each other and are highly interdependent
4. The dynamics operating within the self and family operate in fairly predictable ways, which can be determined by the assessment process

(*e.g.*, normal coping style, personality style, and so on)
5. The dynamics operating in the larger social system are the most flexible and subject to change, which can be understood when you consider the potential numbers of persons in the environments to which the patient is exposed

Accordingly, if a person is maladapting to stress, it is important to examine the various subsystems and systems involved for their potential to contribute toward an adaptive response.

Can the patient's physical subsystem be changed? One hopes so, or hospitals would soon be empty. Remember, however, that it is not only the seriousness of illness that causes regression and potential psychological maladaptation; rather, it is the patient's *perception* of the threat of his illness and its implications for his future that are a major cause of maladaptation because of the anxiety they generate.

Can the intrapsychic subsystem be changed? Yes. Although we cannot change it, we can help the patient to function better temporarily by our actions. It is the patient's conscious or unconscious choice that actually changes his maladaptive process. We are catalysts. We are change agents; we are not the changers in the sense that we singlehandedly turn the patient around. The patient's intrapsychic subsystem operates in a way that is *unique* to that patient and does not yield easily to change. If the patient is maladapting, it will be the response of his ego to your interventions that ultimately can produce change in his maladaptation. Lewin has proposed that there are three main steps in the process of change. These can be helpful to keep in mind when you are attempting to bring about any type of change in a patient's belief system or behavior (Welch, 1979). Lewin's model is presented here with a focus on the patient at risk for maladaptation.

The unfreezing stage

The motivation to change must be put in motion. The patient first must become aware that change is needed.

The moving stage

Based on information he receives during the first stage, the patient can choose a particular course of action from alternatives that he alone or he and the change agent have developed together. The course of action is begun.

The refreezing stage

The action instituted by the change is in place and can be evaluated for its effectiveness. Blocks to success can be evaluated. Modifications or changes in the original plan may be needed to ensure the successful outcome of the process.

Can the family system be changed? Yes, it can be modified. It is similar to each person's intrapsychic system because the family is made up of members who all function in their own usually predictable ways. In addition, there are usually predictable family dynamics involved, which you can discover in the assessment process (see Chap. 8: The Family as a System). There can be more flexibility, however, in a group system than in an individual system because of the greater number of dynamics involved.

Can the other social relationships in the patient's environment be changed? Yes. This is the crucial subsystem for a patient who is maladapting. This is the subsystem of people, which includes caregivers. It is important that caregivers be able to see maladaptation occur, assess it, and intervene or request others to intervene. They also must be able to evaluate and monitor the patient's continuing responses to illness *and* the interventions they design to promote adaptation. This subsystem can make the difference if the patient's body, mind, or family are temporarily or permanently lacking the strength to overcome the problem. If no one in this subsystem observes the patient's maladaptation, then it is possible that he will be discharged from the hospital or clinic without intervention. Remember that the longer a patient responds with maladaptive defenses, the more likely that chronic maladaptation will be an ongoing part of his life.

The following chart describes the critical factors that determine the psychosocial outcome of physical illness:

Patient's Response to the Stress of Illness

Stress

Regression

Possible Outcomes

Adaptation (factors in outcome)

Normal coping style
  Patient's intrapsychic defenses are adaptive
  Patient is able to use his normal stress management to cope adequately with stress
  Illness is not life threatening
  Illness is not highly threatening to patient's self-esteem and body image
  Illness is not threatening to normal role functioning

Personality style
  Illness does not cause a major change in the way the patient normally interacts with others and his environment; personality is strong enough to cope with stress

Family coping style
  Family is normally able to adapt to stress
    Illness is not perceived as life threatening or causing major shifts in role of family member
  One or more family members are emotionally detached enough to allow the patient to voice his concerns about himself

Maladaptation (factors in outcome)

Normal coping style
  Ego unconsciously underuses or overuses certain predictable defense mechanisms
  Patient fails or loses his ability to use conscious stress management mechanisms
  Illness is life threatening or is *perceived* as life threatening
  Illness is threatening to self-esteem or body image
  Illness is threatening to normal role functioning

Personality style
  Depending on the type of illness and its particular threat to the patient, any personality style can be at risk because of the stress of major illness

Family coping style
  Family's normal response to stress may be chronically inadequate, or the family may be overwhelmed by the catastrophic illness or death of one of its members

(continued)

Patient's Response to the Stress of Illness (continued)

Other social relationships in environment
  Caregivers appropriately assess and
    therapeutically intervene with maladapting
    patient
  Patient's level of stress is responsive to
    caregivers' interventions
  Patient's work role is not permanently
    threatened
  Patient's relationships outside of the family
    are not permanently threatened
  Patient has friends with whom he can
    explore his concerns about his illness and
    receive support (close friends are sometimes
    able to be more objective than family
    members)

Illness may cause major shift in role
  functioning within family
Patient has no family to support him
Other social relationships in environment
  Caregivers are unable to assess and
    intervene with maladapting patient
  Patient's level of stress is not responsive to
    caregivers' interventions
  Patient's work role is threatened
  Patient's role functioning in social and work
    relationships is chronically or permanently
    threatened
  Patient has inadequate or no social
    relationships for support

When maladaptive factors are present, the nurse should use a theoretical framework that assesses the various subsystems operating within and around the patient. Once the subsystems are assessed, they must be examined for their potential to change so that adaptation is the ultimate outcome. Using such a framework implies the following belief about psychosocial nursing intervention:

1. Professional nursing functions and activities are directed by a therapeutic purpose.
2. Underlying all nursing activity is a genuine caring and concern for the welfare of the patient.
3. Critical analysis of the patient-client and his condition is accompanied by respect for him as an individual whose dignity is always to be maintained.
4. The patient is an integral part of all planning and decision-making.
5. The nurse is the patient's advocate when he cannot be his own.
6. The nurse supports and promotes health and the quality of life. According to a definition adapted from the World Health Organization, health means complete physical, personal, and social well-being, not solely the absence of disease or infirmity.

(Chrisman and Fowler: The systems in change model for nursing practice. In Riehl J, Roy C [eds]: Conceptual Models for Nursing Practice, 2nd ed, p. 75. New York, Appleton-Century-Crofts, 1980)

The model I have developed is based on one of the change model theories of Robert Chin of Boston University (Bennis and colleagues, 1976).

Chin's model has been used in psychology, sociology, anthropology, public health, business administration, social work, theology, and the health professions.

I have conceptualized the theory presented in earlier chapters using the Chin model as a theoretical base (Table 14-1). It is important to emphasize that this model is based on the assumption that all social and physical subsystems are constantly in change. Accordingly, there is varying flexibility and openness in each of the subsystems. The flexibility and openness must first exist in the caregiver if maladaptive risk is to be identified. Next, there must be at least some flexibility in the patient if a maladaptive course is to be changed. The other subsystems whose flexibility will affect the patient's adaptation are the family and the other caregiving disciplines.

Conclusion

This conceptual model of the psychosocial nursing process with hospitalized patients has been presented in order to give you a formal structure on which to develop your nursing assessment, diagnosis, care plan, intervention, and evaluation of outcome with patients who are in the process of psychosocial adjustment to physical illness. It is a model that can help you to connect and actualize the theory presented in earlier chapters.

Although time constraints in the actual clinical setting may prevent you from formally evaluating each of your patients in this step-by-step manner, this framework can help you as you develop your patients' psychosocial care plan using the nursing process.

Table 14-1.
A Nursing Model for Promotion of Psychosocial Adaptation

Assumptions and Approaches to Psychosocial Nursing Process	Action to Promote Psychosocial Adaptation
Content (assessment)	
(actual or potential maladaptive psychosocial state of patient)	
Stability (the patient's current psychosocial status)	The patient's psychosocial state must be assessed so that the nurse knows what factors are contributing to maladaptation or its potential; in addition, there must be an assessment of the potential for change in the patient in his current condition
	Normal coping style: conscious coping devices as well as unconscious defense mechanisms (obtained in history)
	Personality style (Chap. 5)
	Current coping style (nurse should use knowledge of maladaptive defense mechanisms in Chap. 4)
	Major developmental challenges that *this* illness will present for *this* patient: trust, self-esteem, control, and so on (Chap. 6)
	Current family coping style (assess strengths and weaknesses in family members) (Chap. 8)
	Mental status (Chap. 10)
Change (the potential for the nurse to perceive the patient's status and to become involved)	Nurse's awareness of the desired outcome of adaptation in the patient and realistic appraisal of the steps in the nursing process necessary to achieve the goal
Causation (planning: step I)	
(conceptualizing the possibility of promoting psychosocial adaptation)	
Source of change	Patient and nurse who designs intervention (change agents)
Causal force (motivation)	Depends on the willingness of patient, nurse, and support system to promote patient's adaptation
Goals (planning: step II)	
(desired outcome of nursing intervention)	
Direction	Psychosocial adaptation to illness
Set by	Patient and nurse; remember that the stress of illness can result in the patient's ego being temporarily overwhelmed; he may not be able to be fully objective about his potential or current maladaptation
Intervention	
(the process involved in promoting change)	
Confronting symptoms	Intervention mutually agreed on by patient and nurse; if patient is unable psychologically to make this decision, then the nurse can independently design a systems approach that will support an adaptive response in the patient
Goal of intervention	Psychosocial adaptation in patient and members of patient's social system

(continued)

Table 14-1.
A Nursing Model for Promotion of Psychosocial Adaptation
(*continued*)

Assumptions and Approaches to Psychosocial Nursing Process	Action to Promote Psychosocial Adaptation
Change agent(s) (patient and nurse)	
Place	Primarily, intrapsychic system of the patient; in addition, intrapsychic systems of nurse and all other members of the patient's support system are involved: caregivers, family, and friends; actual setting is wherever social interaction takes place: hospital, home, or community
Role	Psychological openness and astuteness of all involved members (including other nursing and medical caregivers)
Evaluation (outcome of change action)	Did the desired change occur in the patient? Was actual or potential maladaptation reversed?

(After Chin R: The utility of system models and developmental models for practitioners. In Bennis W, Benne K, Chin R et al [eds]: The Planning of Change, 3rd ed, p. 102. New York, Holt, Rinehart and Winston, 1976)

15

Crisis Intervention With the Maladapting Patient

The concept of crisis has been discussed in many of the earlier chapters. Major illness can be a crisis-precipitating event in the life of a person and his family. Maladaptation is the result of an inability to work through the threat of this illness. The degree of maladaptation will depend on many factors, which will be presented in the following pages. In Chapter 9: Stress: Its Implications in Physical Illness, crisis was discussed in several contexts. *Crisis* is defined as a state of reaction within a person who is responding to a hazardous event (Rapaport, 1965). Aguilera and Messick (1978) describe a crisis as both a danger and an opportunity. It is a danger because of its potential to overwhelm a patient or his family. It is an opportunity because, when the crisis is overcome, with or without assistance, the person acquires a more adaptive coping potential for future crises.

Remember that the event that leads to a crisis is usually one that is new to a person or family. They have no experience in knowing how to deal with it, and their coping ability with regard to *this* type of threat has never developed (it never was needed before). In working through the crisis, a higher level of coping skills usually develops; these become part of the person's coping repertoire when challenges occur in the future.

When a patient is under severe stress and copes well, adaptation occurs and the potential crisis is resolved. If the patient does not cope well, but intervention by professionals or by supportive family or friends results in stronger coping ability or in his regaining equilibrium, then maladaptation is reversed; adaptation is the outcome and the crisis is worked through and resolved. If the patient does not cope well and no one in his social system is alert to his coping failure, then the patient's unsuccessful continued defensive and coping attempts can result in maladaptation. The patient is unable to help himself and is in crisis.

A crisis can be experienced by one person, and then, because of family system effects, his family can ultimately be affected by the crisis. If family members are able to cope well with the crisis of one member, it is possible that their support can reduce that member's crisis response.

The major factors that determine whether a threatening event will become a crisis are summarized in the chart that appears on the next page.

Crisis Potential of a Threatening Event

Sequence of Developments After a Critical Event

1. Perception of event by person
2. Degree of threat as perceived by person to:
   a. Personal safety
   b. Life goals
   c. Normal role functioning
   d. Family stability
3. His accurate perception of the threat is strongly influenced by:
   a. Normal personality style
   b. Normal ego strength
   c. A developmental issue that is triggered by the event: trust, threat to self-esteem, control, loss, guilt, or intimacy
   d. Coping skills during normal stresses of living
   e. Level of stress in his life during previous year
   f. Availability of support from:
      (1) Family
      (2) Friends
      (3) Caregivers
4. Outcome
   a. Adaptation (coping) or maladaptation (crisis)

Aguilera and Messick (1978) have described the factors that they believe are essential in determining a person's response to a critical event (Fig. 15-1).

Coping Ability in a Crisis

A person's ability to cope with a stressful and threatening event depends on the many factors outlined above. One of the critical factors is the repertoire of coping skills that the person uses to adapt to the crisis. If these coping abilities are temporarily overwhelmed or are not used by a chronically inadequate ego, it is possible to structure some of them into your intervention plan. These coping abilities have been described as follows:

1. Denying or minimizing the seriousness of the illness
2. Seeking relevant information

3. Requesting reassurance and emotional support
4. Learning specific illness-related procedures
5. Setting concrete, limited goals
6. Rehearsing alternative outcomes
7. Finding a general purpose or pattern of meaning in the course of events

(Moos R: Coping with the crisis of physical illness. In Freeman A, Sack R, Berger P [eds]: Psychiatry for the Primary Care Physician, pp. 31-32. © 1979 The Williams & Wilkins Co., Baltimore)

Denying or minimizing the seriousness of the illness. Until the ego is able to accept the implications of the illness fully, it will use many defense mechanisms to protect itself. Denial, projection, displacement, and avoidance are common. Another frequently used defense is isolation; the person intellectually accepts the meaning of the illness but does not feel the emotion related to it.

Seeking relevant information. By learning more about his illness, its cause, treatment, prognosis, and other related information, the patient gains a sense of control. Intellectual understanding relieves some of the anxiety experienced by all patients, especially those with type A or controlling personalities (see Chap. 5: Personality Styles Seen in General Hospital Patients). Nurses can assist in this process but should not overwhelm the patient with excessive information. Initially, only his specific questions should be answered; excessive detail should be avoided. Within a day or two, the patient will probably ask more specific questions. Let his questions be your guide.

Requesting reassurance and emotional support. Many patients automatically look to family, friends, and hospital caregivers for support when they are threatened by illness. Anxiety can be aroused if too much support is given. Patients with the following personality styles can be threatened by too much nurse involvement: the guarded (suspicious), uninvolved, and antisocial personality types. They can be encouraged to share their fears with family members and friends. Occasionally, with highly anxious patients, it may be necessary for a few days to develop more flexible visiting hours or overnight rules so that trusted family members can provide extra emotional support for these patients in order to avoid crisis. Special attention should be given to the patient who withdraws. Observe him carefully for his reaction to a supportive approach.

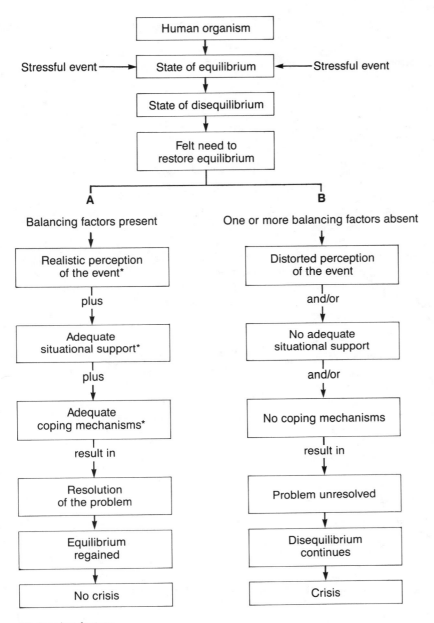

*Balancing factors

Figure 15-1.
Paradigm effect of balancing factors in a stressful event. (Aguilera D, Messick J: Crisis
Intervention: Theory and Methodology, 4th ed, p. 65. St. Louis, CV Mosby, 1982)

Learning specific illness-related procedures.
Patients and families are often threatened by their
lack of skills in providing self-care or care to their
loved ones with newly acquired conditions. Formal
inpatient teaching programs and informal teaching
sessions with staff nurses can help people to
acquire the technical skills required in certain

illnesses such as diabetes or skills involving
catheter care, dressing changes, and so on. The
assistance of visiting nurses during the initial
adjustment stage of home discharge can also be
very helpful to the initially unconfident patient and
family.

Setting concrete, limited goals. For the patient

who is adjusting to a catastrophic illness, or an illness that has a long recuperative period, it is important to help him structure his signs of progress into achievable objectives. For example, the goal of taking the first step is a positive and hopeful goal for an amputee. If this patient sets an initial goal of walking down the aisle with his daughter who will be married in 3 months, you can help him to set another, more easily achievable initial goal that can be mastered in a relatively short time. This approach helps the patient to maintain and continually restore his hope. Hope is an essential element in the rehabilitative process.

Rehearsing alternative outcomes. Rehearsing alternative outcomes is slightly more sophisticated than information seeking. The patient thinks through, in advance, his concerns about his future surgery, recuperation period, and other events that create anxiety in him. In this way he confronts the feared event before it occurs and works through some of the associated anxiety. When the threatening event occurs, some of the anxiety associated with it has already been released or unconsciously defended against by the ego. For example, you can encourage a patient who may be frightened about a cardiac catheterization to talk about his specific concerns and his associated feelings; some of the unpleasant affect is discharged, and you will also be able to correct any misconceptions that may be unnecessarily contributing to his fear.

Finding a general purpose or pattern of meaning. After the initial effects of the illness have been dealt with by the use of the coping skills mentioned above, some thoughtful patients will continue to probe for the reason why the event occurred. Patients often ask, "Why?" It may take several days, weeks, or longer for an existential answer to be arrived at; if this occurs, the patient may develop a peaceful acceptance of the illness. This awareness is usually arrived at through a deep probing of self. Although the patient may ask you and other persons why, it is helpful for you to turn the question back to him gently and ask, "Why do *you* think this happened?" He rarely will find the answer anywhere but inside himself.

A crisis is a sequential event that occurs over a given time. Ballou (1980) has proposed the following four stages to a crisis. They are shown with their accompanying perceptual, emotional, and intellectual components in Table 15-1.

Critical Time for Crisis Resolution

A crisis is a time-limited event. It may last anywhere from a few days to a few weeks (Moos, 1979). A crisis state is a period of disequilibrium. Because the ego is constantly attempting to adapt to intrapsychic or environmental stress, it eventually

Table 15-1.
Stages of Crisis

Stages	Intrapsychic Response	Emotional Response	Intellectual Response
Shock (stress)	Overwhelmed by stressful stimuli	High anxiety; helplessness	Lack of reasoning or problem-solving ability; disorganized
Defensive retreat	Denial or repression of awareness	Apathy or euphoria; low anxiety	Rethinking situation; beginning of defensive distortion of facts
Acknowledgment (renewed stress	Reality can no longer be avoided; increased awareness	Agitated or anergic; depression; grief; high anxiety	Defensive breakdown: (1) disorganization and (2) reorganization using actual or distorted facts in problem solving
Adaptation and change	New reality testing; awareness gradually becomes acceptable	Decrease in anxiety; gradual increase in ability to experience pleasure and sense of internal calm	Integration of new awarenesses into cognitive ego functioning

(After Ballou M: Crisis intervention and the hospital nurse. J Nurs Care 13:18, 1980)

will find a way to relieve itself within a limited time even if the result is maladaptive.

A person who is in crisis is, indeed, in a state of disequilibrium; his normal defense mechanisms are not working in their usual way. Because of this, crisis theorists suggest that he is more able to accept intervention and to develop new types of coping responses than he is under noncrisis conditions (Aguilera and Messick, 1978; Moos, 1979; Parad and Caplan, 1965; Rapaport, 1965; Spiegel, 1979). This belief is the basis of the idea that a crisis can actually be a positive learning experience for a person if the outcome is adaptation rather than maladaptation.

Nursing Process in Crisis Intervention

An essential aspect of crisis intervention by the nurse is that it is a collaborative attempt that involves the nurse *and* the patient as well as the support of the patient's social system. An important factor in crisis intervention is the nurse's openness to his or her patient's response to illness. A nurse can be aware of the patient's psychological dynamics and actually anticipate a crisis if the threatening event has serious implications for the patient's or the family's well-being. Chronic long-term illness or rehabilitation can have as much maladaptive potential as an acute life-threatening illness. Using the various types of data in the psychosocial assessment scale in Chapter 13, you may be able to predict those patients who are most at risk for crisis. Ideally, intervention can begin *before* a crisis actually occurs. An emotional crisis in a patient whose physical equilibrium is unstable presents more overall risk to his physiological status. By intervening and reducing his psychological stress, there is increased probability that you will do the following:

Promote his systemic well-being

Decrease his emotional stress

Frequently, prevent prolonged hospitalization

Reduce his risk of chronic maladaptation

Support his capacity for normal role functioning

Promote adaptive family dynamics, because the averted crisis can no longer disrupt the family

Assessment: Initial Evaluation of Patient's Response

Two types of patient responses can prompt a crisis intervention approach by the nurse: a precrisis situation, in which the threat of illness, the patient's personality style, level of stress he has experienced in the past year, his normal coping ability, and his family dynamics are warning signals that his ability to cope will be under severe stress, and a catastrophic illness or accident, in which the patient and his family have had little or no time to prepare for this serious psychological trauma. When the immediate denial stage passes, intrapsychic crisis in the patient or a system crisis in the family may occur.

Anxiety or depression are the two most common presenting symptoms of poor coping and potential crisis. Ideally, the patient will be able to recognize his own psychological discomfort and work with you as you help him to adapt to the stress of illness. If he is unaware of his maladaptation because of a distorted or lost sense of reality and is unable to help himself even with your support, then psychiatric consultation should be requested.

In the assessment process, it is important that the nurse understand the implications of the illness from the patient's perspective. Too often, as nurses, we believe that we understand the effect that an illness may or may not have on a patient. Actually, what we are doing is viewing the illness through our own eyes, our own value system and life goals, and so on. We actually are projecting our own thoughts and feelings onto the patient's situation. We assume that we are correct. Actually, it is necessary to find out what *this* illness means to *this* patient.

In order to find out how your patient views his illness, use the "tree approach" of information gathering recommended in Chapter 12: Counseling Techniques for Nurses. By demonstrating your caring in your questioning, the patient may feel marked relief. I have been surprised at times by the rapid reduction of anxiety within 5 or 10 minutes of beginning this process with an overwhelmed patient. Do not underestimate your therapeutic value. The counseling techniques recommended in Chapter 12 can assist you in knowing how to talk appropriately with the patient in distress.

A significant clue to the patient's anxiety or depression can be obtained by asking him, "Have you ever known anyone else with this problem?" A large number of patients have indeed known of someone; the person usually had severe complications that resulted in death or permanent disability. The person can be anyone: the distant cousin of a high-school classmate or a relative who may have died 30 years ago (in a much different medical environment). Ask the patient to describe the circumstances. Often, you will learn that the person had a complex illness with a different etiology than the patient's own. There also may have been many other factors present that are not present in your patient's illness.

Frequently, there will be the opportunity for you to correct the patient's misconceptions and identification with the other person. His fears may be dramatically lowered. The following case example helps to illustrate this technique.

Case Example*

Sarah is a 64-year-old woman with diabetes. An injury to her ankle resulted in a chronic ulcer that would not heal. A below-the-knee amputation was recommended, but Sarah adamantly refused to consider it. The urging of caregivers to have the surgery resulted in a high level of anxiety. Her surgeons were fearful that ultimately they would have to remove more of her leg if further tissue deterioration occurred. Finally, psychiatric liaison consultation was requested to "persuade" the patient that amputation was in her best interest.

It was soon discovered that 15 years earlier, Sarah's uncle had been in an automobile accident. He had been in acute shock from severe hemorrhage; kidney failure and severe metabolic distress had resulted. Because of peripheral vascular failure, three of his limbs were amputated, one at a time, in an attempt to save his life. Eventually, he died. Sarah was convinced that the removal of her foot could lead to the same end for herself. With explanation, she was able to understand that her circumstances were different in many ways from those of her uncle. By nightfall she decided to proceed with the amputation recommended by the surgeons.

Sometimes in our work with patients we believe that a high level of psychiatric assessment skills is necessary to understand what is wrong with patients. It is possible that nurses may devalue their own ability to help a troubled patient because

of this misconception. Actually, the patient may be able to tell you why he is reacting in such a way. Surprisingly, we fail to ask him what *he* thinks is causing him to react as he is to the illness. Many times he knows the answer, but until he talks about it and explores it out loud with a caring person it remains an abstract terror to him.

Until you understand *why* the patient is threatened by a particular illness, you will not be able to develop a therapeutic intervention. There are no specific interventions that are guaranteed for certain types of maladaptation. Your detective work in the assessment process and your understanding of the dynamics underlying his distress will help you as you design an intervention for this particular patient.

Planning the Intervention

During the planning stage you will have a chance to evaluate the patient's reality testing about his reaction to his illness. For example, it may be obvious to you, his other caregivers, and his family that his coping is not at an adaptive level. Initially, he may not be aware of his own inadequate coping. When this is so, this stage of crisis intervention can be a challenge, yet not an impossible one. Ballou has recommended the following techniques when the patient is defending himself from awareness of his own responses:

1. Reflecting the patient's feelings
2. Summarizing the content of messages
3. Helping the patient clarify feelings
4. Gently asking the patient to explain the consequences of his or her intended behavior
5. Not personalizing angry or hopeless feelings expressed by the patient but acknowledging his or her right to feel
6. Not avoiding dependency that might be manifest

(Ballou M: Crisis intervention and the hospital nurse. J Nurs Care 13:18, 1980)

In recommendation numbers 5 and 6, Ballou is preparing you for the possibility that the patient may *temporarily* direct some of his frustration and discouragement at you as if *you* were at fault. Remember that these are projections of the patient's own helplessness. Try not to feel helpless or responsible for them, however. Instead, attempt to recognize where your feelings of helplessness originate. Also, try to recognize where these feelings originate in the patient. This can be valuable information for you. These feelings the

---

*Another example of this type of maladaptive identification appears in Chap. 4.

patient has will pass when his coping ability returns. As described in Chapter 14 it is not possible for you to *make* a person cope. In addition to projecting his own feelings onto you, he may temporarily need to rely on your strength until his own returns. This neediness and dependency may last only a day or two.

In your admission assessment of the patient you may have determined that he has a dependent personality style. If he does, it is wise not to allow overdependence on you to continue beyond a day or two. If his dependency becomes a problem for you or other nursing staff members, there is potential for yet another crisis to occur about dependency issues: the unwillingness of nurses to continue meeting unreasonable demands. If marked dependency is occurring beyond 2 days of the crisis, the limit-setting approach outlined in Chapter 16: Nursing Intervention With the Emotionally Complex Patient can help to reduce the anxiety of both the patient and the nursing staff.

Another important consideration in the planning stage of the intervention process is to evaluate the response of the family or of the patient's significant other person to the patient's illness. Such a person or persons may be coping well and have the potential to support the patient while his coping ability is temporarily weakened. Another possibility is that their fear and immobilization may be undermining the patient's ability to cope.

No matter how competently you intervene with the patient, some families are set in their ways. Their family dynamics have been operating for decades and generations. Your intervention may be quite different from anything they are familiar with. This may be yet another threat to family equilibrium. Until you assess their response to their loved one's illness, provide reality testing for them, and obtain support for them if your own time constraints prevent you from becoming actively involved, they may continue to undermine the patient's adaptive capacity. You may have to modify your approach.

Depending on the support services available in your hospital, some sources of support for families are a family therapist with a medical, nursing, or social work background, a psychiatric liaison clinical nursing specialist, a clinical nursing specialist in the specialty field that the patient's illness is classified in (oncology, cardiac disease, obstetrics, and so on), a hospital social worker, or a member of the hospital pastoral care team. If there are no hospital support services you can call on, then ask the family if its priest, minister, or rabbi could help. In addition, most families usually have extended family members who are respected as "elders" who can help during difficult family times.

In planning the intervention, ask the patient about persons whom he trusts and can confide in. If he describes positive relationships with one or more family members or friends and they live within traveling distance of the hospital, include these persons in your plan. One of your recommendations can be as simple as encouraging the patient to share his concerns honestly with them.

Developing the actual steps you will use in your nursing intervention should involve the patient. In most cases, even when he is initially unaware of his maladaptation, your concern and reality testing will usually result in his willingness to work with you. When you and the patient agree about the reasons why he is not coping well, ask him how he thinks you and other staff members can help him. Ask him directly, "Is there something I can do to help?" or "Is there something we [the nurses] can do to help you with this?" or "What do you need from us in order to help you through this time?" The patient may be able to tell you directly. Incorporate his ideas in your plan. Then share with him your own ideas. Some of your proposals may appeal to him more than others. Allow him to describe the merit or lack of merit he would anticipate from the options you present to him. This step is called reviewing the alternatives. The patient should choose the approaches that he believes would be most helpful.

Once you and he have decided on an intervention plan, its success will depend on its use by as many nurses on the unit as possible. This is called a systems approach. It will provide a consistency and security that can be very supportive to a patient whose ego defenses are weakened or overwhelmed. Your plan must be charted on the nursing Kardex and its rationale and use verbally encouraged with the other staff members.

Nurses rarely share their crisis intervention plan with the house officers and attending physicians who are also caring for the patient. They mistakenly believe that physicians are not interested or would not be bothered to use their recommendations. The way that you approach them can make a difference in their receptivity to your ideas. Describe specific examples of the patient's symptoms of psychosocial maladaptation: unusual levels of anxiety, depression, noncompliance or other behaviors; shut down of communication with his spouse; frequent use of analgesics with excessive sleep as a way of avoiding the reality of situation; or similar types of objective data.

Rather than suggesting to the physician that he or she should follow your recommendations, describe the approach you have devised and provide the rationale for your choice. If it is having a positive effect, share your observations. It is then the physician's choice whether or not to use a similar approach. Many physicians are open to nurses' psychosocial recommendations and respect their opinions if they are articulate in presenting supporting data.

Intervention

The key to successful crisis intervention in the general hospital is consistency in the caregiver and in the caregiving system in maintaining the crisis intervention plan that is developed. This will promote the patient's reality-testing ability. Most important, it will allow the patient to trust you and his environment *at a time when his trust in himself may be faltering.*

The goal of crisis intervention is to help the patient regain his *precrisis level of functioning* (Aguilera and Messick, 1978). This is an important point to remember. Sometimes we may expect more than that of ourselves, and this can undermine our confidence in actively intervening with a maladapting patient. For example, a patient may have a type A (controlling) personality and become highly anxious because of the circumstances of his hospitalization. The goal of crisis intervention will be to assist him to understand the source of his anxiety and to gain more of a sense of control of his environment by intervention with the caregiving system. The outcome of intervention will be that his personality style is unchanged. His maladaptive anxiety, however, will perhaps be reduced.

Remember that when you begin to see a reduction in the patient's maladaptation, it is important that you continue the intervention process. The continuity of your approach will be an essential factor in resolving the crisis.

Evaluation of Intervention

The final stage of the nursing crisis intervention process is evaluating the outcome of your intervention. *This is an ongoing process* that should begin in the planning stage. During each interaction with the patient, you should continue to evaluate his mental status, looking specifically for a reduction in his anxiety, depression, or other maladaptive responses that were the original clues that he could not cope with his illness. If you do not see a decrease in his maladaptation response

within 24 hours, be prepared to develop another approach to use with him. You may continue to use your original plan if you and he believe it is helping. A second type of intervention plan can be used as an extra support during the critical period. The choice of a second type of approach should be arrived at using the same process as the original intervention plan. An important factor in a complex crisis situation is the nurse's flexibility in objectively evaluating the patient's response to his or her interventions. The nurse should be prepared to alter the original plan and be creative in developing different alternatives.

When Nursing Crisis Intervention Is Not Enough

On occasion, there are patients whose personality structures are unable to tolerate normal levels of stress in their everyday lives. Accordingly, the stress that accompanies illness and hospitalization can quickly become very threatening. When this occurs, it is not a reflection on the adequacy of the caregiving system. Nurses should try not to personalize the patient's maladaptive reaction. Instead, they can view the patient's maladaptation as the consequence of developmental and environmental factors that were in process before hospital admission. Strong clues in the patient's admission psychosocial history as well as his interactions with hospital personnel can indicate a high crisis potential for this patient.

There will be other patients whose hospital courses are marked by major setbacks and complications, and your interventions will be of great importance to them. As yet another setback occurs, however, it may be "the straw that breaks the camel's back." You may feel unable to deal with the patient's response. Another complex crisis situation is when the patient's coping failure is due to the effects of an organic brain syndrome (OBS). Because of actual deficits in brain functioning, the patient's normal defenses are weakened.

There also will be times when the patient's maladaptive response, such as noncompliance or dependency, results in nurses' inability to be objective. Their frustration level prevents them from being able to solve problems and be a support to the patient.

In all these circumstances, as well as others that contain multiple complicated factors, it is important to be able to recognize that you need assistance in knowing how to care for certain patients. In such cases, be open to the need for formal psychiatric consultation. Attending physicians and house officers are usually alert to the patient who is not coping well and will themselves initiate formal psychiatric consultation to assist the patient. If they are not aware of the maladaptive response, they will usually be receptive to the specific data that a nurse presents about a patient's inability to cope. At such a time you can recommend psychiatric consultation. The final decision is theirs, but physicians can be strongly influenced by an articulate nurse who has astutely assessed his or her patient.

If a psychiatric consultant is called in to work with the patient, it is important that you continue to maintain your involvement with him. You are a very important support person to the patient because you spend more time with him, and he usually has established trust in you.

Most psychiatric consultants are willing to share their impressions of patients with nursing staff members. (If they are psychiatric liaison consultants, they usually will seek you out to share their recommendations.) Talking to the consultant can be especially helpful if you are concerned that your approach to the patient may not be the most ideal or if you want to obtain specific recommendations about what you can do to help the patient.

Potential for Crisis

Many nursing textbooks address the critical developmental periods and situational events that can precipitate crisis. These periods and events usually occur in nonhospital environments and may initially seem to be unrelated to hospitalization and illness. Actually, as Chapter 9 intimated, it is possible that there is an association between developmental or situational crises and the eventual development of physical illness (Holmes and Rahe, 1967).

It is rare for nurses or physicians to include in their original assessment a question about the level of stress that patients experienced during the year before their illness developed. When I talk with patients, I frequently find that they are experiencing a developmental crisis. It may have been further compounded by a situational crisis *before* their physical illness developed. It is as if the illness were precipitated by these psychosocial or environmental strains.

The psyche (the mind) and the soma (the body) are constantly interacting; they are not two subsystems operating independently of each other. I am convinced that there are times when the ego is no longer able to mediate and defend against intrapsychic stress. Through an action probably related to neurotransmitters, it is possible that the temporary overwhelming of the ego results in failure of one of the body's subsystems. Physiological defense mechanisms are affected, and the body's ability to maintain homeostasis is temporarily overcome.

It is possible that the development of physical illness provides the severely stressed person with a means to restore his psychological equilibrium. Stop and think for a moment. What happens when someone becomes ill?

He has a temporary break from his normal work or school pressures.

He is able to withdraw temporarily from his extended social system, which has multiple social dynamics and inherent stresses.

He retreats to the safety of his family or to trusted support persons at home.

Family members and support persons rally and provide the ill person with extra physical as well as emotional care.

Work on job-related decisions, proposals, projects, or term papers is temporarily halted.

Any ongoing conflict in which he is involved is discontinued. The illness temporarily unsettles the adversary.

Often, the illness and its effect of removing the patient from the active psychosocial crisis present an opportunity for him to regain his sense of life goals, priorities, and personal objectivity.

Actually, illness that develops out of these circumstances may be adaptive. Although nurses cannot be expected to help resolve preillness crises that the patient is still reacting to unconsciously when he is hospitalized, it is important to be aware of the possibility of their existence. Take the time to find out how seriously this preillness stressor is affecting the patient. For example, a 52-year-old woman who is admitted with chronic obstructive pulmonary disease may tell you that she has been upset because her 25-year-old schizophrenic son has been in frequent crises because of his refusal to take medication. By using a problem-solving approach with this patient, you and she may devise some different approaches that she can use to help improve her difficult situation. It is also possible that there are no solutions. By helping her to work through to the reality of the situation, however, she may experience a lessening of guilt. She may feel a sense of relief that perhaps there really is no solution and she is not ultimately responsible.

By understanding the patient's preillness stressors, you will find out what postdischarge stressors are waiting at home. The patient can then feel some hope about a chronic problem that may have seemed hopeless. A referral to a social worker to address the family problem may promote both the patient's psychological and physiological adaptation.

When patients are hospitalized and have been experiencing high levels of stress from developmental or situational crises, they are more vulnerable to an inhospital crisis reaction to an illness-related problem. For example, if you discover during the assessment process that a single woman has been admitted with chest pain of undetermined origin, has been retired from her job for 2 years, has developed few outside interests, and reports being chronically depressed since her retirement, part of your nursing intervention with her can be to discuss her preillness living situation and postdischarge plans for seeking meaningful interests.

Too many times we admit patients, obtain extensive physical histories, give them elaborate physical workups, treat their physical ills, and discharge them without being aware of their psychosocial circumstances. It is not unusual for patients such as the women described above to be readmitted 2 months later with similar symptoms.

Whether your patient is in crisis or in a precrisis state, take the time to find out what else is going on in his life. His illness may in part have been caused by it.

Stress and Family Crisis

Stress is the greatest threat to healthy functioning of a family, both physically and socially (Telleen, 1980). Stress has been identified as the link between both psychiatric and physical illness (Dean and Lin, 1977). The most important factor in a family's ability to tolerate stress is the coping ability of the family members. The actual use of coping responses was identified as more important than other factors, such as a sense of control or positive self-esteem, in studying the persistent life strains of marriage and parenting (Pearlin and Schooler, 1978).

The events that cause the most strain in families are listed below:

Persistent life strains or deficits. Long-term types of problems that a person faces in his life role, such as marriage to a partner who has a chronic illness or being a parent or sibling of a premature infant who requires long-term hospitalization

Crises. Suddenly occurring, upsetting events that threaten emotional and physical well-being and require maximum coping ability, such as accidental catastrophic injury to self or family member or sudden death of family member

Transitions. The time following a crisis when adjustments are slowly made and equilibrium is regained, such as a young adolescent discharged after a severe head injury who requires an extended period of treatment to regain his previous level of functioning or a middle-aged mother who requires intermittent courses of chemotherapy after surgery for cancer

Without intervention with the family, members will continue to promote the patient's sickness, whether it is a heightened reaction to gastrointestinal symptoms of Crohn's disease or to symptoms of alcoholism. A systems approach that addresses the family's interactional style and enlightens members about the ways they feed into and promote a continuation of the patient's problems is an essential aspect of the management of critical events that are related to chronic physical or mental disease states.

Developmental Crises

Developmental crises occur as the result of poor adaptation to the emotional, physical, or social challenges of the normal process of growth and aging. Because of the prevalence of material in other textbooks on the major adjustments required during the various developmental stages, this chapter will briefly present the stages and their critical adaptive challenges (Aguilera and Messick, 1978; Erikson, 1963; Kalkman and Davis, 1980; Kyes and Hofling, 1980; Piaget and Inhelder, 1969). Be aware that the system effects within a family cause all family members to be affected by the developmental struggles of its members. For example, an adolescent's struggle to separate from his family has a marked effect on his mother, father, and siblings.

Developmental Stages

Infancy and Early Childhood (0–3 years)

Major issues (progressive from birth): trust, dependency, awareness of separateness from mother, development of autonomy

When issues are not resolved: distrust, poor self-confidence, fusion of self with caregiver, poor self-control

Childhood (3–11 years)

Major issues: identification with significant elders, development of initiative, security, and acceptance within family and eventually within peer group, mastery of age-appropriate skills and intellectual challenges

When issues are not resolved: guilt, lack of direction and purpose, self-undermining behavior, feelings of inadequacy

Adolescence (12–20 years)

Major issues: reawakening of Oedipal conflicts (see Chap. 3), idealization of significant others, resolution of loss of childhood, development of sexual identity, acceptance by peer group, psychological separation from family as adolescent develops his own perceptions of the world, physical separation usually occurs a few years later

When issues are not resolved: inability to separate from family and assume independence, sexual confusion, self-consciousness, inability to form relationship with person of opposite sex, poor object relations

Early Adulthood (20–30 years)

Major issues: ability to develop intimacy and commitment within a relationship, commitment to employment, exploration, and clarification of societal norms as they pertain to self

When issues are not resolved: superficiality in relationships with others, poor goal setting, drifting in and out of relationships and employment, lack of responsibility to self and others

Adulthood (30–50 years)

Major issues: maintenance of life goals, creativity, and spontaneity, ability to maintain meaningful relationships, appropriate channeling of emotions

When issues are not resolved: inability to work or to feel pleasure, poor motivation, egocentrism in goalsetting

Late Adulthood (50 years and older)

Major issues: ability to resolve losses of aging and to integrate ongoing losses, maintenance of hope, acceptance of uncertain future

When issues are not resolved: continual wishing to relive past experiences, inability to take pleasure in the present, loss of hope, depression

Situational Crises

Situational crises are crises resulting from stressful events that threaten a person's physiological, psychological, or social equilibrium (Aguilera and Messick, 1978). Many events have the potential to tax severely a person's adaptive capacity. When these experiences coincide with stressful developmental periods, or if two situational crises occur at or near the same time, they can be more disruptive. In addition, some persons have a lower-than-normal ability to adapt to stress and become

at risk for crisis easily. The following events are the most commonly encountered situational crises: separation from family, marriage, childbirth, divorce, life-threatening or chronic illness, and death. They are briefly reviewed below.

Separation From Family

The process of a young person's moving away from his nuclear family into an independent living situation can result in increased anxiety or depression for a young person (or his parents). Whether the departure is caused by a move to another city for employment, the beginning of college, or enlistment into the armed services, the young adult may experience a period of self-doubt and fear about his ability to cope with the many changes he is experiencing. It is possible that his family has difficulty in promoting his autonomy and allowing him to separate gradually from them psychologically during his middle years of adolescence. As a result, his actual physical departure from the home may be more complicated. Parents' expectations or overcautiousness are internalized and eventually may make it more difficult for the young person to individuate (Aguilera and Messick, 1978; Engel, 1963; Kalkman and Davis, 1980).

Marriage

Despite the tendency today for many young people to live away from home and to marry later than their predecessors, there are still many young men and women who do not move out of their parents' homes until they marry. These people also face the issues discussed above. Because of changing social mores and emphasis on the divorce rate, marriage is approached by many young people with more trepidation than was apparent in their parents' generation. This stress is added to the concerns of the couple as they commit themselves to one another and are subject to the normal strains in an intimate relationship. In addition, they usually are confronted by the differences in their value systems and the expectations of their extended families. Often, these aspects of compromise that are essential to a healthy marital relationship are not of significance during their courtship. The idealization of the partner that is common during the courtship and "honeymoon phase" of the early marriage gives way to the realities of coexistence (Engel, 1963; Kalkman and Davis, 1980; Kyes and Hofling, 1980; Rapaport, 1965).

Childbirth

The arrival of a child in a marriage causes a major shift in the interpersonal dynamics between a husband and a wife. A study of 48 American couples' responses to their first child revealed some of the dynamics that contribute to the crisis potential of childbirth. In the study, all the couples were middle class and between 25 and 35 years of age, and all the husbands were college graduates. Thirty-eight of the 46 couples (83%) reported extensive or severe crisis in adjusting to their first child. Of the 38 couples, the following data were obtained (LeMasters, 1965):

1. Thirty-five of the pregnancies were planned or desired.
2. Thirty-four of the couples' marriages were self-rated as good, and 31 of them were rated as good or better by close friends.
3. The personality development of the 76 husbands and wives was considered average or above average. They did not have "neuroses" or other psychiatric disabilities.
4. The 38 couples admitted that they had idealized the parenting role. They had not been prepared for the reality of taking care of an infant:
   a. The major adjustment reported by the mother was to constant fatigue from full-time care of the infant.
   b. The major adjustment of the father was related to the changes in his wife's former roles of sexual partner and income earner.
5. Mothers with professional training (eight) experienced "extensive" or "severe" crisis in every case.

It is important to emphasize that despite the critical effect of childbirth in a young marriage, most couples adapt effectively within a reasonable time.

Divorce

Divorce is a disruptive event. It results in major role shifts and losses within the family. Some of the issues that divorced persons experience are a disruption in role and normal family dynamics; reactions of children and extended family and friends; social stigma; rejection by former spouse, critical acquaintances, and possibly religious affiliation; loneliness; and anxiety about independent functioning. Many individuals also experience a major decrease in their self-esteem (Kyes and Hofling, 1980).

Because of the crisis potential in the process of divorce, there are many self-help groups offered by agencies in most communities. One of the risks inherent in the postadjustment phase of divorce is remarriage to a partner who is similar to the first spouse. It is common for neurotic needs to lead a person unconsciously into a second marriage with dynamics similar to the first (Aguilera and Messick, 1978).

Major Illness

A life-threatening or severe chronic illness poses many challenges to a person and his family: changes in body image and self-esteem, loss of control, issues of dependence and trust, separation from family, and changes in role functioning.

Because of its usually ongoing nature, the illness continually presents new challenges to the person and his family. Coping ability may be constantly tested.

The following chart divides the adaptive tasks of major illness into seven categories.

Major Sets of Adaptive Tasks

Illness related

1. Dealing with pain and incapacitation
2. Dealing with the hospital environment and special treatment procedures
3. Developing adequate relationships with professional staff

General

1. Preserving a reasonable emotional balance
2. Preserving a satisfactory self-image
3. Preserving relationships with family and friends
4. Preparing for an uncertain future

(After Moos R: Coping with the crisis of physical illness. In Freeman A, Sack R, Berger P [eds]: Psychiatry for the Primary Care Physician, p. 28. © 1979 The Williams & Wilkins Co., Baltimore)

With caregivers' increased awareness to the psychological risks of major illness, patients and families can be assisted in adapting to this major life event. The following case example illustrates how developmental and situational crises were further compounded by a physical illness.

Case Example

John is a 67-year-old retired insurance adjustor. He is married and has three children. He was admitted to the hospital after a major myocardial infarct (MI). He had had an earlier, less severe MI at age 59. Five years ago John developed a tumor of the spinal cord. As the result of surgery and radiation, he is paraplegic. John had to retire because of his disability. He has continued an active life and has many interests, including gardening, working with his tools, and traveling.

He had an unusually strong upper torso and arms and was able to move himself inside and outside by wheelchair. He drove a car and functioned independently. His adaptation to his paraplegia was very good. John's wife and family are strongly supportive. John was told by his physicians 1 year ago that the effects of the tumor would eventually result in loss of control of his bladder and bowels as he grew older. He had become increasingly depressed during the 9 months before admission as he envisioned himself eventually being unable to travel or attend the theatre. He believed that he would become an unbearable burden to his wife.

When the critical stage of MI treatment was over and his survival seemed probable, John became acutely depressed. Psychiatric liaison intervention was requested because he was rapidly losing his will to live.

Because of the severity of his myocardial damage, John was convinced that he would be unable to use his arms in order to maneuver himself in and out of his wheelchair. His concern about his impending bowel and bladder incontinence began to overwhelm him. Because he did not want to worry his wife, he withheld these overwhelming concerns from her. He was markedly anxious and was frightened by his inability to cope.

John was indeed in a difficult situation. His nurses and physicians identified with him and soon lost their objectivity, believing that perhaps there was no way out. John had demonstrated during earlier illnesses that he had strong adaptive ability. His adaptation had been weakened by his concerns of the previous several months. The depression was compounded by the severe MI. He was maladapting. Some of the interventions that were developed with John's approval were as follows:

1. Schedule an arm stress test as soon as possible in order to give him definite knowledge of his upper torso stress capability. (Stress test scheduling in the hospital is usually on a first-come, first-served basis. Physicians were asked to justify an earlier placement for this patient because of his critical need to know his future endurance and mobility potential.)
2. When John had talked out his overwhelming fears and when he felt ready to share them with his wife, he was encouraged to talk about them with her. The consultant pointed out his wife's loneliness and her own unspoken fears because she was perhaps trying to protect him.
3. Consultation with a neurological rehabilitation clinical specialist was arranged so that the patient could gain a more realistic perspective of his future bowel and bladder state.

4. Daily sessions with the psychiatric liaison consultant had the following goals:
   a. Continual reality testing with supporting data.
   b. Encouraging patient to express his deepest fears regarding his future course.
   c. Giving patient choices in his care plan whenever appropriate.
5. Ongoing liaison work with nursing and medical staff.
6. A session with John and wife was held on the third day, when his anxiety level was lower and he agreed to a joint session. Intervention to reduce communication barriers that had developed in their normally open relationship was utilized.

When the results of the stress test were available, they provided a great relief for John. They demonstrated that his activity level could be increased gradually to his pre-MI level as soon as he was comfortable. He became less depressed, more relaxed, and optimistic.

Another crisis developed a few days later, however, when a urological consultant recommended "dye studies" to determine his current urological status. (The test had originally been planned by his caregivers to reduce his anxiety level.) Twenty years earlier John had experienced a cardiac arrest as the result of dye used in a kidney study. The moment the urologist mentioned "dye," John shut out everything else the physician said. He was convinced he would die if he underwent such a study. John initially refused the study. He was asked by the psychiatric liaison consultant if he would be willing to allow the urologist to return. He was encouraged to write down specific questions about his concerns. On the physician's return visit, John learned that the dye was nontoxic and would be in his bladder, not his kidneys. John agreed to have the test. The results showed that he had a large retention capacity and strong sphincter control. His bladder condition was very good, and he was elated. He was discharged a few days later. His adaptation potential and that of his wife were positive.

Death

The potential loss of oneself or a loved one is another event that causes major adaptive stress in a person. The effect of death on patients and families will be dealt with in depth in Chapter 19: The Dying Patient and the Family. Usually death is not a sudden, unexpected event. Both the dying person and his family and loved ones have a time before the death during which they can gradually accept the effects of the impending loss. At times, especially when the dying person is a child or a young or middle-aged adult, the strains of adaptation result in crisis. Unexpected deaths sometimes have a greater potential for crisis, however, because the ego has had no time to develop adaptive mechanisms to deal with the sudden loss.

In either case, families with open patterns of communication will usually respond with strong emotions. The members of an open family are receptive to these emotions and solidly support one another. Their interactions are in contrast to families where emotions are repressed and avoided; the typical way that losses are dealt with is to avoid feelings or verbalized thoughts. This is a closed system of family relationship. When emotional dependence is denied in this type of family, the potential for crises within the family as a whole or in members is increased (Bowen, 1976).

Conclusion

The concepts in this chapter are important in understanding how people maintain psychosocial equilibrium during the threat of physical illness. When the stress of illness disrupts equilibrium, it is possible for nursing intervention to help restore it. By identifying the cause(s) of coping failure, an intervention can be designed to help avert or resolve a crisis. The theory presented in this chapter, when combined with the specific intervention approaches recommended in Chapters 16 to 19, can help to promote psychosocial adaptation in both patients and families.

16

Nursing Intervention With the Emotionally Complex Patient

When a person is admitted to the hospital for whatever reason, it is usually an important event in his life and requires a major adaptive effort. His coping ability can be severely challenged. If a person develops an illness that has a chronic treatment course accompanied by exacerbations and remissions, he too will experience psychic stress in adapting to his changed life style. Accordingly, each family member is affected; the normal dynamics of the family are shifted temporarily or permanently by the changes in functioning of one or more of its members.

When the stress of illness is too great for the ego to respond to in an adaptive manner, one or more types of maladaptive responses can occur. When these initial maladaptive responses occur, they do not always evolve into maladaptation. The ego can, through adaptive efforts, reverse the process. Perceptive caregivers, intervening when maladaptive responses begin to occur, can also help to reverse the process. When patients present unusual psychosocial nursing care challenges, they are most appropriately called emotionally complex patients. Some of the most common types of maladaptive responses are unusual levels of anxiety and depression, suicidal thinking, sexual dysfunction, overdependency, lack of motivation, and noncompliance. (Remember that anxiety and depression are normal responses to stress. Only when they become prolonged or severe are they considered maladaptive.) The degree of emotional stress that occurs as the result of inadequate ego defenses depends on factors that have been described in earlier chapters. They are normal personality style and coping ability, the patient's perception of the illness and the degree of threat it involves, and the availability and strength of a support system (in addition to family members and friends, hospital caregivers are part of the support system).

The major types of maladaptation will be described in this chapter. A brief description of the dynamics of each will be included, as will recommendations for interventions. In all instances, if symptoms of maladaptation persist despite your interventions or are severe, psychiatric consultation should be requested in order to ensure the patient's current emotional comfort and future adaptation. Another important justification for psychiatric consultation is to reduce the stress of caregivers in the prolonged care of a difficult patient. The consultant may be able to recommend alternative approaches to use with the patient that will be more helpful to all concerned.

The Anxious Patient

Anxiety, an unpleasant feeling of dread, is caused by an unconscious conflict between an underlying drive and the reality of the environment; the anxious person is unaware of the specific cause of his feelings. Anxiety is a different emotion from fear. *Fear* is an unpleasant feeling caused by a threat in the environment that is specific and can be identified (Kaplan and Sadock, 1981).

Of the two emotions, fear is more easily relieved. If a person knows the specific cause of his emotional distress, it is possible for him or others to take action to reduce it. The emotion of fear results from a person's familiarity and learned responses to previous negative experiences in his life. For example, a woman may have had an appendectomy at age 25 and, as a result, developed a severe systemic staphylococcal infection. When she enters the hospital for a cholecystectomy at age 50, she may fear a similar occurrence. When a fear is identified it is helpful for the nurse to ask open-end questions using the "tree" approach described in Chapter 12. As the fear is described, the accompanying unpleasant emotion is gradually released. The patient will usually report feeling surprisingly relieved.

Anxiety, on the other hand, is not as easily explained. Another 50-year-old woman who has a high level of preoperative anxiety may have no history of a negative experience with surgery. She and her caregivers may be unable to identify that the cause of her anxiety is due to her strong need for control. The experience of anesthesia and surgery involves giving over complete control of one's body to another. Her feeling of dread may be related to an unconscious fear of dying or her unconscious need to maintain constant control of repressed sexual or aggressive drives.

All normal persons experience fear and anxiety at various times during hospitalization. Some persons with specific personality types are more likely to respond to illness with anxiety. They are the controlled, suspicious, dramatizing, and superior personalities. When you observe patients with traits of those personalities, you can help to decrease their potential for anxiety by interacting with them in specific ways. Their anxiety is primarily due to their lack of trust in their own drives as well as their lack of trust in the environment. The environment includes the specific diagnostic tests and treatments they must undergo to become well. Their environment also includes you and other caregivers. They are not easily able to trust you.

Nursing Intervention

For all persons responding with anxiety to the stress of hospitalization, a professional but warm approach is preferable to one that is hovering and overly caring. First ask the patient if he has an idea what is causing his anxiety. When encouraged to explore the cause of their anxiety, many patients are able to discover the cause. Once they are able to identify the source of their anxiety, their level of discomfort often decreases. Whether or not the patient is able to identify the source of his anxiety with your supportive questioning, it can be helpful to him if you proceed in the following manner.

The patient will be more able to develop trust and a corresponding decrease in anxiety if you explain to him the reasons for the various types of diagnostic tests, treatments, and medications he is receiving. Reassurance should be given in a firm but caring way. Prolonged explanations should be avoided. Alternative choices should be explained to him, and he should be allowed to make as many decisions about his care as possible. Discussion between caregivers about his illness and treatment should not occur within his hearing. This is especially important in intensive care areas, where patients are more prone to anxiety about survival, where patients may appear to be semiconscious or unconscious but are still able to hear discussions about themselves, and where private conversations about patients' conditions are more difficult because of the proximity of beds and open space (Berger, 1979; Donnelly, 1979; Horvath, 1979; Sheehan, 1978).

Nursing Treatment Approaches to Reduce Anxiety

There are two treatment approaches that many nurses have begun to use in their work with the anxious patient as well as the patient in pain: relaxation technique and therapeutic touch. They involve processes by which the patient's anxiety response can potentially be reversed. In addition to possibly reducing the level of intrapsychic discomfort, there is an accompanying change in the patient's physiological state.

The sympathetic division of the autonomic nervous system is activated by anxiety. This causes an increase in heart rate, blood pressure, respiration, and blood supply in the active muscles. When the anxiety level is reduced, a state of both psychological and physical equilibrium returns. These techniques can be used by all nurses. In order to increase your comfort in using them, it can be helpful to use them initially with friends and co-workers.

Relaxation

Several types of relaxation techniques can be used. A simple and effective one is described below. First, it is important to talk with the patient and explore with him the cause of his anxiety. This helps him to establish trust in you and opens the possibility of therapeutic intervention. (Do sit down. You will be more relaxed, and he will feel more secure that you won't be running off.) Ask him if he is interested in learning a relaxation technique that he will be able to learn to do by himself and can provide relief for his anxiety (or pain). Give him a brief overview of what you will be asking him to do. Ask if he has any questions, then proceed slowly in a quiet, calm voice.

> Mr. Branchini, before we begin, I want you to think of a very special occasion or time in your life when you felt very peaceful, happy, and comfortable. Close your eyes now and focus on it. Visualize it in your mind and remember the feelings you felt at that time. Keep the memory in your mind as I talk.

Usually you will see the patient's facial muscles relax. Where there was a worried look, the face may become peaceful.

> Now I want you to lie very still and to make sure that your arms, legs, back, and neck are all in comfortable positions.

Reposition the pillow under the patient's neck and feel for tenseness in the neck muscles. Make sure that the neck is well supported.

> Now take five deep, slow breaths and let them out very slowly. Let your chest relax. Relax your stomach. Let your stomach help you breathe. Now I will ask you to tighten your muscles, then relax them. We'll start with your feet and work through your body up to your head. First point your toes forcefully, now relax them.

In your own mind think of all the pressure points where your patient's body touches the bed: heels, calves, thighs, buttocks, the back, arms, neck and head, and so on. Essentially, all the large muscle groups are included. In addition, the joints are a part of this relaxation approach. Think for a minute how much tension can be experienced in the joints (the ankles, knees, hips, wrists, elbows, shoulders, and neck). When a person is anxious or

in pain, both the muscles and joints are more tense than normal. As you work with the patient, gradually focus on the various parts of the body, progressing upward through the back, arms, neck, and head. Interject reminders to relax as follows:

> Now tighten your ankles; hold them tight; now relax them. Now we're moving up to your calves; tighten them; hold them tight; now relax them; you can feel them being very heavy, very relaxed. You can feel the mattress pressing up against them. Now tighten your knees; hold it; now relax them; they feel very loose.

Continue in this manner. Every now and then, tell the patient that he can feel the mattress pressing up against his back, elbows, or some other body part you are currently focusing on. This promotes a feeling of lightness or floating in the patient. This approach takes approximately 15 minutes to do with the patient. Ideally, it is recommended to talk the patient through the approach twice on the first day, then encourage him to do it twice more, perhaps before dinner and at bedtime. Tell him that you will inquire the next day how it worked for him and will review his technique with him.

The most therapeutic aspect of this method is the effect that the patient can achieve when he uses it by himself four times a day. The most advantageous times can be decided on by you and the patient. Many patients find it helpful to use it on awakening in the morning, before lunch, before dinner, and when going to bed in the evening.

The outcome of this relaxation technique is that patients report that their level of tension is reduced not only during the actual relaxation period, but during the interim period as well when they use it on a regular basis. It is an ideal approach for patients who are anxious or experiencing chronic illness such as angina, cancer, or respiratory disease.

Therapeutic Touch

Therapeutic touch is a treatment approach that involves a special form of communication between nurse and patient. It is beneficial for patients who are anxious or in pain (Boguslawski, 1980; Heidt, 1981; Sandroff, 1980). It can produce a state of physiological relaxation that is measurable by encephalography (EEG), heart rate, temperature, and skin responses (Krieger and colleagues, 1979). No formal scientific explanation is available to explain the cause of the effect. Some of the explanations that have been proposed have a sense of mysticism about them according to Western cultural beliefs; they are very compatible with centuries-old Eastern philosophies, however. It is believed that all humans give off energies and forces that have interpersonal potential (Boguslawski, 1980).

Another theory proposes that the relief experienced may be related to body endorphins and enkephalins. These two substances have opiate-like properties and are believed to be involved in a biochemical pain mediation process (Boguslawski, 1980). Initially, the procedure should be explained to the patient and his willingness to be treated obtained. An essential aspect of therapeutic touch is the nurse's ability to "center." Centering occurs when the nurse "lets go" of his or her psychic energy. There is an accompanying meditative sense of being at a different level of awareness; it is dominated by calmness and serenity. Once the nurse is centered, the actual therapeutic touch treatment takes only a few minutes to perform. The use of this technique can best be learned by attending a therapeutic touch workshop or reading about the subject. Dolores Krieger (1979), a leader in the field, has written a book on the subject.

Medication Management of Anxiety

Moderate and high levels of fear and anxiety result in somatic symptoms (Donnelly, 1979). When a patient's physiological and emotional equilibrium are compromised, it is important to share your observations with his physician. It is possible that he or she may not be aware of the level of anxiety that the patient is experiencing. With specific examples to document your request, anxiety-reducing medication may be ordered for the patient.

If antianxiety medication is ordered, the nurse should observe the effect of the medication over the first 24 hours. If the dose of medication seems to be too high or too low, your reported observations can help to determine a more therapeutic dose.

Generally speaking, for the patient who is nonpsychotic, sedation should be achieved with the use of the minor tranquilizers. Some of the more commonly prescribed minor tranquilizers are diazepam (Valium), chlordiazepoxide hydrochloride (Librium), oxazepam (Serax), and lorazepam (Ativan). Other medications used for sedation in general hospital patients are phenobarbital, meprobamate (Miltown, Equanil), hydroxyzine

pamoate (Vistaril), and diphenhydramine hydrochloride (Benadryl) (Levenson, 1981).

Major tranquilizers have many physiological side-effects and are thus contraindicated for many general hospital patients whose physical conditions are already compromised. The use of major tranquilizers in physically ill persons is usually restricted to patients with preexisting functional psychiatric disorders such as schizophrenia or manic depressive illness, patients with organic brain syndrome (OBS) whose physical and emotional well-being is at risk, and patients who become psychotic for any reason.

The most generally prescribed major tranquilizer for this type of patient is haloperidol (Haldol) (Horvath, 1979). Although side-effects can and do occur with its use, it is less potentially toxic to the physically ill person than some of the other major tranquilizers. It should not be used for an unnecessary time, however. Of all the major tranquilizers, it carries the highest risk of causing *tardive dyskinesia*, a permanent neurological condition with severe side-effects. For example, if it is being used for a patient with OBS, it should be discontinued when the patient's mental status returns to normal. Some of the other major tranquilizers are chlorpromazine (Thorazine), thiondazine (Mellaril), prochlorperazine (Compazine), perphenazine (Trilafon), trifluoperazine (Stelazine), fluphenazine (Prolixin), thiothixene (Navane), and loxapine succinate (Loxitane) (Levenson, 1981).

An important consideration is that sedation is used to control the patient's anxiety until his ego is able to defend itself adequately. Sedation should be instituted with the idea that it will be tapered down and discontinued as soon as possible. Prolonged use should be avoided because of its negative effect on the ability of the ego to defend itself with adaptive mechanisms; the longer the patient's anxiety level is relieved by medication, the longer the normal ego defensive functioning is at rest.

A case example follows.

Case Example

John is a 55-year-old factory foreman with malignant hypertension. Psychiatric consultation was requested by a frustrated group of house officers because John was becoming increasingly suspicious of the efforts of all caregivers, including his nurses. He was refusing all medication, diagnostic tests, and treatments. His reaction to their interventions was bordering on frank paranoia at the time of the consultation.

On entering the patient's room, the consultant remained somewhat aloof and unsmiling. A chair was drawn up to the foot of the patient's bed so that a distance was maintained between the chair and the bed. The chair was positioned so that it did not obstruct the patient's access to the door; the patient was between the door and the consultant. (A seated person is less threatening than a standing person to a suspicious patient.) These choices in approach were designed to minimize anxiety about an unknown person.

Rather than opening the evaluation session with a few general comments and then moving into an evaluation approach, the consultant spent half the session asking the patient about his work and family so that the patient could talk about himself and gradually feel more comfortable. It was especially important for his listener to be nonjudgmental.

The patient warmed to the consultant as he became more involved in describing in detail his knowledge about his work and his control over his subordinates. He also took pride in describing his role in his family.

Once the patient became more relaxed, the consultant began to ask him how he felt about his illness and then about his care in the hospital. Gradually he described his anger about people "telling me what to do." Some of his concerns about their recommendations demonstrated his paranoid thinking. Eventually, the consultant's questions helped him to explore these concerns in such a way that he eventually recognized his lack of trust.

He was asked what it was specifically that concerned him. He described the technical discussions of his condition that his physicians held daily at his bedside; he did not understand what they were talking about. He felt frightened by their complex words. In addition, he was concerned about taking medication prescribed by someone who had not identified himself or herself. He worried that the pharmacy might send the wrong pills. He was afraid that the different types of medications might poison his body; indeed, he had had a negative reaction years before to the synergistic action of three different medications. He didn't know who "really" was in charge of his care. He believed that his physicians thought he was "stupid." He also described a need to somehow be in charge of his own care.

As a way of helping him to understand the difficulty of allowing him to be in charge of his own care, the consultant used the information the patient had shared earlier about his work in the factory and the complexity of his role of foreman. The patient's job was described to him by the consultant as one that was responsible and required a thorough knowledge of many aspects of the assembly line. The patient agreed enthusiastically. The consultant asked him to imagine one of his physicians doing that job. He laughed gleefully. He was then asked if perhaps he would be in a similar position if he tried to do the work of his physician. He gradually realized that it would be similar.

In planning interventions to avert a crisis in this patient, the following recommendations were given:

1. One physician, preferably the chief resident (John was a service patient), should sit with the patient daily and briefly update him on the results of tests already performed, review the reasons for tests ordered for that day and tell him what to expect, explain the reasons for and the action of the various medications ordered for him, and discuss any new treatment or changes in existing treatment. Last, the patient's opinion of the information should be asked.
2. Whenever possible, the patient should be given choices about his care.
3. Discussions about the patient beyond his level of comprehension should take place several rooms away from the patient's doorway. If discussion occurs in the patient's room, he should be included. Complex medical words should not be used.

The house officers and nursing staff began using the recommendations that morning. John's level of comfort gradually increased, as did that of his caregivers.

The Depressed Patient

Depression is another common reaction to illness that can become maladaptive if prolonged or severe. Most general hospital patients who experience depression are responding to a major loss (Donnelly, 1979). Conditions that can cause a depressive reaction are illnesses that will result in a change in role within the family or in the work setting, chronic illnesses, especially those with a debilitating course, amputations, conditions such as stroke, brain injuries, or spinal cord injuries that require a prolonged rehabilitation period and that may result in permanently decreased functioning ability, and terminal illness. The changes in body image that result from these conditions represent a significant loss to many persons.

Often, when a psychiatric consultation is requested for a general hospital patient who is believed to be depressed as the result of illness, it is discovered that he was depressed before his hospital admission. He is frequently responding to an unresolved earlier loss that is then compounded by the illness. Some of the losses that are frequently mentioned by patients are those described in the Holmes and Rahe scale (see Chap. 9). They include loss of a spouse to death or divorce, loss of a member of the immediate family through death or a move out of the home, retirement, or changes in job status.

Depression is observed in two notable ways: changes in feelings and changes in thought content. The major cause of these changes in patients who are physically ill is due to loss of self-esteem (Donnelly, 1979). Self-esteem is related to the value that a lost person or object represented to the patient. His self-esteem was nourished by this emotional investment; when the person or object is lost, a very important source of the patient's self-esteem is decreased as well.

The observable feelings that a depressed person demonstrates are sadness, apathy, and loss of energy. He also experiences a loss of relatedness to other people; he withdraws. Although most patients are listless when depressed, some may experience high levels of anxiety and be agitated. Guilt is experienced, sometimes overwhelmingly. The thought content of the depressed person is evident in what he says. He expresses feelings of failure. These statements are usually associated with a patient's health, wealth, and sense of personal worth and value to others (Donnelly, 1979). Depressed persons are often hopeless that things will ever improve for themselves and feel helpless about being able to do anything about it. If their feelings of hopelessness and helplessness become acute or are prolonged, they may eventually think about or actually attempt suicide. The patient who discusses suicide or attempts it is discussed in the next section of this chapter.

Physical (neurovegetative) changes usually accompany depression. The most common changes are loss of appetite or, in some persons,

increased appetite, constipation, fatigue, pallor, and possibly headaches. Sleep disorders are common. Usually the depressed person will report difficulty falling asleep or remaining asleep; he may also wake up early and be unable to go back to sleep. Some patients will sleep longer than normal. There frequently is a reported decrease in energy level, as well as a decrease in sexual interest and functioning (Kyes and Hofling, 1980).

When a patient's depression is related to a major loss of any type, he will experience grief and undergo a bereavement process. The stages that he will go through before the loss is resolved are the same as those outlined in Chapter 19. If the loss is severe, the *normal* person may take approximately a year before emotional equilibrium returns.

It is worth noting that decreased mental alertness in the elderly, which often is mistaken for "hardening of the arteries" or other dementia-type states, may actually be a depressive reaction. This is especially so when the elderly person experiences decreased socialization and is isolated from normal human encounters. He usually has experienced multiple losses: death of spouse and friends, loss of job-related challenges and social contacts through retirement, and loss of normal physical and intellectual functioning due to aging and illness. Accordingly, his self-esteem can be seriously diminished, and he is at risk for depression. Many elderly persons in nursing homes who are thought to be demented show gradual improvement when they become members of groups that promote talking and sharing of feelings. So too do isolated persons living at home when they take part in adult day-care programs with opportunities for increased socialization.

Nursing Intervention

If you discover that a patient was moderately or acutely depressed before admission, or if the patient becomes acutely depressed during his hospitalization for any reason, a formal psychiatric consultation should be recommended.

When you observe a patient who seems depressed, it is often helpful to say directly, "Mrs. Albert, you seem depressed. Can you tell me how you're feeling?" This tells the patient that her discomfort is apparent and that you are available to listen. If the patient should begin to cry immediately, do not move to touch her or comfort her at that time. Instead, remain sitting nearby. Immediate touching or speaking soothingly before you know what is wrong frequently slows down or stops the patient from telling you what is bothering her.

The most important posture of the nurse is to be caring but quiet. A depressed patient who is lacking in energy and feeling isolated from people usually responds with more withdrawal to a talkative person who utters platitudes. The various counseling techniques presented in Chapter 12: Counseling Techniques for Nurses, can be helpful with depressed patients. The "tree" approach, for example, allows the patient to lead the conversation; your responses should relate to the information he has just shared with you.

The value of this approach can be realized if you think about what it is like to experience a major problem in your life. When you are having a difficult time, do you look for someone who quickly tells you how to solve every aspect of your problem? Or do you instead look for someone who will quietly allow you to talk it out? The other person's occasional questions can draw out different aspects that can help you to work through some of your distressing feelings and thoughts.

When talking with a depressed person, withhold your opinions. Frequently a depressed patient will ask a nurse what he should do or what the nurse thinks about his problem. In these situations, it is usually more insight producing for the patient if you turn the question quietly back to him, asking, "What do you think you should do?" or "How do you feel about ———?"

One of the times that your opinion can be given to a depressed patient is when he has inaccurate information about his illness and various aspects of treatment or rehabilitation. This inaccurate information, if pessimistic, can actually contribute to his depression. Your clarification with realistic information can potentially promote a more hopeful outlook for him.

Ideally, a depressed patient should be cared for with a primary nursing approach so that he can establish trust in an ongoing relationship with his nurse. A team nursing approach, which uses different nurses, may prevent him from verbalizing his deepest feelings. In an ongoing, supportive relationship the patient may be able to work through many of his concerns.

The Use of Antidepressant Medication in Physically Ill Hospital Patients

Because nurses on occasion see patients who are receiving antidepressant medication, they may believe that such medication can be helpful to all depressed patients. Actually, although such intervention is useful in many instances, it is not commonly used in depressed, hospitalized patients with physical illness. There are many reasons for this. The antidepressant medications used today have multiple physiological side-effects that occur with therapeutic dose levels. If these physical effects occurred in a patient with a complex physical illness, they would only complicate the clinical picture. The physician would not know if the physical symptoms were caused by the admitting disease, a new physical condition, or the medication.

Some of the commonly prescribed tricyclic antidepressants are imipramine (Tofranil), desipramine (Norpramin), amitriptyline (Elavil), and doxepin (Sinequan) (Levenson, 1981). The tricyclics have an anticholinergic effect on all body systems. For this reason, they are often contraindicated in a patient with physical illness.

Another group of antidepressants are the monoamine oxidase inhibitors (MAO inhibitors). Three MAO inhibitor antidepressants are isocarboxazid (Marplan), phenelzine (Nardil), and tranylcypromine (Parnate) (Levenson, 1981). They are not as clinically effective with most depressions as the tricyclics, but they act more rapidly. They also produce serious physical side-effects.

An important reason why antidepressants are not used with acutely depressed patients is that tricyclics take from 2 to 4 weeks to become clinically effective (Donnelly, 1979). At this time there is no rapid-acting antidepressant available. An antidepressant that may have a shorter onset of action than the tricyclics has recently been introduced. It is maprotaline (Ludiamil). It has a lower incidence of cardiovascular side-effects than most of the drugs listed above (*Physician's Desk Reference*, 1982).

The Suicidal Patient

Whenever a person is seriously depressed or is depressed because of a chronic illness that has a progressive downhill course, thoughts about wanting to die may be common. When they are with seriously depressed persons, some nurses feel uncertain of what they should say. They are afraid that they should not respond to a patient's broad hints that he wants to die. They also believe they should not ask the patient if he wants to die. They may fear that they might put the idea in the patient's head; if the patient went ahead and committed suicide, they would feel responsible, or the patient might say "yes" and they would not know how to respond.

As described above, the outcome of illness can result in changes in self-esteem because of its multiple effects on body image, self-image, role functioning, and overall quality of life. When depression is noted by nurses working in outpatient clinics or visiting nurse agencies, they may be the only health care professionals in contact with the patient. Nurses in hospital settings who observe patients for several hours may be closer to patients than any other caregiver. In these instances it is important to evaluate the suicide risk of moderately or severely depressed patients.

Certain populations are more at risk for suicide than others. In your assessment of a patient's suicide potential, the following information is helpful. These risk factors should be used only as a guide; actually, anyone, if hopeless enough, can commit suicide (Dubin and Stolberg, 1981, p. 69):

Populations at Increased Risk for Suicide

Older, single, divorced, or widowed men

Caucasians

Protestants

The unemployed

Patients in poor physical health

Patients who leave suicide notes

Patients living alone

Patients with an anniversary death or loss

Patients with sudden changes in life situation

In multiple studies of patients who completed or attempted suicide, the most significant finding of risk factors was that the patient had recently lost a significant relationship (Adam, 1978).

Another important aspect of the assessment of the suicidal plan is the level of risk involved. Generally, plans that involve ingestion, cutting, or stabbing have a lower risk of lethality; drowning, asphyxiation, and strangulation carry a moderate risk; and jumping and shooting are high-risk suicidal choices (Weisman and Worder, 1972). It is emphasized, however, that *any* of the suicidal choices listed above can be lethal.

Table 16-1 contains a comprehensive list of suicidal risk factors and ranks them according to degree of risk.

Nursing Intervention

Whenever a patient talks hopelessly about the future, gives general hints that "you won't have to worry about me much longer," or overtly states "I'd like to get it all over with," it is important to find out what he is thinking. If you prefer, you can avoid using the word suicide in your question. Instead, you can ask, "You sound discouraged, Bob. Do you ever wish you were dead?" or "Do you ever think about ending it all?"

Although these questions might sound provocative to use with a seriously depressed person, they actually can prove to be a relief for him. He may have been thinking about suicide and been frightened by the intrusive and unwanted thoughts. Usually when this happens, the patient suffers alone because he does not dare to tell anyone. When an astute person notices his distress and asks him if he ever has such thoughts, it is a relief for him to unburden himself.

If the patient acknowledges that he has been thinking about killing himself, there are many questions you can ask him, using the suicidal risk factors printed above as a guide. One of the most important ones is, "How would you kill yourself?" If he describes a specific plan, his risk is far more significant than the patient who has vague, unspecified thoughts. His intentions are serious, and psychiatric intervention is essential with no delay.

Another important question that can help you to identify the level of suicide risk in a patient who acknowledges suicidal thinking is, "Is anything keeping you from going ahead with your plan?" If the patient gives you reasons why he does not want to go ahead with his plan, then his risk can be high, but not as high as the person who can give you *no* reason why he should continue to live. Some reasons usually described are, "My family needs me" or "I have an important event or project to complete in the future."

Whenever you assess a patient's suicidal potential as high, notify the physician immediately with a strong recommendation for immediate psychiatric referral. The patient in an inhospital or outpatient setting should be observed constantly until the consultant arrives. The person in an outpatient setting should not be allowed to leave until he is seen by a psychiatric consultant.

If the patient has a moderate suicide potential based on your assessment, the physician should be notified immediately and the patient should be monitored on a one-to-one nursing care basis. Psychiatric consultation is recommended for this patient as well in order to rule out a serious suicide risk.

The patient who has a low risk for suicide should not be underestimated. His risk can shift with any change in his circumstances. The phy-

Table 16-1.
Assessing the Degree of Suicidal Risk

| Behavior or Symptom | Intensity of Risk | | |
	Low	Moderate	High
Anxiety	Mild	Moderate	High, or panic state
Depression	Mild	Moderate	Severe
Isolation-withdrawal	Vague feelings of depression, no withdrawal	Some feelings of helplessness, hopelessness, and withdrawal	Hopeless, helpless, withdrawn and self-deprecating
Daily functioning	Fairly good in most activities	Moderately good in some activities	Not good in any activities
Resources	Several	Some	Few or none
Coping strategies and devices being used	Generally constructive	Some that are constructive	Predominately destructive
Significant others	Several who are available	Few or only one available	Only one, or none available
Psychiatric help in past	None, or positive attitude toward	Yes, and moderately satisfied with	Negative view of help received
Life style	Stable	Moderately stable or unstable	Unstable
Alcohol and drug use	Infrequently to excess	Frequently to excess	Continual abuse
Previous suicide attempts	None, or of low lethality	None to one or more of moderate lethality	None to multiple attempts of high lethality
Disorientation and disorganization	None	Some	Marked
Hostility	Little or none	Some	Marked
Suicidal plan	Vague, fleeting thoughts but no plan	Frequent thoughts, occasional ideas about a plan	Frequent or constant thoughts with a specific plan

(Hatton D, Valente S, Rink A: Suicide Assessment and Intervention, p. 56. New York, Appleton-Century-Crofts, 1977)

sician should again be notified. In all cases, your assessment and the patient's verbatim statements should be recorded. Specific notation about the time and date the physician was notified are important.

At times, some physicians are not responsive to nurses' reports of patients' suicidal ideation or planning. If this type of negativism occurs, it is important to maintain observation of the patient and to pursue that physician or another physician who is attending the patient until an order for psychiatric consultation is obtained. Despite an attending physician's refusal to heed your assessment, the legal responsibility of an attempted or successful suicide will, at least partially, belong to the nurses on duty at the time.

If a patient is found to be actively suicidal, plans should be made for transfer to a psychiatric unit where his safety can be ensured. If, because of complex nursing care, he must remain on a medical or surgical nursing unit, the psychiatric consultant should be asked for specific nursing

care recommendations. He or she should be reminded that the nurses in attendance are not trained to care for the suicidal patient. Frequently, in this type of situation, staff nurses become very anxious about caring for the patient. Whenever possible, a psychiatric clinical specialist from the psychiatric unit or a liaison nurse, if one is available, should be asked to work with the nursing staff in developing a care plan for the patient. In any case, until the patient is assessed by a psychiatric consultant, constant one-to-one nursing care should be instituted.

The Unmotivated Patient

Nursing care of the unmotivated patient is a challenge. It seems that other caregiving disciplines such as medicine, the dietary department, and physical therapy often look to nursing to know how to help the patient "want to get better." Immobility occurs when there are no physical impediments to rehabilitation. Instead, psychological attitudes are preventing the patient's return to fuller role functioning. Whether the patient has experienced a stroke, major surgery, or a heart attack, there comes a point when treatment for his acute illness subsides and it becomes the patient's responsibility to "get himself going."

One of the most helpful clues to the unmotivated patient's response to illness is to find out how he has responded to major stressful life events in the past. Was he an active, eager person who responded to life's challenges with energy? Or did he respond to major setbacks with depression and inertia? Without many exceptions, the patient who has maladapted in his past when a very stressful event occurred is likely to respond in a similar manner with a major illness. If the patient's lack of motivation is not typical for him, it is possible that he is experiencing a reactive depression. In either case, if his lack of motivation is prolonged, his capacity for return to normal functioning is in jeopardy; if nursing intervention does not bring about a change in his motivation, psychiatric consultation should be recommended to the attending physician. As a nurse, your interventions will continue to be very important in the overall goal of his returning to normal functioning.

Nursing Intervention

The recommendations for working with depressed patients can be beneficial with the unmotivated patient. His lack of motivation is frequently associated with his anticipation of many losses: physical mobility, role functioning, sexual functioning, and so on. Often it is difficult for this patient to identify and talk about his fears. It may be helpful for the patient if you can empathize and ask whether he is worried about his ability to get back to work or to take care of his family.

Another important intervention is to do a low level of goal setting on a daily basis. By setting a goal that is easily and quickly achievable, the patient's sense of hope may be more quickly mobilized. Long-range goals with this type of patient serve to further undermine his adaptive ability. A mutual goal set by the patient and you in an informal contract, such as walking to the chair or washing his own legs or eating half of the food on the tray, makes the patient feel good. His desire to attain another goal is reinforced by the positive feelings he is experiencing.

If psychiatric consultation occurs, try to talk with the consultant or ask that specific recommendations for nursing intervention be noted so that you can follow a similar approach. Chart those recommendations on the Kardex so that a systems approach is ensured.

The Alcoholic Patient

Approximately 10 million persons in the United States are alcoholics. This is approximately 7% of the population over 18 years (Estes and associates, 1980). The incidence of alcoholism in hospitalized patients is much higher than in the general population because of the pathological effect of alcohol on multiple body systems. Some of the conditions that are caused by the effects of prolonged, excessive alcohol consumption are alcoholic hepatitis, Laennec's cirrhosis, pancreatitis in the absence of cholelithiasis, chronic gastritis, hematological disorders such as certain anemias and clotting disorders, cerebral degeneration in the absence of Alzheimer's disease or arteriosclerosis, beriberi, and pellagra. Many accident victims or victims of gunshot wounds are alcoholic. Alcoholic patients also have a risk of greater infections, cardiac arrhythymia, and cigarette or other burns (Estes and associates, 1980).

Nursing Intervention

The immediate concern of the nurse caring for the alcoholic patient is the observance of symptoms of alcohol withdrawal. Some alcoholic patients are easily identified by caregivers because of their debilitated appearance or strong odor of alcohol or because they have been hospitalized before. Measures designed to alleviate the symptoms of withdrawal are usually ordered for these patients on admission.

The alcoholic patient who presents a major challenge to the nurse is the one who does not identify his alcohol dependence during the admission process. His first symptoms of withdrawal can proceed to more severe symptoms if caregivers miss the warning signs. Table 16-2 presents the time periods and symptoms of the progressive stages of the alcohol withdrawal process.

If you suspect that a patient's increased restlessness, anxiety, and changes in physiological status may be alcohol related, contact his physician. For example, a patient who is admitted for emergency surgery may begin to demonstrate alcohol withdrawal symptoms on his first postoperative day. At times, the diagnosis of alcohol withdrawal can be difficult for the physician to differentiate from other physiological or functional

Table 16-2.
Timetable of Alcohol Withdrawal

Name of Stage	Time Since Last Drink	Symptoms
Alcoholic tremulousness (may subside after 3 or 4 days with no intervention or may progress to a more severe stage)	Within 12 hours	Movement disorder; coarse, general tremor; perceptual changes; gastrointestinal upset; sleep disturbance; Anxiety, hypervigilance
Alcoholic hallucinosis (can last 1 or 2 days and subside or become more severe)	Within 12 to 24 hours	Perceptual distortion moving to frank auditory or visual hallucinations
Alcoholic seizures	Within 12 to 48 hours	Grand mal seizures in multiple sets of up to 6 seizures
Delirium tremens (approximately 10% of persons die; when persons have medical complications, morbidity is 25%)	Within 3 to 4 days	Tachycardia; blood pressure changes; sweating; fever; marked changes in mental status: hallucinations, delusions, terror, agitation

(Information adapted from Berger and colleagues, 1979; Cassem, 1978; Pattison and Kaufman, 1979; Woodell, 1979)

psychiatric disorders. The most common pharmacological treatment for the alcohol withdrawal syndromes is use of the minor tranquilizers, such as chlordiazepoxide (Librium) or diazepam (Valium). At times, haloperidol (Haldol) may be ordered for extreme combativeness or agitation due to hallucinations (Berger and coauthors, 1979; Cassem, 1978).

If symptoms of alcohol withdrawal occur, the patient's bed should be left in a lowered position. The potential for self-injury may ultimately make restraints necessary. Restraints should not be used for long periods, however. The patient's sedation should be maintained at a level that eliminates the need for constant, full restraints (Cassem, 1978). Whenever possible, the patient should be moved to a room in view of the nurses' station.

The danger of accidental or purposeful injury or death, especially for the patient experiencing alcoholic hallucinosis, cannot be overemphasized. Persons in alcohol withdrawal can experience rapid shifts of mood or delusional or hallucinatory states (Cassem, 1978). Their actions can be swift and tragic. Constant surveillance should be maintained until the patient's safety is ensured.

Another aspect of nursing care is reality testing with the patient once the acute medical condition or withdrawal state is controlled by hospital treatment. Because of the high incidence of alcohol-related illness in hospitals, many larger institutions employ alcohol counselors to intervene with prealcoholic or alcoholic patients. In the past, alcoholic patients often were treated for their alcohol-related systemic diseases, but there was

no attempt to treat the alcoholism itself. As a result, many patients frequently entered and were discharged from hospitals at a high cost to the hospital, welfare agencies, and private insurance companies. The inclusion of alcohol counselors on the treatment team provides an extra resource for the nurse who is working with an alcoholic patient.

A high level of denial is common in alcoholic patients (and, in the earlier stages, in their families as well). If the patient is formally identified as an alcoholic, intervention by the alcohol counselor early in the hospital course may result in the patient's seeking help for his condition after discharge. If an alcohol counselor is not available, the responsibility for patient counseling and education will fall on the physician and the nurse. The reality issues of alcoholism and its negative effects will become even more important for them to emphasize. Firm statements of fact and direct confrontation are often necessary. The defense mechanisms of the alcoholic patient are strong. He uses denial, avoidance, rationalization, and projection (Yearwood and Yates, 1979). Caregivers should avoid excessive persistence in confrontation. It will usually result in strengthening of the patient's defenses.

Follow-up counseling or referral to an alcohol-treatment program is usually recommended. If so, the appointment for the follow-up care should be arranged by the patient, not the caregiver. The patient must ultimately help himself. Efforts by caregivers to perform this service frequently end up in frustration for all concerned. Massachusetts General Hospital has established the policy that the alcoholic patient be informed of the various community resources available to him, including Alcoholics Anonymous. A responsible family member should also be informed about these resources. Arrangements for follow-up treatment are then the patient's responsibility (Cassem, 1978).

The Patient With Sexual Dysfunction as the Result of Physical Illness

This section will present information on two types of sexual dysfunction in which nurses' interventions are important. Changes in sexual functioning have two main causes: actual changes in physiological functioning that impair the physical process, or changes in self-esteem, body image, and self-image that psychogenically contribute to impaired physical functioning. The first is the sexual dysfunction potential of patients with particular diseases that can contribute to changes in sexual functioning. Nurses in hospital settings can educate and talk with patients about various aspects of living with illnesses that may permanently or temporarily affect their normal sexual functioning. Nurses in outpatient or visiting nurse agencies can assess the patient's response to diseases or particular medications that are known to cause decreased sexual functioning. Another type of sexual dysfunction that will be discussed is the sexual acting-out behavior of hospitalized patients.

The Effect of Illness on Sexuality

As discussed above, many diseases result in permanent changes in a person's body image and the way that he relates to other people. The initial effect of these changes can cause a decrease in self-esteem. If the patient's reaction to the changes in his body functioning is maladaptive, the result can be a chronically poor self-image and low self-esteem. All aspects of his life will be affected. Because of the relationship between body image, self-esteem, and sexual functioning, it can be expected that the patient's normal level of sexual functioning will be decreased. Sensitive discussion by the nurse with patients whose conditions are known to cause changes in body image can be valuable. Misunderstandings brought about by caregivers' lack of attention to this essential aspect of humanness can contribute to a decrease in quality of life for the patient and his partner.

Conditions that can contribute to changes in sexual functioning are cardiovascular disease, cancer, amputations, kidney failure, arthritis, and accidental injury resulting in blindness, deafness, or disfigurement. In addition, several physical conditions result in erectile dysfunction. This impotence results in inability to have sexual intercourse and can contribute to psychosexual dysfunction for both males and females. Although it is not generally described in the literature, women can be equally affected by conditions that result in incomplete filling of blood vessels in the genitalia. In the female, as well as in the male, there is an erectile phase that is preliminary to orgasm. Diabetes mellitus of less than 1 year was associated with a 70% rate of impotence; 1 to 5 years of diabetes mellitus resulted in impotence in 43% of the men; and more than 5 years of the illness caused 45% of the men to be impotent (Rubin and Babbott, 1958). The higher incidence of impotence in the first year was not explained in their study. It is possible that as the patient adapts to his new illness and the changes it has created, he experiences a higher level of stress and anxiety. These can contribute to decreased sexual functioning ability.

Fifty percent of colostomy patients whose surgeries are due to cancer of the rectum, which requires sectioning of the autonomic nervous plexuses, have a problem with impotence. This is so also for half the patients with combined abdominal-perineal operations or with prostatic surgeries (Bossert and Freeman, 1979).

Other patients who report impotence are those who have aortoiliac bifurcation grafts for aneurysms of the abdominal aorta or severe atherosclerotic vascular disease of the aorta or iliac vessels (Bossert and Freeman, 1979).

In addition to the information in this chapter, refer to Chapters 18 and 19 for more information on potential sexual dysfunctioning in specific illnesses or conditions.

Although a person may ultimately adapt to the changes in body image and sexual functioning caused by these illnesses, he will undergo a process that, at times, is stressful and frustrating. If the beginning of his process is marked by the ability to discuss concerns with a caregiver who is able to give him honest and reliable answers, his potential for adaptation can be facilitated.

Discussion about sexual functioning should be delayed until the acute phase of hospital treatment is passed. For example, a patient who has had a colostomy will be more focused on his recovery from major surgery and his response to the colostomy itself. When he is preparing for discharge, thoughts about changes in sexual functioning are more likely to be present.

Nursing Discussion of Sexual Dysfunction

Although sex is one of the main sources of pleasurable feelings for most persons, discussion of it is taboo in most Western cultures. As a result, medical and nursing students have, until recently, had little content about sexuality in health and disease in their curricula. This has resulted in a disservice to them and their patients (Hicks, 1980; Meyer, 1979).

As a result of this taboo, lack of knowledge, feelings of inadequacy, and perhaps uncertainty about the need for such discussion, few caregivers are comfortable about entering discussions about sexuality with their patients. When the risk of long-term sexual maladaptation can be potentially reduced, however, perhaps caregivers can begin to risk such involvement.

A few thoughts that might be helpful in working through some of the normal hesitation experienced by nurses are that the patient will rarely react with shock to your discussion. Instead, he will probably be relieved that someone is giving him the chance to talk about his concerns. If he does not have any questions, he will tell you so at this time and there may be no further discussion. Sometimes, patients who initially have no questions will open the discussion with you again in a few days.

Nursing Intervention

A direct and honest approach with patients is usually helpful to them as well as to the nurse who may initially feel uneasy. Opening questions about the patient's general feelings about his condition can result in a natural progression to discussion of sexuality. For example, you might ask, "Mrs. Andrews, how do you feel about your amputation? Do you have any concerns about it? Do you have any concerns that it could have an effect on your relationship with your husband? Do you think it will have an effect on the way you feel about yourself sexually?"

These questions may seem very personal, and indeed they are. They can be very helpful to the thoughtful patient, however, who may already be worrying about her changed appearance and the effect it might have on her husband. If the patient is not psychologically ready to discuss these matters with you, defense mechanisms such as denial, avoidance, and repression will prevent the discussion from proceeding. He will let you know verbally or nonverbally that he is not ready or has no concerns.

The latter is an important point. It is helpful to remember that the goal of a patient's overall rehabilitation is to return him to his preillness level of functioning. The same is true for sexual rehabilitation. If the patient had little or no sexual interest before becoming ill, he will have little or no sexual interest afterward. If a patient tells you he has no concerns, his statement should be accepted.

Most important for your own comfort, when you enter into a discussion about sexual functioning with a patient, acknowledge to yourself that you do not know the answers to all the questions a patient might ask. (Probably no one does.) Instead, be prepared, and offer to find out the answers from someone who does or refer him to someone who is more knowledgeable. Usually physicians in rehabilitation programs or physical therapists can be of assistance. Hospital librarians are also good resource people. They can review the literature and provide you with information.

Effect of Medications on Sexual Functioning

Many commonly prescribed drugs have pharmacological actions that temporarily decrease the normal physiological action of the sexual organs or their nerve supply. Specific information about the cause of physiological effects can be obtained by referring to a pharmacology textbook. The following list presents the names of drugs that can contribute to sexual dysfunction. The most common side-effect is impotence. Other side-effects are decreased sexual drive and ejaculatory disorders.

*Medications That Can Cause Changes in Sexual Functioning**

Antihypertensive Drugs
    Guanethidine (Ismelin)
    Reserpine (Serpasil)
    Guanethidine (Inversine)
    Trimethaphan (Arfonad)
Diuretics
    Spironolactone (Aldactone)

*After Woods J: Drug effects on human sexual behavior. In Woods N (ed): Human Sexuality in Health and Illness, 2d ed. St. Louis, CV Mosby, 1979.

Antidepressants
  Tricyclic type
    Imipramine (Tofranil)
    Desipramine (Norpramin, Pertofrane)
    Amitriptyline (Elavil)
    Nortriptyline (Aventyl)
    Protriptyline (Vivactil)
  MAO inhibitor type
    Phenelzine sulfate (Nardil)
    Tranylcypromine sulfate (Parnate)
    Pargyline (Eutonyl)
Sedatives and tranquilizers
  Major tranquilizers
    Chlorpromazine (Thorazine)
    Prochlorperazine (Compazine)
    Thioridazine (Mellaril)
    Mesoridazine (Serentil)
  Minor tranquilizers
    Chlordiazepoxide (Librium)
    Diazepam (Valium)
  Antispasmodics
    Methantheline (Banthine)
    Glycopyrrolate methobromide (Robinul)
    Hexocyclium (Tral)
  Antihistamines
    Diphenhydramine (Benadryl)
    Promethazine (Phenergan)
    Chlorpheniramine (Chlor-Trimeton)

In the last decade, health care literature has increasingly addressed the sexual needs of patients whose physical conditions cause a change in their normal functioning. Many authors discuss the sexual functioning of patients with specific diseases or conditions. These books can be enlightening for caregivers as well as for patients.

Several books addressing many aspects of sexual adaptation to illness are listed below. They also would be appropriate for intelligent patients and their partners whose anxiety about changes in sexual functioning is due to lack of information. The information included could help alleviate concerns and produce better insight and more hope for a return to rewarding functioning.

Mions F, Swenson M: Sexuality: A Nursing Perspective. New York, McGraw-Hill, 1980

Siemens S, Brandzel RC: Sexuality: Nursing Assessment and Intervention. Philadelphia, JB Lippincott, 1982

Woods N: Human Sexuality in Health and Illness, St. Louis, CV Mosby, 1979

Sexual Acting Out in Hospitalized Patients

Other types of sexual dysfunction that cause nurses concern are sexual aggressiveness or other types of socially unacceptable sexual behavior. In most instances, it is male patients who act out with female caregivers. Likewise, the seductive female patient can be a care challenge for male caregivers. Behaviors that can occur in the hospital are sexually provocative statements or overt sexual gestures such as the patient's attempting to touch the nurse's breasts or hips. Genitalia may be exposed, or masturbation may occur.

In some cases, these behaviors are due to changes in social judgment due to functional psychiatric illness or acute OBS. Usually, however, the causes result from patients' needs "to obtain validation of their sexuality, to gain control of a situation in which they are dependent, or to attract attention" (Woods, 1979, p. 278). Some male cardiac patients, for example, experience great anxiety about their sexuality after myocardial infarct (MI). This can result in acting-out behavior with staff nurses. Their behavior is due to threats to their masculine identity and their need to seek reactions to their sexuality (Cassem and Hackett, 1971).

Sexual acting out by patients frequently results in uncomfortable feelings of anxiety for the nurse. Nurses will often share their unpleasant experience with their peers. Quickly, the other nurses label the patient as someone who is "bad" and should be avoided. The nurses' feelings often are related to their own sexual anxieties and fears about sexual functioning.

Nursing Intervention

If sexual acting out occurs, it can be precipitated by a variety of causes described above. The outcome, however, is ultimately due to the patient's inability to control his impulses. In order to decrease the discomfort of all concerned, it is important that a unified nursing intervention approach be used. At a change of shift report when all caregivers are present, the problem can be identified and discussed briefly so that all nurses will respond in a manner that can help the patient to regain control. The most important responses of the nurse are as follows:

1. Do not avoid the patient.
2. Maintain a professional attitude with the patient rather than allowing anxiety or embarrassment to prevail.

3. Enforce limits on the patient's unacceptable behavior. As soon as he says or does anything unacceptable, he should be told firmly that it *is* unacceptable.

It can be helpful to temporarily assign senior nursing staff members to the care of a sexually acting-out patient. Until his behavior is modified by the actions recommended above, a young and pretty nurse may, by her presence, precipitate unpleasant sexual anxiety in the patient and provoke continued acting out. Many times, the use of a limit-setting approach with sexually acting-out patients is effective. The limit-setting approach is described below. If the limit-setting approach needs further reinforcement, the attending physician can be asked to speak with the patient about his unacceptable sexual behavior. At a different time, the head nurse can speak with the patient and explain that his behavior is unacceptable. In all instances, and on a regular basis, a staff member should take the time to sit with the patient and explore his concerns about the anticipated effects of this illness on his sexuality. Frequently he has many. He may or may not be able to talk about them. The acceptance by the nurse that he may have concerns and that they are normal can help to relieve some of the anxiety that may be causing his behavior.

The Demanding or Noncompliant Patient

Some patients, especially those with illnesses that require long hospitalizations, eventually tax the patience of nurses and other caregivers because of their seemingly incessant need for care. There are many types of patients in this category. They may be persons who normally have strong dependency needs or have regressed to a very dependent state because their normal defenses have been overwhelmed by the stress of prolonged illness. Other personality types who may cause excessive demands on nurses are antisocial, manipulative, or controlling patients. Noncompliant patients also present a problem in nursing care. Information about the underlying dynamics of many of these personalities can be obtained in Chapter 5: Personality Styles Seen in General Hospital Patients.

Nursing Intervention

With demanding or noncompliant patients, the use of a limit-setting approach can be a relief for all concerned. Stop and think for a moment about a patient you have cared for who fits into one of the categories above. During the first week of his hospitalization, his demands or noncompliance may have been tolerated by the staff; their interactions with the patient were adequate. By the second week, however, the patient may wear out the most dedicated nurse by his repeated demands on his or her time and patience. Ultimately, this type of patient often is an unwelcome assignment; his call bells are avoided, and he becomes the object of staff joking in the nurses' conference room.

When a patient care situation has deteriorated to this point or has the potential to do so, the implementation of a limit-setting approach can help to reverse the outcome.

A Limit-Setting Systems Approach to Use With Complicated Patients

It is important to realize that the patient's behavior in the hospital setting springs from unconscious needs and drives. The patient may be aware that his behavior is aggravating to the nurses. He can see annoyance in their faces. He can hear frustration in their voices. He can feel impatience in their touch. He may be helpless to change his behavior, however. It is normal for all persons to regress when subjected to extreme stress; regression is an unconscious protective device of the ego. The patient is usually unaware of his behavior. The stress of hospitalization may have aggravated and accentuated some of his annoying tendencies; some of his behavior may be due to regression; or he may normally behave in such a manner in all interpersonal relationships.

Asking such a patient to change his behavior will not usually work. Remember that his behavior is a reflection of his early childhood experiences and all aspects of his socialization process. Trying to change a patient simply by asking him to change is like expecting a swift river to stop its course suddenly. The only way to change the course of a river is by channeling its forces by external means. So too with a very difficult, demanding patient.

Limit Setting: A Relief for the Patient and the Nurse

Most nurses are caring and sensitive to their patients' needs. Most patients respond positively to their caring and, in fact, may be reluctant to ask for help in the busy environment of the general hospital. A small minority of patients, however, are unable to curb their need for unusual amounts of nursing care. These patients experience this need as a strong urge for someone, *anyone* to respond to them and try to relieve the uncomfortable tension they feel inside.

Their own ability to delay their desire for *instant* need gratification is temporarily not working or has never worked. Their reasons for calling the nurse may be many. They may ask for medication, a fluff of the pillow, a glass of water, or special favors, but it *is the underlying uncomfortable tension* that motivates the request. This tension is caused by many dynamics operating as a result of the multiple forces that shaped the patient's personality during his formative years.

Frequently, these are people who can be compared to a toddler in his need for attention. A young child, when distressed, cannot be reasoned with. He wants his mother *now*. The emotional needs of such a patient cause high levels of internal tension. As a result his ability to hear what caregivers are saying when they ask him to stop his negative behavior is very limited. He may be able to hear what nurses are saying but be unable to control his various needs.

Limit setting is a nursing approach by which patients participate with their nurse in the planning process of reducing their undesirable behavior. Many nurses consider limit setting a form of punishment for the patient and are hesitant to use it as a way of curbing his undesired behavior. Accordingly, they think about it only as a "last resort": when the patient is nearly out of control and they are totally frustrated. Instead, perceptive nurses should identify the problem patient as soon as his untypical behavior begins to be noticeable to them. Negative comments about him in report are usually an important clue, as well as the thought "Oh, no" when his call light goes on. Other clues are observations of negative behavior such as extreme dependence or demandingness with nursing staff, family, or friends.

You and other members of your nursing unit may decide that a limit-setting approach is indicated for a difficult, demanding patient or a noncompliant patient whose unreasonable behavior is causing moderate to severe stress for the majority of nursing staff members.

These should be your guide in designing a limit-setting nursing plan. Limit setting is actually a type of behavior modification (see Chap. 3: Major Theories of Personality Development). Keep in mind that limit setting and behavior modification are not fancy terms for withholding care; rather, they are a way of rewarding desirable behavior. If you are able to identify a predominant personality style used by the patient, refer to Chapter 5:

Personality Styles Seen in General Hospital Patients. In that chapter you will find specific interventions to use with different types of personalities.

Limit setting should not imply unkind behavior on the nurses' part. It is important to remember that by imposing reasonable and caring limits on a patient *before* he becomes a nursing nightmare, he will be spared from his own feeling of being out of control. He will also be protected from the negative behavior of nurses, which can result if his behavior causes morale problems for them (Flaskerud and colleagues, 1979). Another negative aspect of allowing the patient's behavior to continue unchecked is that nurses frequently feel guilty when they avoid patients or lack patience with them.

The Limit-Setting Nursing Process
The steps involved in limit setting begin with the nursing process.

1. *Assess the patient and diagnose the problem he is presenting.* In designing the limit-setting approach you will use, it is advisable to assess the patient and his unique personality characteristics and circumstances with one or two other caregivers. A small group will provide more objectivity. Remember, the reason you are designing a limit-setting plan is that, in many cases, the patient is beginning to be a nuisance. You may be frustrated with the patient and lack objectivity about the reasonableness of your plan. *It also is in the patient's best interest to help him behave in a more adaptive manner.*

2. *Plan a limit-setting intervention designed to meet the patient's unique situation.* A helpful recommendation in formulating the limit-setting approach with a very difficult patient is to schedule a formal meeting of 1 hour with an objective person who does not usually work on your unit. This could be a psychiatric liaison nurse whose preparation has specifically prepared him or her to deal with this type of problem. If your hospital does not employ such a clinical specialist, a psychiatric nurse or nursing supervisor may also provide valuable assistance.

Make an agreement with the patient about the new approach. It is essential to successful limit setting that the patient be a part of the planning process. Explain to the patient that specific parts of his behavior are occasionally troublesome to you in giving his care. Because these troublesome types of behavior are ego-syntonic, the patient is not aware of them in most cases. *Ego-syntonic* refers to the acceptability of a person's ideas or impulses to himself (Hinsie and Campbell, 1977). They are compatible with his value system. He is only aware of the negative response in caregivers.

It is important to tell the patient kindly and in a low-key, nonthreatening manner *what* it is that bothers you and other nurses. You can then describe the plan you have outlined with the advantages to him. You can tell him that after the plan is implemented he should notice a more positive manner in his nurses. He should also feel more secure because he will know what to expect of his nurses.

Then, most important, allow him to discuss the plan with you and encourage him to air his positive and negative feelings about it. Be attentive to his negative views and revise your plan so that it is acceptable to him. This type of compromise is very important. Without it, the patient may feel angry because his thoughts and feelings were disregarded, and his compliance to the plan will never develop; his behavior may even deteriorate.

This type of agreement to the limit-setting plan is a promise that if *you* do what you say you will do, then the patient will do what *he* says he will do. It is a contract. It is an agreement between people to carry out their promises to one another. If one member breaks the contract, it is frequently because the expectations involved were unrealistic to begin with or because the resolutions of one member or both were weakened by other needs, conscious or unconscious. The only time that this type of contracting can be eliminated is if you have a patient whose emotional or intellectual functioning is so impaired that he is unable to understand you or to be reasoned with.

3. *Implement the limit-setting approach.* Outline the agreed-on nursing plan in the nursing Kardex and nursing care plan. This is the most essential step in guaranteeing the success of a limit-setting approach. This outline will provide specific care information to members of the nursing staff on all three shifts. If, for example, only some members of one shift use this approach with the patient, there will be no modification of the patient's negative behavior, and frustration may occur. When *all* members of a caregiving team use the same approach in caring for a patient, a systems approach is in process.

Maintain consistency on all shifts and with all personnel. If, for example, your patient's problem is one of deep suspicion, advise all other caregivers, physicians, social workers, dietitians, x-ray personnel, and others of the best approach to use with him. It will decrease the patient's anxiety as well as their own.

4. *Evaluate the effects of the limit-setting intervention. Modify the original plan if indicated.* The success of a limit-setting intervention depends on the patient's response to the intervention and the nurse's sensitivity to the patient's response. Ongoing evaluation may indicate that the patient is not responding as anticipated. If this occurs, the nurse and patient should discuss what aspect(s) of the plan are unacceptable to the patient, and compromises acceptable to both should be agreed on. In addition to ongoing evaluation by the nurses on all shifts, the patient should have an opportunity to tell his primary nurse what he needs from the nursing staff. The primary nurse and the patient can then compromise and agree about the patient's and nurses' expectations of each other. Actually, it is a case of "I'll help you if you'll help me." This should be done formally, every day. When given the opportunity to express his needs, the patient's level of anxiety and demandingness will often decrease. When we treat this patient as if he were an adult, his behavior may respond accordingly.

Without a limit-setting approach, the patients' hospital behavior may continue in a demanding, dependent, child-like manner, resulting in a serious decline in morale for the patient *and* his nurses. The following outline summarizes the steps in the nursing process of limit setting.

Steps in the Limit-Setting Nursing Process

A. Assessment
 1. Identify and define the patient's problems:
  a. Physical
  b. Psychosocial
 2. Establish a nursing diagnosis or diagnoses
B. Planning
 1. Set objectives to resolve the problem identified in the nursing diagnosis(es):
  a. Immediate
  b. Intermediate
  c. Long range
 2. Contract with the patient (*i.e.*, make an agreement with the patient about what he needs from the nursing staff and what the nursing staff needs from him)

C. Implementation
   1. Provide care integrated with limit-setting intervention
D. Evaluation
   1. Appraise the outcome of the intervention daily with the patient
   2. If necessary, modify or change the original intervention in a planning session with the patient

The following case example about a potentially very difficult situation may explain the value of this approach:

Case Example

Tom is a 29-year-old patient with sickle cell anemia. His admission history revealed that he had multiple hospital admissions during a complicated course of the disease. Each year previously he was admitted several times for exacerbations of his illness. His earlier admissions were at other area hospitals, and this was his first admission at a different hospital. An alert nurse noted that the intern suspected substance abuse in the patient's history. She combined this undocumented possibility with observations of the patient's whining behavior, his lack of compliance to no smoking regulations because of in-room oxygen use, and unreasonable demands on the dietary department.

By the patient's second day of admission, he had already aroused general negativism in the nursing staff. His nurse arranged for a conference to discuss a limit-setting nursing plan. The possible limit-setting approaches were discussed in a 45-minute nursing conference. Discussion of the plan with the patient took approximately 15 minutes, and he was agreeable to it after his own expectations of care were discussed and agreed on by his primary nurse. Within the first day after the limit-setting plan was started, the patient became more compliant and was less demanding of the nursing staff. Each day during his morning care, he and his primary nurse talked about his nursing care to determine if any changes were needed. The patient had never experienced this approach, which involved his own input into the care he wanted. He responded well.

On Tom's fourth day in the hospital, the unit received a call from a social worker employed by the state to work in a sickle cell patient support program. He said that the patient was well known to him and warned that he was a "very difficult" patient. He arranged to come to the hospital at the end of the patient's admission to discuss the patient. When he came to the hospital and talked to the patient, he reported, "This is the best hospital admission he's ever had. Usually the nurses are tearing their hair out and everyone's had it. I don't know what you've done, but he's very pleased with his care, which is unheard of for him. In the past he has frequently signed himself out."

Perhaps this example will help you to see that a limit-setting approach is not time consuming to implement and can yield positive results for all concerned.

The Medication-Dependent Patient

Another type of patient who causes concerns for nurses is the person who develops a dependency on narcotic pain medication. This patient (and the information presented below) should not be confused with the patient who is admitted to the hospital with an already existing drug-addiction problem. The patient described below is someone who experiences pain as the result of a medical or surgical condition. His requests for analgesia do not taper off within an expected time but remain constant and consistent.

It is common for hospital patients who develop medication dependency to have many dependent personality traits. The underlying dynamics and recommendations for interventions with dependent persons are described in Chapter 5: Personality Styles Seen in General Hospital Patients. Another type of patient who may have an increased tendency to become dependent on medication is the one with a dramatizing, emotionally involved captivating personality, also described in Chapter 5. Medication-dependent patients' requests for medication are prompted by their need to relieve distressing feelings of tension. The psychic dependence that results is due to their need to change their state of consciousness in order to cope more effectively (Pattison and Kaufman, 1979).

Nurses and physicians begin to suspect dependence on pain medication when the patient's medication schedule shows that he is receiving his analgesia at the exact intervals of time allowed. Nurses are frequently asked for "an earlier shot" about 15 to 30 minutes before the medication is allowed to be given. Incidentally, this loosening of rules should be avoided. It not only can jeopardize the patient's physiological equilibrium, but it establishes a precedent that frequently becomes a major issue. Once an allowance has been made, the patient will not forget it. He may persistently and annoyingly ask for further concessions regarding medication.

When the normal period for acute and moderate pain goes beyond what is expected for the patient's surgery or medical condition, and consistent requests for pain medication continue, caregivers' suspicions become more definite. Frequently, for a few more days high doses of analgesia are maintained. After that, there may be discussions between the physician and nurses about what alternatives are open to them to reduce the levels of pain medication.

Placebo Use

At times, health care professionals decide to use a placebo. The use of placebos is a subject that creates much controversy. A *placebo* is any medication used to relieve symptoms, not by pharmacological action but because of the patient's expectation of pain relief (Hinsie and Campbell, 1977). Research by Levine and colleagues (1978) suggests that when a person receives a placebo there is a neurological reaction in which enkephalins and endorphins are released by the brain. These neurotransmitters are known to be causative agents in pain relief when narcotic analgesics are administered to patients. Continued research is needed to further explore the action of these substances in placebo response. The advantages and disadvantages of placebo use will not be discussed here because of the complex issues involved and the lack of a clear-cut opinion about them. However, if placebos are ordered by a physician, these general guidelines may help to ensure a more positive outcome for the patient.

It is not unusual for placebos to be used with patients whose prolonged use of narcotic analgesia raises caregivers' concerns. Frequently, when placebo use with patients is done deceptively, a whole new series of problems develops that compounds and worsens the situation. For that reason, the recommendations of one of the nation's respected liaison psychiatrists on the use of placebos will be presented below. Although nurses cannot order the use of placebos, their observations about such use are frequently listened to by physicians.

Frequently, saline is substituted for the patient's normal pain medication. An order for a placebo may be written by a physician to be given on an alternate basis with normal pain medication; the idea is to test the patient's response to saline. If he reports relief, does this confirm that his complaints of pain were a trick in order to receive pain medication? Usually not. Numerous clinical studies have found that one third of *all* patients experiencing real pain respond to placebos with reported relief (Hackett, 1978b). This is true of the population at large and is true also for this type of patient. His response to a placebo does not mean that he has no pain. Actually, the use of deceptive types of placebos is seriously frowned on by the most experienced pain experts (Engel, 1968; Hackett, 1978b; Marks and Sachar, 1973; Merskey and Spear, 1967). The main reason is that the patient is being deceived, and he usually discovers the deception. What does this do to his ability to trust *any* caregivers during the remainder of his hospitalization?

The approach strongly recommended for all patients is for the physician to discuss concerns about overuse of narcotics with the patient, explain that one third of all patients respond to placebos, and say that for the next few days a variety of medications will be used to test the patient's response to them. In this way, all deception is avoided, and, in fact, the patient frequently becomes more cooperative about his analgesia requests. It is highly advised that the use of normal saline be avoided altogether. Instead, mild anxiety-relieving medication such as diazepam or oxazepam should be substituted (Hackett, 1978). After a trial placebo course of several days, the patient can be informed of the results in order to avoid his feelings of being deceived or powerless.

The Organic Brain Syndrome Patient

The causes and specific symptoms for different types of OBS were presented in Chapter 11. There are two main categories of organic brain syndrome: delirium and dementia. The nursing approaches to these two patients are different because the patients present two different types of problems. The symptoms can be compared by referring to Table 16-3.

Nursing Intervention

There are general guidelines that can promote orientation in both demented and delirious patients and help them to regain a sense of control:

1. The patient should have the same nurse rather than a series of caregivers.
2. Do not change the patient's room unless it is absolutely necessary. Familiar surroundings can help him to maintain orientation.
3. He should be regularly checked by nursing staff.
4. Hang a large calendar in the patient's room. Ask the family to bring in a clock. Both can help to keep him oriented to time. A few personal belongings will also be useful.
5. Seat the patient in the hall near the nursing station.
6. At night, use a night light in the room. Leave the window shade up enough to allow some light to come in from the street.
7. Explain all procedures and requests of patients slowly, introducing one idea at a time.
8. Use the patient's first name, especially with delirious patients.
9. Safeguard patient's safety at all times.
   a. Obtain order for mechanical restraints when necessary.
   b. Obtain order for sedation when necessary. Do not overuse sedation.
   c. The bed should always be left in the lowest position because of the danger of falls due to disorientation.

Mechanical Restraints

At times, in order to protect the safety of the patient during episodes of acute delirium or dementia, it may be necessary to use mechanical restraints. It is important that they be used only when absolutely necessary and until pharmacological restraints, such as one of the major tranquilizers, become effective in sedating the patient so that he is no longer a danger to himself or others.

Mechanical restraints include camisoles, wrist restraints, and ankle restraints. They should be used only with a physician's order. The use of restraints is frightening to a patient. Even though he may not appear to understand, tell him what you are doing and that the restraints will protect him from hurting himself. Emphasize that they are temporary. They should be applied with care in order not to injure a patient who may be combative. In severe situations, it may be necessary to bring in extra personnel, such as orderlies and security guards, to assist you. Make sure that you assign them their tasks in advance so that confusion about who is doing what does not result in injury to the patient or to the caregivers.

Cuff restraints should be adequately padded so that no injury to the skin or extremities occurs. Good skin care is essential. The restraints should

Table 16-3.
Two Types of Organic Brain Syndrome

Variables	Delirium	Dementia
Onset	Usually rapid; waxes and wanes abruptly	Usually slow: 1 month or more
Level of awareness	Increased or decreased	Normal or decreased
Orientation	Disoriented	Usually not affected until late in course
Appearance and behavior	May be semicomatose; agitated	Usually slowed responses
Speech and communication	Incoherence; degree of change based on severity of delirium	Usually slowed because of cognitive deficits
Mood	Labile; anxiety or panic common	Constricted affect or depression
Thinking process	Markedly altered	Mildly altered; decreased intellectual ability
Memory	Partial or full loss of recent memory; remote memory intact	Partial loss of both recent and remote memory
Perception	Usually markedly altered	Usually intact or mildly affected
Abstract thinking and judgment	Markedly decreased	Mildly decreased
Sleep-wakefulness cycle	Disrupted	Usually not affected
Treatment	Identify and remove underlying cause; symptomatic treatment	Symptomatic treatment
Prognosis	Reversible in most cases	Usually irreversible

(Information adapted from Kaplan and Sadock, 1981; Langsley, 1979; Lipowski, 1979; Lishman, 1978; Solomon and Patch, 1974)

be released every 2 hours to allow for exercising of the restrained limbs (Stuart and Sundeen, 1979).

Nursing Intervention With the Delirious Patient

Working with a delirious patient can be a frightening experience for most nurses. An important point to remember in caring for the delirious patient is that he usually is able to remember the events that occurred during his delirium. He remembers what he said, did, and thought about. He also will remember how you responded to him. The delirious patient who is out of control as a result of his disturbed thinking and perceptual processes is a danger both to himself and to you. By being attentive to the signs of increasing restlessness and anxiety, especially in clinical areas where organic psychoses are common, such as intensive care units, it may be possible to avert a full-blown psychotic delirium by notifying the physician. An essential aspect of caring for the patient with an acute delirious-type OBS is to note the exact time of your nursing assessment of mental state. The patient with acute OBS can demonstrate rapid shifts in his mental status. He can be semicomatose at one time and within 10 minutes become panicky and unmanageable as the result of a delusional or hallucinatory episode. When an etiology is established, treatment of the underlying condition or withdrawal of the toxic drug can begin.

The most preferable drug for uncontrolled delirious patients is haloperidol (Surman, 1978). The dose and schedule should follow the recommendations of a standard pharmacology reference for use with uncontrollable patients. Until the delirium is reduced and the patient becomes more calm and able to be reasoned with, physical restraints may be necessary. They should be used with caution and only when absolutely necessary. Frequently there may be a paranoid element early in the delirium. With such patients, the following recommendations will help to avoid more serious confrontation:

1. Remain near the foot of the bed.
2. Do not touch the patient to comfort him.
3. Accept his statements quietly, no matter how bizarre. It is not advisable to agree with him, simply to acknowledge his statements by a nod of the head.

Nursing Intervention With the Demented Patient

The patient with senile dementia will be most comfortable in familiar environments. In mild cases, generally the major deficits are in the areas of memory and thinking style. With emotionally supportive caregiving, these patients' sense of comfort and security is enhanced. Feelings of panic with progressive dementia are common. They are caused by the patient's sudden awareness that he does not know where he is or where he is going. Emotion regulation, due to a weakening of defensive ego functioning, is inadequate at times and is one of the main factors in the panic state or other episodes of dysphoria.

Adult day-care programs can prove to be excellent resources as the dementia becomes more severe and families develop concern about their loved one's safety when alone. Poor social judgment, decreased concentration, and impoverished thinking usually require that the person have supervision available. Another beneficial aspect of adult day-care programs is that the patient's decreased mental functioning may be partially due to depressive symptoms. The opportunity for increased socialization, peer support, and purposeful activities can decrease the feelings of loss so often present in the elderly. Unresolved loss is an important dynamic in elderly persons' depression.

When patients with mild to moderate dementia are admitted to the hospital, it is not uncommon for them to be confused during the first few days because of unfamiliar surroundings. It may be necessary to orient them frequently to where they are and why they are in the hospital. Their anxiety level may be high. Slow, gentle explanations will promote their security. Within a few days they should be more relaxed. A night light and special reminders to call you rather than getting up on their own at night can help to decrease the possibility of falls due to disorientation.

When dementia becomes severe, the patient will require constant monitoring. It may be necessary to restrain the patient because his disorientation is acute. Ideally, restraints should only be used when absolutely necessary because they often cause the patient to feel more terror.

Sensory Disturbances

Sensory Deprivation

Sensory deprivation is a mental state caused by a reduction of stimuli from the environment. The ego, which is normally activated by these stimuli, is affected when they are no longer present. It loses its normal reality testing and thought processing abilities. As a result, many types of reactions can occur: regression, confusion, disorientation, primitive emotional responses, and the potential for hallucination. The different types of patients for whom sensory deprivation can bring about maladaptive psychosocial consequences are as follows:

- Ophthalmology patients whose eyes are bandaged
- Orthopaedic patients who are immobilized for extended periods
- Geriatric patients in nursing homes who lack social and environmental stimuli
- Any patient whose treatment includes extensive bed rest: intensive care unit patients, burn patients, and so on (Kaplan and Sadock, 1981)

Nursing Intervention

An awareness of the potential for sensory deprivation, and creative nursing care designed to promote psychological stimulation, is the best treatment approach with these patients. Frequent interpersonal contact with the patient by the nurse is important. Touching the patient promotes his sense of value as a person and increases his "connectedness" with the environment.

Contact with auxiliary hospital personnel, such as pastoral care and occupational or recreation therapy staff, should be offered to the patient if hospitalization will be prolonged. If these services are not offered at your hospital, it may be possible for a volunteer from the hospital or the patient's church or temple to spend time with the patient.

Sensory Overload

Sensory overload is the opposite of sensory deprivation. In it, the ego is bombarded by sensory stimuli of all types: sounds, pain, constant interaction with people, and a disturbed sleep-waking cycle. Eventually the ego can be temporarily overwhelmed. Patients in intensive care units often experience sensory overload. The ego will attempt to adapt to a high level of sensory stimuli by using the defense mechanism of denial. The ego can be weakened by excessive coping attempts or an altered mental state due to organic causes, or it may normally be weak. When this occurs, ego ability to maintain denial may be eroded, and sensory overload occurs.

The symptoms of sensory overload can appear similar to a mild delirium. In fact, if the patient is in an intensive care unit, there may be interacting components of both OBS and sensory deprivation. He will become confused and mildly disoriented, recent memory will deteriorate, and illusory phenomenon may occur; for instance, the patient may think that there are "bugs crawling on the wall" when he is looking at the design in the wallpaper. Hypnagogic states may also occur when the patient drifts in and out of sleep and is unable to distinguish dreams from reality.

Nursing Intervention

The patient experiencing sensory overload will need nursing intervention to reduce the number of sensory stimuli. Lights should be dimmed and shades drawn in his unit if possible. Contacts with nonessential hospital personnel should be kept to a minimum. Family members whose efforts are well meaning should be encouraged to keep visits to the restricted time period. A schedule that limits nursing care to specific periods can allow the patient to sleep for brief periods. If the patient falls asleep, the nurse as advocate can intervene with other caregivers and family members who want to awaken him. Medication for pain, anxiety, and sleep should be carefully administered to avoid excessive disruption of psychological equilibrium. If the patient is in the intensive care unit, he should be moved to a regular nursing unit as soon as his condition permits.

Conclusion

The stress of illness is a challenge for *all* humans. Regardless of normal intrapsychic functioning, if a stressor is severe enough, emotional complications can occur. This type of intrapsychic maladaptation can have an effect on many other subsystems, including the family and caregivers. Depending on the type of emotional distress that the patient is experiencing, there are many different nursing approaches and interventions that can help to restore his or her psychosocial equilibrium. The theory in this chapter can be used in each phase of the nursing process. By understanding the dynamics of the specific type of emotional complication you are observing, your interventions can be more appropriately designed to reduce the level of psychosocial stress being experienced by the patient, his family, *and* the nurse(s) caring for them.

In order to help in the process of using a model to evaluate the psychosocial effects of illness on patients and their families, this chapter will present 11 conditions that have a known psychosocial risk. The major psychosocial issues of illness for each condition will be reviewed. The dynamics of each of these issues were covered in Chapter 6. They are trust, self-esteem, control, loss, guilt, and intimacy. Recommendations for specific nursing approaches that can reduce the risk of psychosocial maladaptation will be included.

The conditions were chosen because of their prevalence in inpatient and outpatient care settings, the severe and acute adaptive challenge that is attached to these illnesses, and the specific needs of women in the care setting that nurses have been increasingly addressing in the past decade. The conditions that will be presented in this chapter are infertility, exceptional child or child with congenital anomalies, hysterectomy and menopause, disfiguring conditions such as amputation, mastectomy, and ostomy, and isolation for communicable diseases or immunosuppressive conditions.

Note that in the array of medical and nursing textbooks published today, the tendency to skim over the psychosocial effects of illness continues to be the norm. Nursing has traditionally identified the psychosocial component of illness as being within its practice scope (Kim and Moritz, 1982). The increasing use of the categories of nursing diagnosis points out the lack of specific research with definite findings on patients' short- and long-term adaptation to illness. Whenever possible, this chapter will include specific references about the psychosocial effects of illness. At other times, unresearched yet frequently observed psychosocial outcomes of illness will be presented for their potential value in assisting the nurse in the assessment, diagnosis, and intervention process.

17

Psychosocial Aspects of Specific Physical Conditions

Infertility

In today's society, an increasing number of young couples have decided to delay indefinitely or never to have children. Accordingly, there is greater social acceptance of childless couples. For some people who are unable to conceive a child, however, the lack of a child becomes a crisis that touches every aspect of a couple's relationship. This includes their psychosocial functioning in the greater social context; it also can cause major stresses in intrapsychic functioning (Taymor and Bresnick, 1978). The changes in their own relationship, as well as those in relationships with other persons, are outward manifestations of intrapsychic stress. The result of frustration due to inability to conceive frequently results in increased depression, anxiety, obsession, guilt, and isolation in one or both partners. A fall in self-esteem is one of the first shifts in the psychodynamic process. Using systems theory, it is possible to understand the vicious cycle that results from infertility. Anxiety is a commonly identified factor in infertility (Kleegman and Kaufman, 1966; Taymor, 1978). Whether anxiety causes infertility or is the result of infertility is a continuous debate.

Psychosocial Issues

Trust
The husband and wife who desire a child and are unable to conceive can have conscious or unconscious responses to many trust issues. On an individual basis, each member of the couple can begin to doubt his or her own ability to function normally. Trust in normal body functioning is something that most persons take for granted until it is undermined in some way. Trust in one another, which is the foundation of any long-term and committed relationship, can also be affected. This is especially so if one or the other member projects possible inadequacies onto the other; serious conflict, which often is maladaptively avoided, can be the result.

Another aspect of trust that becomes important for the couple is their belief in their physician. The care of infertile couples requires that the physician become aware of all areas of a couple's sexual functioning. It is especially important that the physician be capable of an empathic relationship. If his or her personality is coolly clinical and aloof, the couple frequently begins to feel "observed" and inadequate. The psychological distress that accompanies their loss of trust in their physician can promote hopelessness that their problem ever will be resolved.

Self-esteem
The desire for a child is a psychological investment that develops as the result of socialization from earliest childhood. For some, the ability to produce a child becomes deeply ingrained in the self-concept. When infertility occurs, the self-image can be seriously undermined. The maintenance of self-esteem is partially due to a person's being able to fulfill his role expectations. When this ability is lost or hope of fulfilling it is lost, self-esteem falls.

The result is a sense of failure for some; they become self-rejecting. This self-rejection can result in anticipated rejection by their extended families, especially by their own mothers, or by their larger social environment. Some infertile young couples eventually begin to withdraw from their normal circle of friends, most of whom have children. This type of isolation can further erode self-esteem.

Control
The inability to obtain something that is desired results in a feeling of loss of control. Conception or contraception is usually within a couples' control. Infertility results in a sense of loss of control. Normal sexual functioning is ideally free and spontaneous. It is usually subject only to the scrutiny of the persons involved. Not so for the infertile couple in infertility treatment. Their sexual technique, frequency, and indeed their own bodies are subject to the control of the treating physician. Part of the treatment process frequently requires pharmacological intervention with various hormone preparations for one or both partners. The taking of medication raises control issues for many people.

Loss
A childless couple is responding to many losses, consciously and unconsciously (Taymor and Bresnick, 1978). The most obvious is the possibility that they may never have a child. It is the desire to avoid this loss that provides the motivation for prolonged infertility care. They frequently alternate between feelings of hope that a child can be conceived and feelings of loss when despair overcomes their hope. It is difficult for this loss to be accepted because of the uncertain state in which infertile couples live. Ambivalence and mood swings are not uncommon as a result of this uncertainty.

Guilt
Guilt can contribute to psychosocial maladaptation in the childless couple in a variety of ways. Some of the causes may be that one or both of the partners may have been active sexually with other partners earlier. They may believe that their infertility is some type of "punishment." If a contraceptive agent, such as birth control pills, is implicated in lack of ovulation, the woman may feel increased guilt. This may also occur if the results of abortion are found to be a contributing factor. Pelvic inflammatory disease is sometimes found to be the cause of infertility. If this is attributed to past or present venereal disease, the woman may feel at fault.

Intimacy

Intimacy in a couple's relationship is the degree of openness, honesty, and trust that they experience together. Problems in communication that result from infertility or the treatment process can develop or serve to undermine further an already conflicted relationship. The level of intimacy that each partner experiences in all aspects of the relationship—emotional, intellectual, and physical—can deteriorate as the infertility treatment period progresses without positive results.

Nursing Approaches

The issues and their maladaptive outcomes outlined above are not necessarily permanent or as crisis producing as they may initially sound. Infertile couples will experience some or all of the distressing psychosocial effects described above as part of the normal process of being infertile. Because of the shame that is experienced by many infertile couples about their physical condition, they rarely discuss it with others. Their communication with each other often is affected as each member tries to protect the other. This adaptive attempt, however, can result ultimately in a shutdown of their communication.

Couple Support Group

An ideal approach to the psychosocial stress of infertility can be participation by husbands and wives in a group experience with other infertile couples. Rather than offering the group on a "needed" basis, it can be included as part of the overall infertility treatment process. Frequently, when people must acknowledge that they "need" a group, their typical response is to deny that they are having any difficulty.

The advantages of a peer group are that feelings of uniqueness, inadequacy, and isolation are decreased. Since all members are experiencing many of the same emotions, they find support and approval. One of the advantages of a couples' group is that feelings and thoughts that a husband or wife may be afraid to express to the spouse may be identified, discussed, and defused in a group environment. Frequently, the members find great relief when they realize that they and their spouses are similar to other members of the group. Self-acceptance can be promoted by an awareness that one's feelings are normal.

When marked psychosocial disturbance occurs in one or both members of the couple as the result of infertility, the couple should be referred to a mental health professional with knowledge of individual psychodynamics who is skilled in couple or family therapy. On occasion, the referral of the maladaptive member of the couple for individual treatment further isolates the functional spouse and promotes further deterioration of the relationship. The couple's relationship is already under stress because of infertility. Ideally, it should be supported; barriers to communication should be avoided.

Exceptional Child or Child With Congenital Anomalies

One of the most anticipated events in the lives of most couples is the arrival of a child. For most, the child is the embodiment of future hopes and dreams (Kennell, 1978). When a child is born who is less than perfect because of a congenital anomaly, the parents undergo a major adaptive challenge.

The stages in the adaptive process are the same regardless of the type of defect: shock, denial, sadness and anger, disequilibrium, and reorganization (Drotar and colleagues, 1975). The time sequence of the various stages depends, however, on the type of defect involved. For example, the shock and denial stages for the parents of a child with a cleft lip-cleft palate anomaly are usually briefer than those for parents of a Down's syndrome infant.

Anomalies, especially of the head, are more difficult initially for parents to adjust to. Eventually, any type of anomaly presents a major adaptive challenge. The major factors that will help to determine adaption vs. maladaption are the normal coping styles of each of the parents, their openness of communication, the long-term implications of the anomaly, whether the anomaly is hereditary, the financial burden that the anomaly may cause, and the availability and use of other persons for support (Kennell, 1978; Waechter, 1977).

Psychosocial Issues

Trust

The care given by nursing and medical caregivers to the infant and parents during the few days after birth can have far-reaching consequences on the adaptation of each of the parents as well as on the developing child. There may be other children in the family. The ultimate adaptation of each of the members can depend on the way that the new parents are helped to integrate the cognitive awareness of all aspects of the new baby's condition.

If caregivers are open, honest, and *caring* in their discussions with the new parents, trust in the caregivers' recommendations will be promoted. Unfortunately, caregivers may be evasive because of their own inability to deal with this type of tragedy. Another possibility is that they may mistakenly believe that the situation is "too much" for the parents to deal with and thus avoid any discussion that allows the parents to talk about their feelings regarding their child.

When caregivers give tender care to an infant with an anomaly, it promotes the parents' acceptance of their child. Without parents' acceptance of the infant, the essential bonding process between parent and child is disturbed (Waechter, 1977). The bonding process is one of the underlying dynamics in the infant's ability to trust his caregivers and, eventually, the environment at large.

Self-esteem

The self-esteem of parents can be suddenly affected when their anticipation of a perfect child is disrupted. They view the birth anomaly as a reflection of their own inadequacies. Ultimately, an acute or prolonged depressive episode may occur if these feelings are not relieved. Unrelieved feelings of decreased self-esteem, as well as overall inability to resolve the changes brought about by the arrival of a child with a birth anomaly, contribute to higher rates of marital disruption and alcoholism (Waechter, 1977). Self-esteem is also affected if the child's condition is found to be caused by a genetic disorder passed on by one or both parents.

Control

Many parents report a feeling of loss of control in their lives as they look ahead to the years of care that the new infant may require. This continues to happen to parents who have been caring for a child with an anomaly for some time. A condition such as cystic fibrosis may result in frequent exacerbations of acute illness. Other conditions may require a series of complex surgeries over several years.

Loss

Loss is a major issue of the parent of any child with a congenital anomaly. Before birth, the image of the anticipated child is perfect. One of the first stages of the acceptance process is for the parents to mourn the loss of their "perfect" child. This must occur before they are able to work through the stages toward accepting the child who in one or more ways is missing an element of perfection (Waechter, 1977).

If the child's condition is the result of a genetic abnormality, another aspect of loss can occur. In such a case, the implications for future children can have a profound effect on parents' hopes of ever being able to deliver a normal child. If the youngster has Tay-Sachs disease, for example, the parents also face the loss of the child through death. Parents of children with abnormalities of the major organs also report constant fears that their children will die soon, even when medical opinions contradict the possibility (Waechter, 1977).

Yet another difficult experience is the reawakening of loss that couples undergo as the child grows and develops. At each of the developmental milestone stages of the normal infant—crawling, walking, teething, feeding, toilet training, entering school, playing sports, and so on—the parents are reminded that their child is different. A mild to moderate grief response is normal as each of these awarenesses is gradually integrated.

Anger, which is a normal response to loss, is a common emotion in these parents. Again, this anger will come and go and be reawakened as the grief processes, described above, are underway. The anger will usually be expressed in the manner that the person customarily used to cope before the arrival of the child. It is also possible that it may be the result of maladaption due to the original unresolved crisis of the baby's birth. The anger may be directed at the self, with self-destructive behavior, or it may be repressed and result in depression. It can also be directed toward the spouse or others by projection or displacement. Potentially, it can be released in more adaptive ways with some other aggression-releasing activity, such as working or active involvement in sports.

Guilt

Guilt can become a problem for many parents of children with anomalies. They may consciously or unconsciously believe that the child is the result of earlier sins of omission or commission (Kennell, 1978; Waechter, 1977). Guilt can be difficult too when the parent or parents are discovered to be genetic carriers of specific types of conditions.

Some parents impose unrealistic expectations on themselves in their care of the child. These unrelenting guilt feelings can prevent parents from developing a more realistic balance that allows them to experience some relief from the care giving process. Relationships with other children in the family can also be impaired when guilt is excessive, and at times unnecessary care prevents normal interaction. Negative acting-out behavior in siblings is not unusual in such instances.

Intimacy

One of the risks of birth anomalies is that they can ultimately cause a shutdown in communication between husband and wife, between one or both parents and the child, between siblings and parents, between members of the extended family, and between the parents and their normal social relationships. This is the result of many types of social dynamics:

1. One person is trying to protect the other; the issue is avoided.
2. People are afraid that they or others will be unable to control their emotions; loss of control and shame could result.
3. Those who are not immediately affected feel guilty that they have not been similarly affected.
4. One or both parents may deny the implications of the child's condition and need for treatment. It is also possible that each of the spouses can be at different stages in the acceptance process and are unable to communicate with one another. The result in the nondenying partner is avoidance and anger toward the denying spouse.

Nursing Approaches

One of the most important factors in parents' adaptive acceptance of their child is openness on the part of all caregivers about the child. If a primary nurse will be working with the family, he or she should confer with the physician about plans for treatment and the prognosis of the infant. Evasion, inaccurate responses, or uncommitted care by caregivers can be highly significant to parents (Waechter, 1977).

Regarding truth telling with parents, it is not necessary to give the treatment plan for the next 10 years in minute detail, but it can be helpful to give a broad overview. Positive aspects of the treatment approach are important to the concerned parents. As the initial shock wears off, and they are more able to tolerate a realistic understanding of the effects of the infant's condition, the parents will ask more specific questions.

Obstetrical caregivers can ask patients questions that allow them to talk about their feelings about their new infant. It also can be helpful to new parents of a child with an abnormality to be aware of the normal responses of other parents in similar circumstances. This exploration should ideally take place with both parents present. It can help them to accept distressing feelings and responses if and when they should occur. The information that can be helpful to them includes Kübler-Ross's stages of acceptance of loss, outlined in Chapter 6: Major Psychosocial Issues of Patients With Physical Illness and Bowlby's stages in the bereavement process, discussed in Chapter 19: The Dying Patient and the Family.

In addition to an explanation about the normal emotional responses to their child, it is helpful to explain some of the unwelcome changes in couple social dynamics that appear above. By explaining this information to both parents at this stressful time when listening ability may be interspersed with denial, it is more likely that in the future the couple will be able to recognize, understand, and resolve changes in their relationship adaptively.

Nurses in outpatient gynecology and pediatric settings can assess the ongoing adaptation of families by asking a question such as, "How are you and Mr. Adams handling Timmy's spina bifida?" When problems are occurring, this type of question can open a floodgate. Counseling by the nurse with a follow-up visit can be a relief for the mother. Arranging meetings with other families who have children with similar conditions can also be helpful. If more severe relationship problems are occurring, referral to a family therapist should take place to prevent the severe types of family maladaption that can develop.

Hysterectomy and Menopause

In Western societies there are many myths about the psychological consequences of hysterectomy and menopause. These myths may cause women to approach these events with dread. Often, the negative experiences of one or two women acquaintances are accepted by their premenopausal peers or relatives as "the way it is." In this section, the results of research on menopause and its psychological effects will be presented so that caregivers can form a conceptual base to use with patients in clinical practice.

Development of a Feminine Body Image

During the toddler stage, most little girls play "mother." They imitate their mothers' parenting style. They talk about "someday, when I have a baby, I'll do such and such." During the important identification stage of the Oedipal period, there is a heightened curiosity about sexual functioning in children of both sexes about their parents of the same sex. Young girls incorporate their mother's expressed opinions and nonverbal responses to all sexual matters. The curiosity about their own and others' sexual functioning remains high in young girls during the latency stage of psychosexual development. By the time a female adolescent begins sexual development, many of her concepts about her own immature breasts and uterus, as well as her own potential sexuality, are formed. These are primarily the result of socialization by her mother and other female members of the family.

Children often overhear comments by aunts, grandmothers, and older sisters about sexual matters. The father's normal interactions with her mother and herself also contribute to a young girl's view of sexuality. If he is affectionate, loving, and respectful of his wife and female family members, the child's feminine self-image is enhanced. On the other hand, derogatory sexual comments, careless sexual behavior with no regard for its effect on young children, or physical abuse of the mother by her partner contribute to a poor sexual self-image for a young girl.

The presence and functions of the breasts and uterus become integrated into the self-concept of the adolescent female. They are the crux of her womanliness. Depending on her socialization process, a young girl's emotional investment in her uterus's child-bearing potential can be great or small. If a woman has little interest in raising a family, the effects of menopause or hysterectomy will be adapted to in a similar manner to any other change in her life. If, however, there is or was great emotional investment in child-bearing ability, hysterectomy, at any age, including menopausal and postmenopausal ages, can be psychologically threatening.

Unlike the functioning of most body systems, which occurs quietly and is usually out of the conscious realm, the functioning of a woman's reproductive system during her fertile years is usually a phenomenon that she thinks about often. This is due to a woman's consciousness of the stages in the menstrual cycle. Moodiness, achiness, swelling, and other menstruation-related symptoms may be evaluated and regarded as normal or abnormal based on a woman's calculations of when her period last occurred or is expected.

Many women talk about their periods as being a nuisance or, worse, being physiologically or emotionally draining. On the other hand, they are also an affirmation of their womanliness. Although it is rarely acknowledged consciously, the ongoing rhythm of the menstrual cycle is psychologically comforting to many women. The loss of this cycle, which has been a conscious part of normal body functioning, body image, and self-image for 30 or more years, may normally be accompanied by feelings of sadness.

Factors in the Psychological Outcome of Hysterectomy

Hysterectomy is one of the most frequently performed surgeries in the United States. Over 725,000 women underwent this procedure in 1974 (Finck, 1979). The emotional care of the posthysterectomy woman is less than optimal in many acute care and outpatient settings (Krueger and associates, 1979). Forty percent of patients who undergo gynecological surgery experience varying degrees of depression. In a small majority of those patients it sometimes lasts for several months (Kroger, 1962). Anxiety, compulsive overeating, and a decrease in sexual desire and functioning have been identified as common outcomes of the surgery (Keith, 1980). It is possible that these symptoms may be a consequence of the psychological effects of the loss of the uterus and its symbolism to women. These symptoms have not been directly attributed to the endocrine changes in the posthysterectomy woman (Notman, 1979). The following predisposing factors have been identified as significant to psychosocial maladaptation following hysterectomy. There is no special significance to the order in which these factors are presented (Roeske, 1979).

1. Poor feminine self-image (*e.g.*, unconfident and self-demeaning self-beliefs)
2. Poor history of ability to tolerate stress:
   a. For example, history of many depressive reactions
   b. History of psychiatric illness
3. History of multiple physical problems:
   a. Subjective pain in pelvis, abdomen, and back
   b. Multiple surgeries and hospital admissions
4. Less than 35 years old
5. Desire for more children
6. Chronically poor marital relationship
7. Cultural or religious prohibitions within social environment

8. Negativity of spouse or sexual partner about surgery
9. Woman's expectation that surgery will result in negative changes in sexual functioning
10. Lack of meaningful career or hobbies

Although a woman may hear only a few strongly negative statements about the psychological effects of hysterectomy, they may color her thinking and cause her to generalize these views. They may form the basis for fears that hysterectomy can cause mental illness.

Because of curiosity about the relationship between hysterectomy and mental illness, many studies were done in Great Britain in the 1960s. In Great Britain, where medical care is socialized, the referral for psychiatric treatment is not affected by concern for its cost to the person. In the United States, insurance coverage for psychiatric treatment ranges from nonexistent to limited with the insurance plans covering most people; the cost of psychiatric care may prevent many woman from obtaining help. Accordingly, the referral rates of British gynecological patients for psychiatric follow-up study are more reflective of actual psychiatric symptomatology than those in the United States.

The results of the most comprehensive study reported in the literature appear below. Seven hundred and twenty-nine hysterectomy patients were compared to a comparable number of women cholecystectomy patients for the incidence of psychological sequelae following their surgeries. The findings were as follows (Barker, 1968):

1. Seven percent of the hysterectomy patients were referred for psychiatric care:
   a. This was two and one-half times the rate of cholecystectomy patients.
   b. This was three times higher than the psychiatric referral rate of the general population.
2. Depression was the most frequent symptom of psychiatric distress.
3. The peak period for psychiatric referral was 2 years after the surgery.
4. The psychiatric referral rate was twice as high in women with no presurgical symptoms of pelvic pathology.
5. Fifty-seven percent of all patients with previous psychiatric histories were rereferred.
6. Patients with marital disruption were referred six times more frequently than those with no marital instability.

These findings point out that a relatively small number of women experience psychological mal-adaptation after hysterectomy. Of those who do, many have previous histories of psychological maladaptation in their intrapsychic or marital functioning. Accordingly, few women with no previous history of emotional dysfunction *spontaneously* develop psychological sequelae after this surgery.

Psychosocial Response to Menopause

One of the important facts about menopause is that it coincides with middle age. The occurrence of menopause is but one aspect of the adaptive and developmental challenges of women in this age range. Frequently, the dysphoric feelings experienced by women during their 40s are attributed to the menopause process. Actually, they can be due to the *normal* response to the multiple losses that women are experiencing during middle adulthood. Some of these losses are listed below (Ballinger, 1976; Brown, 1976; Bungay and colleagues, 1980; Fink, 1980; Hammond, 1976; Notman, 1979; Severne, 1979):

1. Children who had previously lived at home leave to attend college, establish separate residences as young adults, or be married.
2. Loss of active mothering role as result of above.
3. Awareness of loss of intimacy in marital relationship may become evident as husband and wife are alone for the first time since they were newly married.
4. Loss of youthful appearance.
5. Gradual loss of physical functioning when contrasted to that of young adulthood.
6. Change in relationship to parents. Often, a senile dementia in the parent(s) results in role reversal. The adult child becomes the caretaker of the parent.
7. Death of parents.
8. Awareness of lost opportunities with the passing of youth.
9. Job advancement opportunities may be given to younger women.
10. Increasing awareness of finality of own life and those of loved ones.
11. Loss of menses and ability to have children.

It seems obvious that the loss of menses, in the context of the other changes that a woman is experiencing, is only one factor that can contribute to a chronic or acute episode of psychological distress.

Often, neurovegetative changes in functioning are associated with menopause. Some of these changes are decreased interest in sex, lack of energy, changes in eating and sleeping patterns, and chronic constipation. *Remember that these are symptoms of depression.* From an endocrine viewpoint, the *only* significant physical change is "hot flashes." The development of hot flashes is related to the decreased supply of circulating estrogen. This causes transient changes in vasomotor functioning that are experienced as unexpected feelings of warmth or as chill, palpitations, and parasthesias (Severne, 1977). These symptoms diminish and disappear following menopause.

A longitudinal study of 922 married Belgian women aged 46 to 55 years revealed that the women who reported the most distress from menopause were unemployed women from the lower classes. Women from the upper classes and all women who were employed reported fewer difficulties with the menopausal period. (International Health Foundation, 1973, 1977). Problems that are attributable to menopause are the result of "overvaluing, undervaluing, or imposing of other attributes on the function of reproduction" (Brown, 1976, p. 112).

The controversy of estrogen supplementation for menopausal and postmenopausal women continues among caregivers and laywomen. Generally, the use of estrogen, when given in an appropriate dose, provides the following therapeutic effects:

1. Decrease in vasomotor symptoms of menopause (Severne, 1977).
2. Decrease in development of osteoporosis. *Osteoporosis* is a metabolic bone disorder that causes crippling effects in postmenopausal women who have never taken estrogen. The density of the bones decreases. Fractures are common, and collapse of the vertebra can occur. Over 5 million post-menopausal women in the United States have this condition (Brunner and Suddarth, 1975).
3. Prolongation of sexual functioning into later years. The loss of estrogen after menopause results in changes in vaginal tissue structure, lubrication, and normal functioning ability (Sarrel, 1980).

The therapeutic dose of estrogen varies widely in women. Arriving at the proper estrogen level for a given woman involves the woman and her physician being flexible and trying varying doses so that proper evaluation for their overall effect can occur.

A positive note on the menopausal, postmenopausal, or posthysterectomy years is that many women have an increased interest in their own sexual pleasure. This has been widely attributed to their loss of fear of pregnancy. Another less recognized possibility is that the normal premenopausal female has a certain level of circulatory female hormones and a lesser amount of circulating male hormone, testosterone. One of the effects of testosterone is that it promotes sexual interest and drive. As the menopause approaches, the level of estrogen produced by the ovaries decreases. Although the level of testosterone does not change, its effects are not as strongly neutralized by estrogen. The result may be a stronger libido (Fink, 1980).

Finally, a study done of women by Gail Sheehy, published in 1978, revealed some surprising findings. In a study of the quality of life of women in the decades of 20 to 30, 30 to 40, 40 to 50, 50 to 60, and 60 to 70, she found that women in the 50 to 60 range reported a higher level of happiness and overall quality of life than women in any other decade except for the young 20s. In fact, the happiness level of women increases markedly in the 50s and 60s.

Psychosocial Issues

Because of the material presented above, the following section will be abbreviated.

Trust
Trust in self and others relating to acceptance and lack of rejection are major conscious and unconscious issues.

Self-esteem
Self-esteem can be threatened during female middle adulthood because of the physical and relationship losses described above.

Control
Many of the events of midlife can cause a woman to feel that she has little control over what is happening to her. If she is a person who has spent 20 years at home in the mothering role, the departure of children, signs of her own physical decline as well as those of parents and other elderly relatives, and changes in the overall social environment may cause feelings of helplessness. The period of middle age for persons with families has been called "the sandwiched generation." The needs of children and elderly parents can cause a

woman to feel that her own needs are unimportant or nonexistent.

Loss
The losses of the middle-aged woman are described above.

Guilt
The time of middle age may result in conflict in some women, particularly those who heavily invested their time and emotional energy in meeting the needs of others during their earlier years. Women with self-sacrificing characteristics may feel unneeded as children leave home. Indeed, they may be threatened and continue to hold on as their children approach adulthood and attempt to separate from the family. One of the underlying dynamics of this tendency is guilt. The emotionally healthy middle-aged woman, after many years of attending to her family's needs, finally has time to develop herself as a person, continue or develop a deeper, more intimate relationship with her husband, begin or resume her education, obtain meaningful employment, and pursue new interests. Guilt-ridden women can have difficulty allowing themselves these pleasures.

Intimacy
Intimacy in the marital relationship and in friendships as well can be especially meaningful during middle adulthood. The ability to commit oneself to a relationship is an important indicator of maturity in the young adult (Erikson, 1963). Because of involvement in educational and career pursuits, the resulting mobility caused by these pursuits, striving for upward social mobility, developing value systems, and a mildly egocentric tendency that is relatively normal in the young adult, the ability to form committed, intimate relationships is sometimes delayed until middle adulthood (Levenson, 1978; Sheehy, 1974, 1981).

Nursing Approaches

Nurses on gynecology surgery units can encourage posthysterectomy patients to discuss their concerns about themselves and their emotional, intellectual, and sexual relationships with their husbands. Corrections of false concepts and education about the realities of adjustment to hysterectomy are important.

Many hysterectomy patients report that, although they had no desire for more children, the removal of the uterus caused a finality that was experienced as a major loss. Women may experience a grief process with the Kübler-Ross or Bowlby responses of mild to severe distress depending on their ages and emotional investment in child bearing.

There is another important education point that should be raised in caring for patients with vaginal hysterectomies. The majority of women experience a loss of vaginal sensation for up to 6 months. This is the result of nerve trauma caused by the surgery. Eventually, sensation should return to normal (Moran, 1979). An unprepared woman can become distraught that her normal sexual functioning may be permanently impaired if she is not reassured that this is a normal outcome of the surgery. She should be encouraged to ask her surgeon about this effect.

Although some women who undergo abdominal hysterectomy experience a change in sexual desire and functioning, it is probable that this change is due to inadequate preoperative education or underlying conflict in the marital relationship. Frequently, when the patient is given adequate information and has the opportunity to discuss her concerns, these problems will decrease and gradually her normal sexual activity pattern will return. Reassurances that normal sexual desire and activity should not be impaired by the surgery can be most advantageous if given by the physician when surgery is decided on.

Another very important time when a hysterectomy patient is amenable to this information and frequently will have questions is during the few days before discharge. It is often comfortable for a patient to discuss her sexuality with a knowledgeable nurse. You can suggest that any changes in desire or lubrication can possibly be caused by her own shyness at resuming sexual relations. She should be encouraged to discuss her concerns with her partner in order to ensure extra understanding if she is experiencing increased anxiety. The use of estrogen cream or water-soluble jellies intravaginally can reduce initial discomfort during intercourse. Generally, the posthysterectomy woman can look forward to unchanged sexual pleasure after her surgery.

In the outpatient setting, nurses can be sensitive to the physical symptoms of depression that may signal signs of maladaptation to midlife, whether the woman has had a hysterectomy or is in her menopausal years. If chronic or acute dysphoric feelings of depression or anxiety are troubling to a woman, she should be referred for psychotherapy or counseling.

Disfiguring Conditions

A disease process can be cured by surgery that removes the disease. At times it is necessary to remove more than the exact site of pathology. Whenever the result is visible to the patient and others and results in a changed body image, it can be classified as disfiguring surgery.

Amputation

Amputation is a surgical procedure that usually results in psychological trauma for the patient. The loss of a limb or part of a limb requires major adaptive ability as the multiple losses are grieved. Shifts in body image and self-image are the outcome of the grieving process as the amputee gradually lets go of former abilities, functions, and self-images. Self-esteem may undergo rapid changes as awareness of new losses occur. Emotional lability, the emotional swings that are common in the grieving process, are closely related to the variations in self-esteem experienced by the patient (Bossert and Freeman, 1979).

The patient who undergoes amputation of one or more limbs is usually introduced to the rehabilitation process as soon as his physical condition following surgery is stabilized. Whenever possible, most experts in the field of rehabilitation medicine recommend that a bandaging device should be directly applied in the operating room if no complications are present to allow a more rapid process of adjustment to a prosthetic device. These devices, either rigid or semirigid, reduce swelling and pain in the postoperative period. If such a device is used, it is frequently possible to have a temporary prosthesis available within 4 to 5 days after surgery. The use of a prosthesis as soon as possible within the postsurgical period can provide hope for the patient who may fear the loss of mobility.

Psychosocial Issues

The initial surgical recommendation that the limb should be removed results in many doubts for the patient. His ability to trust a surgeon, who in most cases is a stranger, that his recommendation is valid can be a major challenge. It may in fact delay the removal of a diseased limb. If a patient is highly suspicious or anxious about such a recommendation, and his overall physical condition is deteriorating as the result of systemic toxic invasion, it is advisable to do the following:

1. Seek immediate psychiatric liaison consultation to determine the patient's reasons for refusing surgery.
2. Avoid doing the surgery unless the patient's life is jeopardized until some resolution of the patient's psychic stress is achieved. Without such resolution, the patient's adaptation following surgery can be severely compromised. He may experience a paranoid psychotic reaction, marked anxiety, severe depression, and concomitant physical complications as the result of severe mental stress. Another outcome of a patient's being coerced into an unwanted amputation is a complex rehabilitation process.

Trust
One of the most difficult adjustments of the person who has had one or both legs amputated is to develop trust in his caregivers that they will hold him securely and not allow him to fall. He also must trust in the recommendations and plans of rehabilitation physicians (physiatrists) and physical therapists. Rehabilitation is always a painful process because of the use of stumps that have not yet fully healed or give the patient phantom limb pain.

Self-esteem
The amputee, whether he has lost part of a hand, arm, foot, or leg, frequently experiences a severe drop in self-esteem. Unless his previous coping ability was high and he had very positive self-esteem and a strong support network, he may expect rejection by others. He frequently doubts that he will be able to return to full functioning, even with a prosthetic device. These ideas, accurate or not, diminish his self-esteem. In addition, the multiple and gradual awarenesses of loss of former abilities may also have a deep effect on a person's sense of worth and self-image.

Control
Feelings of powerlessness are common and result in a major adaptive effort in order to overcome them. When the patient thinks about his future functioning, he frequently believes that he will be unable to control himself in many circumstances that normally he would have had no difficulty encountering.

Feelings of anger and frustration in amputees are common as the slow rehabilitation process is underway. The patient may fear loss of control of himself because of anger. Many male amputees also fear that they may cry uncontrollably. They may have been socialized into feeling that crying in men is not acceptable. Permission by caregivers that such feelings are normal and acceptable to them can allow amputees to grieve their loss adaptively both in the hospital and after discharge, when the grief process will continue.

When excessive control of emotions occurs, the repression frequently causes a disruption in the normal grief response. Maladaptive or unresolved grief reactions can result.

Loss

The amputee faces many types of loss, including actual loss of the physical part(s) and loss of function of the limb(s). Depending on the limb(s) affected, the availability of a prosthesis, and adaptation to the prosthesis, the patient may no longer be able to walk, run, write, play sports, drive, or operate complex machinery. The patient also loses previous self-image and body image and role function if he is no longer able to work in his former occupation.

Guilt

Guilt feelings in amputees whose surgeries were necessitated by traumatic injury may occur if their accidents were due to their own carelessness. Guilt may also be experienced by people with circulatory problems whose poor personal hygiene or carelessness may have contributed to the deterioration of the affected limb.

Intimacy

One of the common fears of an amputee is rejection by his or her sexual partner because of the missing part. This subject, often avoided by patients, is of intense concern for many (Bossert and Freeman, 1979). The patient frequently is too embarrassed to discuss his concerns about his own sexuality, but it should be part of the rehabilitative effort of caregivers to open discussion and encourage him to talk about his fears. The ability to share his feelings may be decreased as the patient tries to resolve many of his concerns privately. Sharing them with another, even a normally trusted partner, may initially be too risky because of his vulnerability.

Nursing Approaches

One of the most important roles of the nurse in caring for the amputee is to allow him to talk about the many feelings he is experiencing as the result of his surgery. The counseling techniques described

in Chapter 12 and specifically the section on leading skills can be helpful. The setting of realistic, short-term goals is an important therapeutic approach. Honest, encouraging feedback can provide much-needed support.

Patient education should include information on the normal emotional responses to loss (either the Kübler-Ross or Bowlby stages can be used). When uncontrollable emotion is expressed, the nurse can sit quietly with the patient. Platitudes should be avoided. They can cause increased feelings of fury or isolation in the patient.

Patients can be encouraged to talk about their feelings about their changed body and how they think others may react to them. Discussion about intimacy within a sexual relationship is also important. As described above, amputees often are concerned about rejection by their partner.

Ostomy

The word *ostomy* is used here to define an abdominal stoma that is the result of a temporary or permanent diversion of the intestinal or urinary tract. The initial psychosocial concerns of patients with either a temporary or permanent ostomy are similar. The differences will be examined under the separate issues below.

One of the major factors that can cause difficulty in a patient's ability to accept his ostomy is the emphasis in U.S. culture on cleanliness, grooming, and the normal privacy of the process of elimination. These values evolve from early childhood experience. Youngsters of 2 and 3 years are socialized to conform to society's expectations regarding toileting. Accordingly, these values are deeply imbued in the personality; self-esteem, body image, and many personality traits are developed in the youngster when he is acquiring his beliefs about elimination. As a result, when an ostomy is necessary, it can be a major adaptive challenge.

The circumstances surrounding the ostomy surgery may have an impact on the patient's response. Is this a sudden, unexpected ostomy (as a result of trauma) that the patient had no time to prepare for psychologically? Is this a temporary ostomy being performed to give the bowel a rest from diverticulitis or another type of bowel disease? Is there a possibility that there is a malignant tumor? In the latter case, the patient's concern about the ostomy will usually be secondary to his major concern for his life.

Psychosocial Issues

Trust

The patient with an ostomy is in an unfamiliar situation. He is frightened. He feels like a child because of his total dependence on you for the care of his stoma and removal of his waste products. Initially, he will be watching you closely for your reaction to the appearance of the stoma, the odor, or the feces or urine. He will also depend on you to teach him how to care for himself. Remember that he has been able to take care of his own elimination process since he was very young. Temporarily, he must give over that function to someone else. He may expect rejection.

Self-esteem

Because an ostomy returns a person to a dependent status and causes a major shift in his internal and external perceptions of his body, he is subject to shame and a feeling of self-rejection. His body image has the potential to change markedly. As a result of this psychic blow to self-esteem and the losses that a patient experiences with an ostomy, he is at risk for depression. A brief depressive episode is not unusual as the ego works to resolve these new circumstances.

Loss

As mentioned above, the ostomy patient loses control over the bowel function. This is experienced as a loss by the patient. In addition, if his surgery involved the removal of a section of bowel, rectum, ureter, or bladder, this represents the loss of a body part. Initially he may also anticipate changes in his life style, ability to travel, sit in a theater near other people, make love with his partner, and so on. Usually these initial expectations can be resolved, and the patient is able to resume his normal activities. Whether he is able to resolve them usually depends far more on his psychosocial adaptation than on his physiological adaptation to the surgery.

Guilt

If the ostomy patient's illness is the result of bowel disease that was aggravated by poor adherence to a prescribed diet, guilt may result. The patient may also experience initial guilt about anticipated changes in his partner's life style. Actually, if the latter occurs, this guilt may represent projections of the patient's own uncertainty about the effects of the ostomy in his own life style. Another time when guilt may be expressed is during the nurse's care of the stoma and feces or urine. He will apologize for the inconvenience, messiness, and so on. The patient is actually looking for reassurance from you when he is making such comments that he (as a person) is still accepted by you.

Control

There are two major factors that can further add to the sense of loss of control that is common for ostomy patients.

1. What is the person's normal personality style? Is he fastidious? Does he have a controlling personality type? (See Chapter 5: Personality Styles Seen in General Hospital Patients.) If so, this patient will be even more threatened by this condition than someone whose approach to life and to new situations is more relaxed and easygoing.

2. Where was the ostomy performed? Was it high in the bowel, in the jejunum, in the lower part of the colon, or in the ureter? Jejunostomies or ureterostomies can be more threatening to people because the contents are watery and unformed. Because of their liquid form, the patient has greater fear of "accidents." On the other hand, if the ostomy is performed near the end of the bowel, the feces are usually well formed. Once the ostomy is healed, it is usually possible to obtain a degree of control of the timing of bowel movements.

Intimacy

One of the major concerns of ostomy patients who have sexual partners is *if* they can function sexually, *how* they can function sexually, and *how* their partner or future partners (in the case of single, young ostomy patients) are going to react to them. The patient can become fearful of developing any relationship with a member of the opposite sex. When these concerns are not addressed in the hospital before discharge, the uncertainty that the patient feels can contribute to an overall failure of interpersonal communication. This can create stress in the relationship, which, if prolonged, can be more difficult to resolve. A shutdown in all aspects of the relationship can occur, even in long-married partners, if these issues are not addressed while the patient is in the early stages of adjustment to his changed body. It is wise to wait to discuss these issues until the patient's initial dismay or denial of the surgery gives way to more acceptance. The ideal time is often when discharge planning and teaching is occurring.

Nursing Approaches

An essential aspect of nursing care of the ostomy patient is your response to him. As discussed above, he will be watching you for the slightest negative clue. If you demonstrate acceptance of him, first as a human being with worth and dignity and second as a person with an ostomy that is acceptable to you, he will be more able to incorporate your acceptance into his own image of himself; your acceptance can form the basis of his own self-acceptance. You can also serve as a role model to his spouse, family members, and friends.

By asking him open-ended questions (see Chapter 12: Counseling Techniques for Nurses), you can encourage him to talk about his feelings and thoughts. By exploring important issues in the hospital, his adaptative process can be better worked through.

The importance of talking with an ostomy patient cannot be overemphasized. On occasion, the spouse or other important support person should be included. Many problems with adaptation can be easily avoided by perceptive nursing care. For example, if you notice that the patient is unwilling to look at his colostomy after a few days of care, talking with him about his feelings is very important. If his behavior is unchanged despite your efforts, he can receive counseling assistance from an enterostomal or psychiatric liaison nurse specialist.

Whenever patients express major concerns about whether they will be able to resume a normal life style, it can be very helpful for them to talk with someone who has an ostomy and is fully participating in life. If your hospital has an ostomy nursing clinical specialist or enterostomal therapist, he or she can help to arrange an ostomy visitor before the patient goes home.

If you do not have an ostomy specialist at your hospital, contact the local chapter of the American Cancer Society for information about how to arrange for an ostomy visitor. Although your patient may not have had an ostomy because of cancer, he can still receive a psychological boost from talking with a person who is well adjusted to his ostomy. If, despite these interventions, you continue to be concerned about actual or potential psychosocial maladaptation, formal psychiatric consultation should be requested.

Mastectomy

Every year, nearly 340,000 women undergo a mastectomy (Haug and colleagues, 1981). Mastectomy is a type of surgery that is especially threatening to a woman's psychosocial equilibrium. Some of the factors that contribute to maladaptive potential are listed below:

1. Usually there is little time to prepare for the actuality of a mastectomy. In fact, the patient may undergo surgery and not know what she will discover on awakening.
2. Mastectomy involves the removal not only of a part of her body, but a part of her body that the woman may perceive as essential to her womanliness. She often will experience strong self-doubt, if not in the hospital, then frequently after she returns home.
3. The results of a mastectomy are unpleasant to see. Unlike other surgeries that leave an observable scar but leave the contour of the body unchanged, mastectomy results in a radically different look and feel to a most personal part of the body.
4. The removal of a breast also signals the presence of cancer and all its accompanying fearful prospects.
5. Women who have a sexual relationship, including women who have been married many years, will fear rejection by their partners. Many women initially do not acknowledge this consciously in the hospital. (Remember, they are also responding to a diagnosis of cancer, which is inherent in mastectomy. The ego cannot immediately accept all the implications of this surgery.) Although not consciously acknowledged in most cases, it is an unconscious fear. Lack of conscious awareness of this fear can cause changes in personality dynamics that can become permanently maladaptive if no intervention takes place. They are demonstrated in a variety of ways.

After mastectomy, a woman's body may heal and the concern may not return. However, the well-being of the patient, her spouse or partner, and ultimately her family can be permanently impaired if maladaptation is not averted or resolved. A study of 41 mastectomy patients revealed that 1 in 4 women become so depressed after surgery that they considered suicide (Jamison and associates, 1978).

Psychosocial Issues

Trust

The ability of the mastectomy patient to trust her physician is important. She is turning over to him not only her current well-being during the diagnostic and surgical intervention phases of her treatment, but also her future well-being. (Many normal women ask themselves how they would respond to a diagnosis of breast cancer. In fact, eight of ten biopsied breast lumps are benign [Tully, 1978]. Accordingly, based on the number of mastectomies reported above, in a given year many women face the very real possibility of a mastectomy.) Many women secretly fear the need for such surgery. When a breast lump is discovered, it frequently heightens a fear that was already present.

Mastectomy patients face two other important trust issues: trusting their own ability to cope with the effects of this surgery, and trusting their partners, families, and friends to accept them and still view them as complete women.

Self-esteem

A mastectomy strikes a major blow to a woman's sense of worth and perception of her own body. Review of the development of a feminine body image (see above) can be helpful in understanding the response of a woman to mastectomy.

A woman who is experiencing a major blow to self-esteem as a result of mastectomy will commonly project her feelings of worthlessness onto her partner. She will say, for example, "You don't love me any more" or "You think I'm ugly now, don't you?" Actually, her partner may not be experiencing any major difficulty with her changed appearance, but alienation in the relationship can occur if her poor self-esteem continues to manifest itself in this maladaptive form.

Control

One of the major control issues is the sense of loss of control and accompanying anxiety the patient feels if she is scheduled for biopsy and mastectomy (if the biopsy is positive) during the same procedure. This issue will be discussed below.

Another important control issue is the woman's fear of losing emotional control. It is normal to have strong feelings of grief and rage after mastectomy. For women who are unaccustomed to such strong feelings, they can be frightening. A woman may respond by suppressing them. If they are too intolerable, they may be repressed. The adaptive process can be slowed maladaptively or stopped altogether. The woman may just feel numb. This numbness is actually a form of crisis, and its significance should not be underestimated.

Loss

The losses experienced by a woman following mastectomy are many. First of all, the presence of

cancer is a threat to her life. As she is gradually adapting to this fearsome possibility, she is also faced daily with the loss of her former body concept, loss of her complete sense of femininity, the actual loss of her breast, loss of attractiveness to her partner, and potential loss of full arm function if rehabilitation is not complete. These are all potentially devastating because they occur all at once. They may occur with no warning if she was in denial before biopsy surgery and woke up to find her breast removed.

Guilt

Women can experience guilt if they delayed even slightly before obtaining a medical opinion of a breast lump. Most women, on discovering a breast lump, may wait before obtaining medical or surgical consultation to "make sure I really felt it." Another form of guilt experienced by many women is that they believe they are no longer physically or sexually attractive to their partners. They may mistakenly believe that their partner is staying with them out of pity. They feel guilty that "he is stuck with me."

Intimacy

The ability to feel good about oneself is an essential aspect of being able to engage in an intimate relationship. Because of the potential for decrease in self-esteem that this surgery causes, it frequently has an effect, even if temporarily, on a woman's ability to feel emotionally and physically close to her partner. As emphasized above, this is not uncommon in even the most secure and long-lasting marriages.

Nursing Approaches

It is recommended that a woman facing possible mastectomy obtain three opinions before her surgery. Because of the potential for psychosocial distress that the surgery presents, it should not be entered into without first examining the treatment options available. The process of obtaining these opinions may take up to a week. The risk of delay of surgical intervention should be seriously weighed with the risk of permanent disfigurement and accompanying psychosocial distress that can result if radical surgery is performed. As recently as a decade ago, it was believed that radical mastectomy was the treatment choice for most breast malignancies.

Today, there are several approaches that, at least initially, appear to offer women an equally good prognosis of arrest of cancer. They are the simple mastectomy or lumpectomy. Subsequent chemotherapy or radiation usually is also standard treatment. Some surgeons are able to perform breast reconstruction at the time of the original surgery depending on the tumor. Other surgeons can perform the surgery in such a way that reconstruction can be performed in the near future. It is also possible for reconstruction to be performed and a nearly normal nipple constructed using the woman's own body tissue.

In most cases, it is preferable for any woman who is undergoing breast biopsy to explore the alternatives open to her and talk them over with someone she trusts (frequently, another woman is able to understand the threat of mastectomy in a different way than her spouse).

Because of the potential for maladaptation from denial and longlasting repression, a combined biopsy and radical mastectomy during the same operation should be avoided. Although it may seem to caregivers that a one-time surgery is safer physically than the double risks of anesthesia, the risks should again be weighed against the possibility of long-term psychosocial maladaptation. Two separate procedures may be more preferable in allowing the patient to begin adapting psychologically to this threatening event, especially if she subsequently discovers that she could have explored her surgical options and had a choice other than a radical mastectomy.

Severe Burns

Caring for a patient with severe burns can present a great challenge for caregivers because of complex psychosocial and physiological interactions (Goodstein and Hurwitz, 1975). Initially, psychotic reactions may occur as the result of OBS due to physiological disequilibrium caused by shock, electrolyte imbalance, and infection. As the patient's sensorium clears, there frequently is the possibility of a depressive reaction because of the prolonged and painful treatment process that lies ahead. If disfiguring burns of the face, neck, chest, arms, or hands have occurred, there is the further impact of decreased self-esteem in the depression response.

There are varying opinions about the necessity of psychiatric consultation as a routine treatment approach to the care of the burn patient. Some authors do not routinely recommend such intervention except when obvious psychosocial maladaptation is occurring (Hamburg and co-workers, 1953; Hamburg and colleagues, 1953; Andreason and associates, 1972). Some liaison psychiatrists recommend working with the patient *and* the burn team (Jorgenson and Brophy, 1975; Goodstein and Hurwitz, 1975). Others recommend working only with the burn team in order to help interpret the patient's responses (Weisz, 1967).

Because the psychosocial issues of the severely burned patient are profound, and because the effects on the family and the caregivers can be severe (Barry, 1978; Chang and Herzog, 1975), including a psychiatric liaison consultant, if available, on the burn team at the beginning of the treatment process can help to reduce the psychological stress of all involved. In addition, the psychiatric consultant may remain a "constant" when house officer rotations change if the patient's treatment, as often happens, occurs over several months (Goodstein and Hurwitz, 1975).

Three different stages have been identified in the recovery of the burn patient: acute, intermediate, and recuperative. The acute stage usually occurs for the first several weeks. It includes a high probability of organic delirium, sleep deprivation, hyperactivity, and overt resistance to medical intervention.

The intermediate stage lasts from several weeks to several months. This stage involves painful debridement, skin grafting, and contracture-avoiding procedures. Depression, discouragement, and dependency are commonly seen. For nursing caregivers the stress of patient care can be high because of the long and difficult care involved on a prolonged daily basis.

The recuperative stage involves the remaining part of the patient's hospitalization and the convalescent period at home before his normal roles are resumed. He may be confronted with permanent physical disabilities and the need for vocational retraining (Jorgenson and Brophy, 1975).

Psychosocial Issues

Trust
The severely burned patient often must assume psychological dependence similar to that of an infant on his environment for a prolonged period. Regression is a normal response to severe burns (Andreason and colleagues, 1972). His level of pain is usually severe. A mismove by any staff member can cause excruciating pain. He frequently is on a Stryker frame or circoelectric bed. Turning on these types of apparatus can cause intense fear of falling and a further increase of pain. A similar type of fear can be experienced when he is being moved from bed to stretcher and from stretcher to a Hubbard tank. Medication availability and its

scheduling for pain and anxiety may become an issue in a patient's ability to trust.

Self-esteem

The self-esteem of burn patients can be severely affected when marked disfigurement occurs. The opportunity for replenishment of self-esteem is decreased because of the long-term disruption of important relationships that normally provide the patient with verbal or nonverbal feedback about his worth.

Control

As described above, the condition of being severely burned necessitates relinquishing control over most, if not all, aspects of life for a prolonged period. Depending on the patient's personality style, this can present a severe adaptive challenge.

Loss

The burn patient faces many losses: loss of his normal appearance, a fear of rejection by others because of his changed appearance, and perhaps the loss of his normal work role. Another aspect of loss that may be present is related to the way the burns occurred. Was he in a fire that destroyed his home or apartment? Did he cause the fire? Was he a survivor of a fire in which others were killed? Did he lose one or more members of his family or a friend?

Guilt

Survivor guilt is the intense guilt experienced when the victim was spared death and others died (Horowitz, 1976). This type of guilt results in the person's wondering why he was spared, feeling unworthy to be alive, and so on. It is also common for victims of fires or accidents to have severe nightmares and night terrors in which the event is reexperienced.

Intimacy

A follow-up study of burn patients has revealed that intimacy problems are present in a larger-than-normal rate following recovery. Increases in family discord, divorce, and juvenile delinquency in burn patients or the children of burn patients have been reported (Chang and Herzog, 1975). The prolonged treatment period results in necessary role shifts in the family. Intimacy between partners is also concurrently diminished.

Nursing Approaches

One of the most important aspects of care of the burn patient is to promote his trust in the care-giving system. If one physician on the surgical team does not develop a one-to-one relationship with the patient that is a painless "I'm here to talk with you, not to hurt you" approach, this should be recommended by the head nurse or primary nurse. It is important for hope to be instilled on an ongoing basis; this is best done by the physician who is coordinating the case (Goodstein and Hurwitz, 1975).

Nursing care can be most effective once the patient establishes trust. Although primary nursing is recommended as the preferable approach to the care of most patients, the burn patient requires many unbroken hours of care. It is not unusual for the nurse in such a situation to develop depression, discouragement, and hopelessness when for weeks and months he or she works daily with the patient. It is not in the best interest of the patient or the nurse for such feelings to be promoted by doggedly adhering to a primary nursing model. For this reason, two or preferably three "primary" nurses should ideally rotate the care. The patient may prefer one of the three and develop a close relationship with him or her. If so, that nurse, when not working directly with the patient, can be with him for a "painless" visit.

Trust issues can be relieved by empathically anticipating the patient's response to moving on apparatus, debridement procedures, and so on. Delayed medication timing should not be allowed to undermine the patient's confidence in the environment. If mild sedation is necessary to relieve constant anxiety, an order for regularly scheduled, rather than as needed minor tranquilizers should be obtained once initial homeostasis is ensured. The effects of pain medication should be closely monitored so that adequate pain relief is obtained.

The patient's self-esteem can be promoted by giving honest answers, instilling hope when realistic, and providing accurate feedback. One of the most helpful aids to hope as reported by patients was the ability to talk to other burn patients who had fully recovered from their burns or were in a stage of treatment ahead of the patient (Hamburg and colleagues, 1953).

Control can be restored to the patient by allowing him, whenever possible, to have choices in his care regimen. An important aspect of the patient's psychological recovery from his burns is the opportunity to work through the anxiety associated with the event that caused the burns. He may need to describe the circumstances of the fire or accident on many occasions. This may seem redundant to staff members, but it is very valuable in the progressive release of the unpleasant conscious feelings surrounding the event. It also promotes the release of frightening repressed feelings that could become a maladaptive dynamic. As the unpleasant affect is released, the troubling nightmares about the event that may be occurring should gradually decrease. Survivor guilt can also be reduced by allowing the patient to relive the event. Reality testing by the nurse when unrealistic self-accusations occur can provide the patient with a more self-accepting orientation.

A very important part of the care of a patient who has experienced prolonged hospitalization is to help him separate and terminate relationships with caregivers. This is best done a few weeks in advance of anticipated discharge. The process can be started with questions such as, "How do you feel about going home in 2 weeks?" or "How do you think it will be when you get home?"

As the days go by, the nurse can share his or her feelings about how it has been caring for the patient, how he or she feels about him, or other similar thoughts. This allows the nurse to begin the termination process (this is a loss for the nurse, after all), and invites the patient to examine his feelings. Remember that the care of this patient involved the development of an intimate and often intense relationship because of the dependency that occurred.

Without the opportunity for each member to express his or her feelings, this loss will not be as easily resolved. The patient, after discharge, may, for example, experience profound sadness and feelings of loss that he may not fully understand. By encouraging him to deal with these feelings while he is still hospitalized, a more adaptive resolution of the separation process can occur.

Isolation for Communicable Diseases and Immunosuppressive Conditions

One of the basic fears of a human being is that he will be rejected and abandoned (Cassem, 1978). When isolation becomes necessary, either to protect others from an infectious patient or a patient from infectious others, the added sense of abandonment will add to the other already present stressful factors of illness. Although guilt feelings may accompany their thoughts, there rarely are nurses who find long-range satisfaction in caring for the patient in isolation for a communicable

disease. This is probably due to the extra precautions and work involved in such care as well as a legitimate fear of contracting the patient's illness. Is it also possible that there is an unconscious identification with such a patient that results in equally unconscious fears of abandonment in the nurse? These feelings about patients with communicable disease are interestingly reflected in the unusually limited attention to the psychosocial adaptation of such patients to their enforced separateness in the nursing and medical literature. Ask yourself the following questions. They may help you to understand the feelings of your isolated patients.

> How would it feel to be in isolation for any reason? Add to that the fears that you would have if you also had some type of infectious disease or immunosuppressive failure.

> How would you feel when your family and friends came to visit?

> How would you feel if a loved one were in isolation?

The major problems experienced by patients in isolation are depression, anxiety, irregular sleep, withdrawal, disorientation, and regression (Kellerman and colleagues, 1977). Many of these problems are directly caused by the psychosocial stress of feeling different and alone. Families of patients in isolation also experience increased stress as the result of their loved one's confinement. Their normal ways of communicating with the patient are changed, primarily because of the lack of their normal physical accessibility to him. They also usually have unspoken fears that they will become infected or will infect him. An invisible but real barrier becomes present in the relationship.

Psychosocial Issues

Trust
Regardless of the cause of isolation, the patient may experience a temporary loss of trust in his body's ability to protect him. Eventually, as his condition improves, these feelings should subside. If his loss of trust is prolonged, especially for the patient with immunosuppressive failure, a maladaptive but reality-based consistent suspiciousness of others can result.

Self-esteem
Related to the loss of trust in the body's ability to defend him, the patient's image of his body and its defenses can be changed. Again, the

process of adaptation should ideally prevent a permanent deterioration of body image from occurring. When a prolonged course of treatment is involved, such as that for pulmonary tuberculosis or the repeated episodes of immunosuppressive failure due to the effects of chemotherapeutic agents, there is more possibility of this type of maladaptation. Another risk to self-esteem is caused by the changes in relationships necessitated by the isolation restrictions.

For some patients, isolation for communicable disease carries with it feelings of "dirtiness," which can contribute to a decrease in sense of worth. Indeed, there can be some reality to these feelings because some infectious diseases are socially unacceptable. They are contracted in ways that are generally disapproved of by society; these include infectious hepatitis caused by mainlining of drugs and venereal diseases.

Control

The major control issue of the patient in isolation is his confinement. Regardless of his wishes, he must adhere to the orders of his caregivers. This can be especially anxiety provoking for the independent person with a controlling type of personality. Anger in such a patient is common. When repressed, it can be the major contributing factor to a depressive reaction (Donnelly, 1979). The patient also can become angry or distressed by the restrictions imposed on his visitors.

Loss

The major loss issue of isolation patients is the loss of normal ways of interacting with their loved ones. Most conditions that require isolation are temporary, so that the ability to be with loved ones will eventually be resumed. If immunosuppressive failure is a permanent or long-term condition requiring prolonged or permanent separation from loved ones, then a grief response can be expected. The patient will not be able to participate in most of the pleasurable activities of life, such as attending special family events, being touched or held, and having spontaneous choices. Such a patient inevitably will be working through his response to his own loss of self by death.

Guilt

The patient with a communicable disease may experience guilt because his own behavior might have contributed to his disease. It is also possible that he may have given it to others. The patient who is undergoing long-term treatment for immunosuppressive failure may feel guilt about his

separation from and effect of his illness on his family. Also, he may feel guilt about the effect of the staggering cost of such treatment on his family's finances.

Intimacy

As mentioned above, the normal ability to maintain intimate relationships emotionally and physically is disrupted by isolation. If long-term isolation occurs, the resulting shifts in family role functioning may cause maladaptation in one or more of the members.

Nursing Approaches

Nurses can promote psychological adaption in isolated patients by occasionally asking the patient how he feels about being isolated. The opportunity to release dysphoric feelings can potentially reduce a buildup of tension and feelings that would normally be maladaptively repressed. Nurses should be attentive to their own comments, which may unnecessarily contribute to patients' feelings of differentness or deficiency.

One of the problems that occurs with isolated patients is their frustration in having to wait for caregivers to bring as-needed medication or to answer their requests for care that requires gowning. Nurses understandably can respond to unexpected calls from patients with annoyance when they are very busy. The care of an isolation patient is time consuming. If annoyance is experienced, however, it is one of those times when care should be taken to avoid revealing it to isolation patients, whose self-esteem and sense of control are already diminished. When an approximate time for isolation has been established, it can be used as a way of promoting optimism in the patient. Any intervention designed to return some control of care to the patient is helpful.

The family members of isolation patients should be informed of their loved one's status in a way that will not weaken the relationship structure. They should be educated about the reason for isolation or about isolation procedures in ways that do not cause fear or anxiety. If you detect unusual concern in the family, encourage them to call you if they want to check on the patient's condition. Whenever possible, a telephone should be available in the patient's room so that contact with family and friends can be ensured. Remember that he does not have access to public telephones. One of the most important roles of the nurse is to serve as a liaison to promote communication and prevent an excessive sense of isolation in the patient.

Conclusion

Living with a condition that makes a person look or feel "different" can be a major challenge. For those patients who have the courage to begin working through the various stages of the Kübler-Ross acceptance process, life can be experienced on a far broader scale. Adaptation to such a condition can promote a quality of life in which a person is able to accept a variety of life's invitations. Family dynamics too can become fuller and richer.

Because of the many types of clinical settings in which nurses work—acute care, outpatient, rehabilitation, industrial health, schools, physicians' offices—they have ongoing opportunities to assess and intervene with people who have maladaptively or incompletely resolved all the aspects of living with various types of physical conditions.

Chronic illness imposes on its victims and their families a severe challenge to adaptation. The challenge is more severe than that of acute illness. Acute illness, by its nature, usually ends in recovery or, occasionally, in death. It occurs within a time-limited period. By remembering the elements of crisis theory, you can see that the defensive ability of the ego may be temporarily disorganized by the event. As the acute crisis of illness subsides, stress decreases. The person's coping ability has an opportunity to restore equilibrium.

Chronic illness usually has no *definite* end after which a normal level of health can be expected to resume. It chronically disrupts self-esteem, body image, social relationships, a person's accustomed roles in family, work, and the community, sexuality, and sense of autonomy. This is disruptive to the patient and his family. There is no aspect of psychosocial functioning that is untouched in any family member. Accordingly, the family system is subject to continual stress. Despite strong attempts at conscious coping, or use of unconscious defensive mechanisms by the ego, the result frequently is less than optimal and may eventually result in family disorganization or disintegration. There are families, however, for whom the experience of being with a chronically ill member promotes strength and unity (Udelman and Udelman, 1980).

18

The Coping Challenge of Chronic Illness

Major Effects of Chronic Illness on Psychosocial Stress of Patients, Families, and Nurses

Chronic illnesses have a course of exacerbations and remissions over several years. Examples of illnesses in this category are heart disease, many forms of cancer, strokes resulting from cerebrovascular accidents, chronic obstructive pulmonary disease, and spinal cord injuries. Eventually, most of these illnesses end in death after several months or years of a gradually deteriorating course.

Mailick (1979) has described three stages in the course of chronic illness. The initial stage involves the diagnosis and treatment plan for the illness. In some illnesses, such as some forms of cancer or multiple sclerosis, this stage can last several months. The next stage involves learning to live with the illness and the many changes it is causing and will continue to cause in the lives of all family members. The final stage is the ending of the episode of illness. Usually, this involves the patient's death. For some conditions, however, such as burns, it can mean recovery. The stages are not discretely progressive. Rather, the patient and his family may work through one stage and then return to it at a later time because of new events. It is important to remember that each family member will proceed at his or her own pace through this process. Some members may never proceed at all; they may remain fixated in the initial stage when the emotions and reactions at the time of diagnosis persist throughout the entire illness.

White (1974) has proposed three variables that are important during the diagnosis stage:

1. *Procuring an appropriate amount of information to guide action* (Mailick, 1979, p. 120). People in the initial phase of a chronic illness should not be given too little or too much information. The subject of how much information is enough has been covered in earlier chapters and is also addressed in the next chapter. Essentially, patients are looking for simple answers to their questions in the beginning. They are not ready to hear an indepth discussion of all the possible treatments, outcomes, and courses of the illness.

   A very important aspect of information-giving by health care professionals is that it ideally should be done in the presence of both the patient and his spouse or other family member (Krupp, 1976). The giving of information at different times to different people can eventually cause conflict as the disease progresses. In the beginning, most persons deny all or part of the information they hear about their own or their loved one's illness. When a physician or nurse relays *identical* information separately, the patient and spouse will usually recall different parts of that same information. Remember, the information they are receiving is usually unwanted, frightening, and threatening. Initially, it is normal under these circumstances for the ego to shut off whatever it cannot tolerate.

   If the patient and his family members are all aware of the same information from the beginning of the illness, there is more possibility of maintaining communication and openess throughout the course of the illness. This is an important component in an adaptive response to chronic illness. If, on the other hand, secrets, "protection" of the other, and disagreements occur about the actual conditions of the illness, its treatment, and its effects, a maladaptive outcome can develop.

2. *Preserving enough autonomy to allow for flexibility of options* (Mailick, 1979, p. 120). An important aspect of the diagnosis stage of chronic illness is that the patient and his family be given the information they need and that they be part of the decision-making process when treatment choices are available.

3. *Maintaining the internal organization of the person and his family* (Mailick, 1979, p. 121). The growing awareness that a person has a serious illness that has a long uncertain course can precipitate a crisis for the patient or one or more family members. The ongoing assessment by the nurse of all family members can provide important clues that family disruption may be occurring. Successful intervention by the nurse at this time can prevent further deterioration. It can also prevent the development of long-term and frequently permanent maladaptive responses. If it is obvious that nursing intervention is not resolving the problem, referral at this time, instead of many months into the illness, to a mental health professional trained in family therapy, rather than individual therapy, is strongly recommended. Most health care professionals can recall families whose members were permanently scarred emotionally by maladaptive responses to disrupting chronic illness.

Patient Response

There are many ways that a person can respond to chronic illness. Initially, all of them are normal as the ego seeks to adapt. If they do not give way to more mature defenses and behavior, then they become maladaptive. Denial, regression, and acting-out behavior are common in both the patient and one or more family members. Some persons seem to embrace the sick role (Krupp, 1976).

Regarding the sick role, some caregivers expect certain types of behavior of patients, especially those whom they see over a prolonged period. Ideally, they may expect a person to be compliant, ready to accept opinions with a minimum of questioning, nonhostile, pleasant, moderately intelligent, and possessing a value system similar to their own. Realistically, how often are these qualities present? The potential for conflict in the caregiving system is increased in the patient with chronic illness because of the long-term relationships inherent in the treatment process.

The emotionally mature patient may compliantly accept his care with few questions. This can be due to his fear of abandonment, especially by his primary physician. The physician is a very important person in the patient's overall ability to cope with illness; he or she is the symbol of hope (Bruhn, 1977). Often, the patient's behavior and that of the family is motivated by attempts to avoid the physician's displeasure and possible rejection.

Family Response

Although the ill member of the family may compliantly accept his care, it is common for the spouse in a normally mature and responsible marital dyad to develop strong anger toward the caregiving system if he or she is excluded from the information and decision-making processes. This is especially so when the sick spouse temporarily regresses to an untypical, childlike, passive, and compliant state without fully understanding the issues of his illness. This type of spouse hostility can be decreased by joint discussions with both members of the couple.

Research on the effects of chronic illness in families has revealed that there frequently are permanent disruptions in postillness family functioning (Crain and colleagues, 1966; Landsman, 1975; Levenstein, 1980; Martin, 1976; Salk and colleagues, 1972; Treuting, 1962). It is important to remember that no family ever has harmonious, supportive, loving relationships between all its members all the time. There are chronic strains within all family groups and new strains of various intensity being introduced at all times. When severe family disruption occurs as the result of chronic illness, it frequently is caused by the intensification of already strained family communication and coping patterns.

A shutdown of communication is a common family response. Repressed grief, depression, and hopelessness occur at varying intervals. During exacerbations of the illness, family members will often repress anger and hostility toward each other in attempts to maintain equilibrium. When remissions occur, these repressed feelings can break through. They may appear inappropriate for the precipitating event. Actually, they are often the result of excessive and sometimes prolonged conscious or unconscious needs to avoid confrontation (Mailick, 1979). Ambivalent feelings about the ill member may occur. Guilt as an outcome of these feelings is common.

Another complicated task required of family members is to be able to relinquish their newly acquired roles if the ill member experiences periods of remission in his illness. When he is feeling better, he will want to resume as many of his former roles within the family as possible. If other members consistently and capably fill these roles, he will question his own value to his family.

Response of the Nurse

Caring for patients with chronic illness can be an adaptive challenge for nurses as well as patients and families. It is natural that nurses identify with chronically ill patients. In this process, they actually feel what it is like to be in the illness role themselves. When nurses are consciously aware of this identification, they are able to empathize objectively and provide warm and ongoing therapeutic care. If, however, the identification process is unconscious, the nurse may take on the patient's feelings, find them difficult to tolerate, and eventually shut down his or her awareness of the patient's feelings and reactions. This becomes an important dynamic in withdrawal and distancing from involvement with patients.

At various times *all* caregivers must pull back from therapeutic involvement with patients; it is an adaptive device of the ego. When it occurs consistently, it can diminish a nurse's capacity to enter into meaningful relationships either with patients or in any other sphere of life. Remaining open and aware of your own feeling and thinking reactions to patients with chronic illness can help you to remain open and aware to your patient's feelings and thoughts as well.

• • •

The remainder of this chapter will address the specific issues of patients with the following chronic diseases: cancer, heart disease, stroke, chronic obstructive pulmonary disease, and spinal cord injuries.

The Patient With Cancer

Psychosocial Issues

Of all diseases in the Western world, one that arouses a strong emotional response in both laypersons and health care professionals is cancer. The reason is because it shows no respect for its victims. Anyone—man, woman, child, bank president, or street cleaner— is vulnerable. Indeed, two out of three families will have members with cancer. During this decade it is estimated that 6,500,000 new cases will be diagnosed, 3,500,000 people will die of cancer, and more than 10,000,000 people will receive medical care for their cancer (American Cancer Society, 1980).

It is the unpredictability of the development of the illness, as well as the alteration in life style of its victims and family members, that creates the excessive accompanying psychosocial stress of its diagnosis and treatment. The need for emotional and social support during the course of illness and treatment cannot be overemphasized. The strain on patients and their families can be excessive because of the interactional effects that this illness has on *all* aspects of psychosocial functioning.

Martin has identified three major variables that affect these multiple aspects of psychosocial functioning:

1. *Tumor characteristics.* These include origin, natural history, degree of malignancy, sensitivity to therapeutic modalities, and stage at time of diagnosis.
2. *Age of patient at time of diagnosis.* For the purpose of discussing the psychosocial aspects of cancer, the human life span will be divided into child, adolescent, young adult, middle adult, and old adult. Each of these age groups is subject to different categories of disease, different emotional problems, and a different set of societal problems. The infant or child is emotionally and socially dependent on society for total nourishment and support. The adolescent is struggling for personal definition and escape from the bondage of dependency. The young adult is looking forward to planning and developing societal relationships. Middle adulthood is full of choices, others depend on this age group, and it can be identified in most instances as life at its least threatening time. Old adults are dependent emotionally and socially. These people are venerated and frequently look forward to the end of their lives and death.
3. *Strength and effectiveness of various available support systems (medical, psychological, and social).* The medical plans for prevention, treatment, and rehabilitation are not always well defined; however, the state of the art at present is identifiable, and effective protocols are being used. In the psychological and social disciplines, there are very few well-defined protocols; each patient and family requires a different format. Thus there is a need for identification of the psychosocial issues that impinge on the cancer patient and his family and for appropriate research formats directed at resolving these issues.

(Cohen J, Cullen J, Martin L: Psychosocial Aspects of Cancer, pp. 4-5. New York, Raven Press, 1982)

Trust

From the beginning of the diagnostic process, the patient with cancer must believe in his physician's ability to treat his cancer. His continuation of hope for recovery is strongly associated with his belief in his physician. When this belief is not present, the result is *objective helplessness*. Objective helplessness is a patient's belief that no help is available to him from people in his environment. Loss of hope accompanies a state of objective helplessness. *Subjective helplessness*, on the other hand, is the patient's feeling-belief that he cannot help himself. He lacks the ability to think for himself or to be assertive or take action on his own behalf (Renneker, 1981). In essence, the patient loses trust in himself.

Trust that other caregivers and family and friends will not abandon them is another important concern of cancer patients. In fact, many people unconsciously withdraw from and avoid relationships with cancer patients because of their own anxiety that occurs when they identify with the patient. The person with cancer gradually becomes aware of the discomfort that others may experience and may temporarily or permanently socially isolate himself from others, including his own family.

Self-esteem

The self-esteem of cancer patients can be threatened in many ways. First of all, a patient may feel that his body has failed him. This can have a profound effect on his self-image and body image. If the cancer results in radical head or neck surgery, mastectomy, colostomy, orchiectomy, or radical pelvic surgery, fears of self-disintegration are more profound (Schain, 1981). In some cases, when loss of self-esteem is accompanied by feelings of self-rejection, these feelings may be projected angrily onto others in the environment. The mastectomy patient, for example, may accuse her husband, "You don't find me attractive anymore."

Control

For cancer patients, many aspects of their lives seem out of control. At times, these feelings can be overwhelming. The discovery of a new lump or shadow on an x-ray film removes any sense of mastery over the disease. The disease seems to control patients rather than their having any control over it (Renneker, 1981).

Loss

The losses experienced by cancer patients are well known to most nurses, who may have lost family members or friends to cancer and have observed the losses of cancer patients first hand. The threat of loss of self has not been well explored in the literature, but it is the ultimate threat for many patients. It can occur gradually as role independence, personal dignity, physical integrity, and a holistic sense of well-being are lost. When remissions occur in the disease process, the patient can experience loss, only to regain what was lost, then lose it again through exacerbations or death.

Guilt

Guilt can be experienced when the cancer patient asks himself, "What did I do to deserve this?" He can feel guilt for the effect that his disease is having on his family members, emotionally and financially. There is another aspect of guilt that can afflict well-educated persons who try to intellectually grapple with the "why" of their cancer. Some theorists are proposing that preexisting personality characteristics may play a part in the development of cancer (Abse and colleagues, 1974; Bahnson, 1981; Grissom and colleagues, 1975; Schmale and Iker, 1966). This causes the introspective patient to wonder how he contributed to his own cancer and to feel guilt that he "allowed" it to happen.

Intimacy

One of the most difficult aspects of living with cancer is the changes that occur in all relationships, intimate or casual. The change in intimate relationships is very complex. The patient may or may not be consciously aware of these changes; many times they are the result of unconscious ego defense mechanisms in both the patient and loved ones. Denial, avoidance, regression, conversion, projection, and withdrawal are common. There frequently is deep repression of anger and hostility. Depressive reactions result in increased isolation; accordingly, the normally supportive closeness of loved ones is lost.

One of the consequences of these changes in interpersonal communication is that the quality of a couple's sexual relationship also suffers. The feelings of fatigue, sluggishness, and malaise that result from chemotherapy or the disease process itself can cause a decrease of libido in a person who normally enjoys sexual intimacy. A third aspect of sexual intimacy was discussed above. If the treatment of cancer requires castration, mastectomy, or any other invasive or disfiguring surgery, the patient may believe that he has no physical appeal to his partner; he feels repulsive.

Nursing Approaches

Cancer patients sometimes feel as if they were on an emotional roller coaster. The nurse can help the cancer patient by envisioning himself or herself in the car directly behind the one occupied by the patient. When the patient is high, he may be feeling genuinely happy for a brief time or may be in denial. At this time, attempts to engage the patient in deep discussion about his "honest" feelings about cancer are inappropriate. The nurse can mirror the patient's feelings in a lighthearted way. When the patient is feeling low, the nurse can respond in a way that says to the patient, "I understand; I'm with you." Leading questions and attentiveness to the patient's emotional and intellectual responses are therapeutic at such a time. Helping the patient to gain a sense of control over as many aspects of care as possible is another therapeutic goal.

A patient may initially not hear various aspects of conversations with his caregivers because of partial denial. Ideally, you can be present when the physician is talking with the patient. If the physician and patient prefer to be alone, you may need to check with physicians to learn what information has been given to the patient. Reinforce this information with the patient; answer his questions simply. As described above, this is ideally done with a spouse or family member in attendance.

It is important to interject at this point a discussion about the need for hope in cancer patients and the similarity in appearance between hope and a low to moderate level of denial. When patients and family express hope, despite clinical evidence that indicates it is not appropriate, we must respect the fact that these expressions are indicators of their lack of readiness to accept the threat that this illness holds for them. Unless the potential for maladaptive outcome is high, I believe that these expressions should not be disturbed by the intervention recommendations for working with patients in maladaptive denial that are described in Chapter 20: The Nurse and the Dying Patient in the section on intervention.

The following case example may clarify this point:

Case Example

Ann is a 43-year-old married mother of four sons aged 8 through 16. She was diagnosed 3 months ago with a malignant, inoperable brain tumor. On her first admission, it was learned that communication patterns within the family have normally been closed, with little acknowledgment of difficulties. During her second admission, her surgeon removed excessive brain tissue to decrease intracranial pressure. Her prognosis of approximately 1 year was unchanged, however. She described that she would be traveling to a major cancer center for a second opinion. She looked well physically, and there was no evidence of depression. She smiled frequently. She remarked that she, her husband, and her children were all "back to normal," and she was hopeful that things will be all right.

Can we call this hope? Or is it denial? Under these circumstances, this family is using its defense of hope-denial to stabilize life and maintain as much normality as possible. I would find it difficult to consider disturbing the equilibrium that they have created with their hope. Certainly, the advancement of disease will, too soon, cause reality to present itself. I believe that as long as a family can find peace and a degree of normality living with a difficult prognosis by maintaining hope, and all members of the family are adapting, it can be *quietly* respected by caregivers. I do not believe, however, that we should excessively support the hope. By doing so, we can provide the basis for the hope eventually developing into maladaptive denial as the symptoms of the disease become more obvious.

Pain control is an important issue for cancer patients. Analgesia should be pain relieving and consistent whenever not physiologically contraindicated. Inadequate medication can undermine a patient's coping ability. He may fear losing control of himself if his pain is too great. This subject is addressed in the next chapter.

Finally, nurses in both inpatient and outpatient settings can perform a valuable service to cancer patients and families by assessing the emotional response of all members to the continuing stress of living with cancer. This can only be done by asking the patient and his spouse *separately* and then together how each is feeling emotionally, how he or she thinks the spouse is coping, and how the family is handling the illness. Frequently, spouses give a more realistic view of the emotional strain of the illness; they usually will not yield this information in the presence of their loved one. When family disruption or maladaption in one family member is chronically present, for example, in a teenager who is destructively acting out, referral to a family therapist is recommended. Family therapy provides the members with a safe, supportive environment in which to examine their own and the overall family's response to the multiple issues of cancer. The potential for maladaptation is decreased. Accordingly, the potential for a good quality of life for all members is increased.

The Patient With Coronary Artery Disease

Patients with arteriosclerotic heart disease fall into three main categories: chronic angina pectoris, acute myocardial infarction (MI), and coronary artery bypass surgery. Although psychosocial effects within the three categories differ and will be addressed separately, the majority of the effects are due to the chronicity of the illness once the acute stage is past.

Psychosocial Issues

Research on the correlation between arteriosclerotic disease and the presence of type A personality demonstrated a significant relationship between the two factors (Rosenman, 1971). Informal observations are reported by cardiologists and cardiac nurses that type A personality characteristics are present in a majority of their cardiac patients. Some of these characteristics are aggressiveness, anxiety, repression of emotions, hyperactivity, competitiveness, intense work involvement, high level of discipline, and involvement in a dominant and socially acceptable occupation (Pancheri and associates, 1978). (The type A personality was described in Chap. 5.)

These types of personality traits, when present, become an important factor in a cardiac patient's ability to adapt to the restrictions on his activity and diet. In addition, the person with a type A personality has a strong need to maintain control. Accordingly, the chronicity and unpredictability of his illness present a difficult challenge. The need to take different types of medications on an ongoing basis may also become a control issue.

The effects of cardiac disease, especially on the spouse, are stressful. Since many cardiac patients are men, research on spouses' response to cardiac illness has focused on the psychosocial effects on the wives of cardiac patients. In a study of 50 male MI patients and their wives, there were discrepancies in their separate interpretations of the psychological outcomes of their illnesses. The husbands acknowledged concerns about financial problems, depression, curtailment of activities, and fear of recurrent attack. They did not view these concerns as major adjustment difficulties, however. Their wives did. They found that their husbands were minimizing their problems (Ezra, 1961).

In exploratory group work with cardiac bypass surgical patients and their wives, I found the same tendency in all the patients. It is repeatedly present in patients I have seen in the clinical setting as well. This response seems to be due to the prolongation of the defense mechanism of denial after MI or bypass surgery. Initially, this denial is an adaptive coping response that helps the patient through the critical and acute care periods. It is possible that the controlling type A personality, in order to avoid the anxiety associated with the many unknowns in his future, maintains a maladaptive level of denial for an indefinite period or until there is more certainty to his long-term prognosis (Soloff, 1977).

Although the majority of patients fully recover physically from heart surgery, the results of research on the psychological consequences of surgery have not been promising. Over one third of 70 patients who participated in one study were found to have "significant psychological hindrances one year after their surgeries." These maladaptive responses were anxiety, depression, poor self-esteem, passive dependency, somatic preoccupation, paranoid tendencies, and withdrawal. They also had impaired marital and sexual functioning (Heller and colleagues, 1974).

A more recent study of 30 patients found that at 1 to 2 years after coronary artery bypass, 83% were unemployed and 57% were sexually impaired. Other maladaptive personality outcomes were low self-esteem, constricted social life, and decreased pleasure from close relationships. A significant number of patients also had increased and persistent dependency needs, serious distortions of body image, and symptomatic depression (Gundle and colleagues, 1980).

The maladaptation problems of the male cardiac patient can contribute to maladaptation in the spouse as well. Research findings have indicated that the effects of maladaptation in spouses after their husbands' MIs can be prolonged. In wives who had no previous history of psychological distress before their husbands' MIs, 38% reported moderate to severe psychological distress during their husbands' hospitalization. Two months after discharge, the rate of moderate to severe psychological distress had risen to 60%. One year after

discharge, 58% of the wives continued to report moderate to severe psychological distress as a result of their husbands' MIs (Mayou and associates, 1978).

There is another noteworthy aspect about the psychological functioning of coronary artery bypass patients. Delirium after surgery occurs in approximately 28% of all patients. The psychiatric symptoms that result are those of a toxic organic brain syndrome (OBS) (see Chap. 11). The contributing factors that have been found to correlate with a delirious response after surgery are severity of recovery room illness, unexpressed anxiety, and active-dominant personality. Of the patients in the study who developed delirium, one fourth of them, or approximately 7% of the total bypass surgical patient population, developed a major psychosis (Kornfeld and colleagues, 1978). The nursing care of patients who are psychotic as the result of an OBS is discussed in Chapters 11 and 17.

Trust

Many aspects of trust are challenges for the cardiac patient. The important ones are trust of his caregivers during the acute post-MI or postbypass surgical period. In either instance, the patient is in a critical care environment that in itself is stressful. His life depends on the knowledge of his physician and nurse caregivers. For the person with an aloof, controlling, or suspicious personality, the unpredictable and tension-filled environment can produce high levels of anxiety. Engel (1976) has found that the most common precipitant of death from cardiac failure is ventricular fibrillation. One of the causes of ventricular fibrillation can be sudden emotional stress. If a patient experiences high levels of anxiety as a result of problems in trusting the environment, he is at greater risk for physiological as well as emotional sequelae.

Another major trust factor for many cardiac patients that has been informally observed is their fear that their hearts may dysfunction at any time. The heart is a vital organ. It is indeed the core of a person. Core is derived from the Latin *cor*, meaning heart (Jenney and colleagues, 1979). Basic lack of trust in his heart can have a major effect on a person's sense of self-esteem and sense of control; it is also a loss that must be resolved.

Self-esteem

A cardiac patient's self-esteem is threatened by his illness. Arteriosclerotic heart disease often develops in the active working man. For many persons, one of the major sources of self-esteem is their work (Taves and associates, 1963). When their work role is threatened, as it often is with heart disease, there is an increased threat to the maintenance of self-esteem. If the patient is a normally independent, hard-driving person, he may find it difficult to assume the passive, compliant patient role that is imposed on him in the intensive care unit and during his hospitalization and rehabilitation. If these characteristics are in direct opposition to his normal traits, his self-image can be temporarily weakened and his self-esteem will be diminished. The disruption of his normal role in the family as head of the household can also undermine his feelings about his own worth.

Control

Some of the control issues of the cardiac patient have already been mentioned above. The major source of the patient's feeling of lack of control is the unpredictable nature of his illness; an angina attack or, worse, an MI can occur at any time. This is frightening to the patient and his family. It also makes him angry and resentful. He cannot lose his temper, however; he tells himself that he must learn to live with it—another control issue. Many cardiac patients repress their emotions because of a desire to avoid angina attacks. As discovered in the bypass surgical group study, the wives of MI victims also try to repress their feelings as a way of avoiding upsetting their husbands. This was reported by each of the wives. Their repressed and conscious anger and growing resentment about their husband's inability to communicate with them may be a contributing factor to the high levels of psychological distress reported by these wives.

Loss

The cardiac patient can experience a major loss when arteriosclerotic heart disease is diagnosed. Until then he has had a normal heart that worked well and could be relied on; his cardiac illness is yet another indication of his loss of youth. His body functioning in most instances could be taken for granted. For the ambitious, goal-oriented person who has always functioned well, the intrapsychic and social system changes caused by his heart disease are experienced consciously or unconsciously as a loss.

The stages of acceptance outlined by Kübler-Ross match the stages that I observed in the male cardiac surgical patients in the group setting and that have also been present in patients seen individually. As in any bereavement process, the final acceptance of the loss can take up to 1 year. The first stage, that of denial, may be prolonged

and, in some people, may never give way to the remaining stages in the acceptance process. The lack of working through of this stage may be due to fear of the feelings of anger or depression of the later stages. The bargaining stage of the acceptance process is marked by ambivalent thoughts that alternate between acceptance and rejection of a changed self-image and a different life style.

Guilt

One of the most important factors in the cardiac patient's rehabilitation is whether he will be able to return to his previous employment (Cay, 1978). This can threaten the financial well-being of his family. Research has found that when financial problems arise because of the illness, the family response is more negative and there is disruption within the family system (Ezra, 1961). Guilt can become a problem when financial worries plague a man and he believes his family is being deprived. He can also experience guilt about his inability to function in many roles that he formerly performed.

Intimacy

As each of the wives reported in the cardiac group study, there was a change in the style of communication that had been normal within the marriage. The result they described was a shutdown in the couple's ability to talk with each other. Eventually the wives began to feel resentful. Their resentment seemed directed at their husband's illness in most cases. It is possible that if their anger were experienced toward their husbands, they would have felt uncomfortable levels of guilt. Avoidance can become an important couple dynamic when this occurs.

The sexual concerns of some cardiac patients are evidenced by provocative sexual acting-out behavior toward the nurses. The greatest fear of these men is impotence (Cassem and Hackett, 1971).

Many cardiac patients and their spouses are concerned that sexual intercourse and orgasm are too taxing on the damaged heart. Anxiety about sexual functioning is common during the rehabilitation process. Research has been carried out on the cardiovascular effects of intercourse. Masters and Johnson (1966) found that there is a gradual increase in both the heart and respiratory rates; the heart rate during orgasm ranges between 100 and 175 beats a minute. Respirations are around 40 a minute.

Hellerstein and Friedman (1970) studied the effects of sexual activity on 48 coronary patients and found that the heart rate range was 90 to 144 beats a minute. The mean rate was 117.4 beats. The mean rate reduced to 97 and 85, respectively, during the first and second minutes after orgasm. Blood pressure rose to 162/89 mm Hg with orgasm and fell to 145/88 mm Hg within 2 minutes.

More than half the patients in the study (58.3%) reported a slight decrease in sexual activity, from 2.1 times a week 1 year before the MI to 1.6 times a week after the attack. The change was attributed to the following reasons: change in sexual desire, woman's decision not to have intercourse, depression, fear, and cardiac symptoms. None of these men were impotent. The remaining 41.7% of the men reported no change in sexual functioning. A study by Rhodes (1974) found that there is no significant difference in heart rate between the various coital positions. These findings were duplicated by Stein (1975). One of the final conclusions of the Hellerstein and Friedman study was that sexual intercourse between partners of 20 or more years (when congestive heart failure was not present) in their own bedroom was similar to the physical effect of walking up one flight of stairs.

Nursing Approaches

During the immediate acute stage of care of the MI or postbypass patient, it is important for nurses to be attentive to the patient's pain and anxiety levels. Response with appropriate levels of medication will promote the patient's trust in the caregiving system. It will also help him to trust in his own ability to control himself in the fearful situation.

As soon as the most acute part of the intensive care experience is over, the patient should be prepared for his eventual transfer to a regular nursing unit. This can be described in positive terms and interpreted to the patient as a sign of his improvement. It is helpful to ask the patient on the day or two before transfer how he feels about being moved out of the unit. It is common for a patient to experience anxiety about being monitored less closely. The chance to talk about his fears can help to decrease them by allowing the unpleasant affect to be released. Another time when anxiety commonly increases is before the patient is discharged home. Raising the question, "How do you feel about going home in 2 days?" can help to decrease anxiety and prepare the patient psychologically for discharge.

The cardiac rehabilitation teaching should be done with both the patient and spouse together whenever possible. As discussed early in the chapter, this can reduce potential areas of conflict. A brief and general presentation of the findings about changes in couple communication, as well as the research findings on the effects of sexual intercourse on the heart, can give the couple information that may help in their adaptation.

Finally, as research with the wives of cardiac patients showed, psychosocial stability may be compromised for extended periods in both partners. When questioning reveals marital or individual dysfunction, nurses in outpatient settings can refer these persons to a family therapist.

The Stroke Patient (Cerebral Vascular Accident)

A cerebral vascular accident (CVA) is a condition that results from vascular insufficiency, embolism, thrombosis, or an intracerebral hemorrhage. These conditions all cause a reduced supply of blood to the brain. Paralysis occurs on the opposite side of the body from the side of the brain affected. The patient's ability to talk can be affected if the left brain is involved. In addition to speech and motor disabilities, altered psychosocial functioning is common (Labi and colleagues, 1980). Short-range changes in mental status can last for 6 to 8 weeks as the result of cerebral edema and temporarily changed tissue functioning. The symptoms of confusion and other OBS changes can gradually subside during this period. By 3 months after the CVA, the changes in emotional, intellectual, and motor functioning that remain will probably be permanent (Charatan and Fisk, 1978).

Psychosocial Issues

Fears common in stroke patients are fear of being permanently crippled and handicapped, fear of another stroke, fear of being dependent on others, and fear of loss of love (Charatan and Fisk, 1978, p. 1403).

Trust
The stroke patient is often partially paralyzed and may also have lost his ability to speak. He is suddenly and swiftly forced into a completely helpless and dependent state with no time to prepare himself mentally. He is totally reliant on others to anticipate his needs. Despite the personality regression that is common in all illness states, it is demoralizing for most patients to be reduced to total dependency similar to that of a very young child.

Self-esteem

The stroke patient's self-esteem is dealt a severe blow. Depression is common as a result. Changed body image and self-image are strong dynamics because of the many losses and changes in body and psychological functioning. The patient is often disgusted with his inability to function and the useless appearance of the affected limbs.

Control

The stroke patient, as a result of the OBS that accompanies his stroke, often experiences changes in the quality of his emotions. They become more primitive. Rage and grief predominate, and lability is common (Charatan and Fisk, 1978). The patient's ego is aware of the changes, however, and he is usually frightened by his loss of normal emotional control. As the physiological state of the brain stabilizes, there can be more return of emotional control.

If there is major loss of motor and speech functions, the patient may feel overwhelmed at times by the anxiety that accompanies such a helpless state in which he has lost full or partial control over all aspects of his life.

Loss

The patient's losses will depend on the degree of permanent impairment caused by the stroke. In addition to the losses mentioned above, other important social losses are: his ability to be independently mobile; impaired physical function, including bladder and bowel control, which could lead to embarassment and fears of disgrace; loss of normal role in the family; loss of ability to work, loss of ability to function normally in social relationships, and so on.

Guilt

The patient frequently feels as if he were a burden to all. He anticipates that nurses, family members, and others will tire of caring for him. He becomes especially watchful for nonverbal and verbal clues that his suspicions are correct. It is not uncommon for some stroke patients to say, "I wish I were dead." Sometimes this is due to their wish that they no longer be a burden to others, especially if they are severely incapacitated by the CVA.

Intimacy

The ability to maintain close relationships in a previous context is often affected. The patient may feel useless to his partner or other family members.

Accordingly, his communication patterns change. This is also affected by the presence of depression. Sexual intercourse, common in happily married elderly persons, may no longer be possible because of paralysis. The stroke patient's sense of worth as a person can be strongly enhanced by a partner who continues to demonstrate his caring by maintaining sexual closeness.

Nursing Approaches

As much as possible, try to anticipate the needs of stroke patients. Although this is the usual recommendation for all patients, it is especially important for the patient who has experienced paralysis or loss of speech. Attentive nursing care can promote self-esteem and lessen feelings of rage about helplessness. It can be very helpful to a patient with speech loss if you attempt to identify what his feelings may be at a given time. For example, when he is feeding himself and the utensils are difficult to manage, you can comment, "It is probably making you angry that eating is so complicated." It can be an emotional relief to have his feelings recognized. It lets him know you understand and opens the possibility for him to talk or write about his feelings with you if he is able. Your question also gives him permission to have these normal feelings. It is not uncommon for him to begin crying when his real feelings are recognized. This is due to the lack of emotional control and lability caused by the OBS mental state as well as the relief of experiencing your understanding.

It can also comfort the patient if you reassure him that some of his excessive emotion is due to the injury to the brain itself. As the swelling decreases in the ensuing weeks, you can tell him that he will be able to regain more control. Similarly, some of the confusion can be expected to decrease gradually. These statements can help to promote hope, and the patient's level of hope will be a strong factor in his ultimate psychosocial adaptation.

Your honest reassurance, combined with opportunities for the patient to express feelings of discouragement and sadness, will avoid excessive buildup of dysphoric feelings. The nursing care plan for the unmotivated patient that appears in Chapter 16 can be helpful for all CVA patients, especially those who lack the impetus for rehabilitation.

The Patient With Chronic Obstructive Pulmonary Disease

Chronic obstructive pulmonary disease is a chronic illness that affects all spheres of a patient's functioning. Because the illness affects the basic function of breathing, it diminishes vitality and produces symptoms that cause psychosocial complications (Dudley and colleagues, 1980). Lustig and coauthors (1972, p. 315) found that these patients as a group were "highly anxious, socially isolated, lonely, and afraid to commit themselves to vocational activities." Dudley and associates (1973) described them as living very emotionally constricted lives. They were afraid to feel angry, depressed, or happy; any change in emotions worsened their pulmonary symptoms.

Psychosocial Issues

Trust
As this disease progresses, the patient becomes more and more dependent on his physician and family. This seems to be so regardless of the patient's normal personality before he developed his chronic illness. Because of the potential for a lengthy final stage of illness, this dependency and complete trust can become a strain for those who are so heavily depended on. The patient is able to sense this and often feels anxiety about abandonment.

Self-esteem
One of the most common outcomes of this illness is that the patient must retire from an active work role as the disease progresses. The major loss of this important source of self-esteem, as well as the loss of many other sources of self-esteem, cause his sense of worth to fall. Accordingly, with this decrease in self-esteem it is not uncommon for depression to be a common clinical finding in the patient with moderate to advanced disease. The body image of the patient is affected by his excessive body preoccupation and emphasis on physical symptoms, which are often considered to be much higher than that observed in patients with other types of illnesses (Agle and Baum, 1977).

Control
The loss of a sense of control over one's ability to breathe has the potential to cause marked anxiety in all persons. Accordingly, anxiety dominates the clinical picture of these patients. Certainly, the patient has very little control over the advancing disease process. It promotes in him the feeling of helplessness. Ultimately, hopelessness may result.

Loss
As described above, the losses of such a patient are many. Part of the reason for the volume of losses he experiences is due to the self-isolation and social withdrawal that is common in patients with this chronic illness. This is a protective device he uses to prevent over-exertion or emotional excitation, which can aggravate episodes of breathing difficulties.

Guilt
In many cases the patient may have brought about his own lung problems with excessive smoking. His breathing difficulties may be work related, and he may have ignored occupational safety regulations. Guilt can be an underlying dynamic to psychosocial maladaptation when his previous actions are the cause of his current problems.

Intimacy
Because of the triggering effect of emotions on pulmonary distress, these patients and their families often "tiptoe" around emotional issues. This represses normal family dynamics. Normal sexual functioning of the patient decreases as the disease progresses. This is usually attributed to shortness of breath and easy fatigability. Agle and Baum (1977) suspect that there may be a significant psychogenic effect on the male patient's sexual functioning.

Nursing Approaches

The nursing care of this patient is centered on reducing physical discomfort and promoting psychosocial adaptation through supportive counseling and rehabilitation teaching of self-help techniques. Support of the family during the chronic stages of hospitalization is another important aspect of care.

It is not unusual for patients with moderate to severe disease to be hospitalized for several weeks or months. Initial nursing attempts to reduce anxiety levels in patients and family members can result in higher levels of adaptation to the prolonged institutionalization experience. If primary nursing is used, it can be less stressful for two or three nurses to share the care. This is recommended because the patient may become excessively dependent.

If the patient's level of depression or anxiety becomes prolonged and maladaptive, psychiatric consultation is recommended as a way of relieving the patient, family, and caregiver from the heavy emotional demands that can develop as time passes and the illness progresses.

The Patient With a Spinal Cord Injury

The effects of a spinal cord injury (SCI) that produces quadriplegia or paraplegia are profound. It is a catastrophic injury that occurs with no warning. There are permanent and all-encompassing consequences for a person for the remainder of his life. These effects will also be experienced by the family. There can be little doubt that the swift, unconscious use of denial by the ego is adaptive during the acute stage of treatment. The patient's life is frequently in jeopardy during this acute period as a result of the accident.

Ultimately, the denial should gradually decrease. It may be observed for a longer period than the denial period commonly seen in cancer patients, for example. Because of the overwhelming threat of paralysis, it may take longer for the ego to relinquish denial, its strongest and most basic defense mechanism. Before denial can be decreased, the patient's ego must have other defense mechanisms ready to assist him in coping with the threat of lifetime paralysis.

Paralysis is a major loss. The adaptation to paralysis occurs as the loss is grieved in a process that has been compared to the Kübler-Ross stages of acceptance (Bracken and Shepard, 1980). Siller (1969) has described the grieving process of the SCI patient as gradually letting go of the ties to hundreds of former functions and abilities that are now lost. This dissolution of each tie is carried out separately by the ego. If the ego were to be fully aware of the massive losses faced by the patient, it could be completely overwhelmed.

During the initial stage of hospitalization, it is possible that an OBS resulting from direct injury to the spinal cord or related etiology can result in atypical emotional or behavioral responses (Guttman, 1976). These responses can sometimes be misinterpreted by caregivers, who may not be aware of their organic etiology; they may incorrectly attribute them to the patient's premorbid personality style and coping failure.

Papers and studies on the relationship between preinjury personality and coping ability after injury have produced sometimes opposing results. Generally, the somewhat passive personality is able to cope better with paralysis than the ambitious and highly motivated type (Siller, 1969; Thorn and colleagues, 1946; Wittkower and colleagues, 1954). In addition, the person with a premorbid history of stable personality and social functioning has less risk of maladaptation (Kerr and Thompson, 1972).

Another important factor in the adaptation process is the availability of a caring and close-knit social group. During the long months and years of invalidism that lie ahead, the support of the patient's family and friends can continue to provide him with a sense of belonging and worth.

Psychosocial Issues

For discussion purposes, the psychosocial issues of quadriplegics will be addressed below. You can deductively substitute the issues of the paraplegic when they seem to fit. In the section on intimacy, the sexual issues of both types of patients will be discussed.

Trust
The quadriplegic patient is totally dependent on caregivers. He is unable to perform any personal functions. His trust in the environment must be absolute. If the caregiving system is inattentive to his needs, or if he develops personality conflicts with caregivers, a high level of anxiety can result. This is true also if he is a person who has had previous difficulties in trusting others.

Self-esteem
The ability to maintain self-esteem comes from many sources: intrapsychic supplies acquired during the early developmental stages, gratifying interpersonal relationships, and various types of role functioning. If the patient had low self-esteem before his accident because of inadequate sources of feedback in the three areas described above, his risk of maladaptation from poor self-esteem is great. The ability of the patient's ego to maintain self-esteem will be weakened because he will be unable to continue preaccident interpersonal relationships and roles. They will be subject to radical changes.

Control

The patient's capacity to control his own life is completely relinquished to others if he is to survive. Such a realization, especially for an independent person, can be overwhelming. The response to such an intellectual awareness can be a number of emotions that can threaten to overpower the ego. The quadriplegic may feel that he will not be able to control his feelings of rage, sadness, loss, hopelessness, and so on. The ego, if able to adapt, will use defense mechanisms to repress these strong feelings or at least reduce them to a level that allows the patient to believe he will not be overcome completely by his reactions.

Loss

The losses that are experienced by this patient, as mentioned above, are profound. They cover every aspect of his life. It is possible that in order to survive such losses and cope with them, the ego must use denial and other basic defenses (see Chapter 4: The Use of Defense Mechanisms in Physical Illness) to a higher degree than that of the average psychologically healthy adult who has no physical impairments.

Guilt

The patient may feel guilt as he observes the effect of his illness on his family. The emotional pain and financial expense that they incur are high. He may also feel self-reproach because of having contributed to his own condition; many SCI persons are young men or women who were injured in automobile or motorcycle accidents, diving accidents, and so on that may have occurred as a result of carelessness. The patient may have been driving a vehicle in which someone else was killed. Survivor guilt can add seriously to the patient's burden.

Intimacy

Close relationships with others are seriously impaired as the result of this injury. The quadriplegic patient is primarily in a taking or receiving type of relationship with others, especially in the acute and recuperative stages of recovery from the accident. He may consciously or unconsciously withdraw from relationships or be unable to maintain his commitment to them emotionally and intellectually. The paraplegic patient who is rehabilitated after his injury will experience change in his mobility and bladder and bowel functioning but will be able to participate more fully in relationships and function in his former roles than the quadri-plegic patient. The capacity for sexual functioning is an important yet frequently ignored part of the rehabilitation of the quadriplegic or paraplegic patient.

Robert Baxter is a quadriplegic; his injury occurred in 1970. During the past several years he has taught courses and seminars and consulted and written about the psychological rehabilitation of the SCI patient. He has counseled hundreds of paraplegics and quadriplegics. Baxter (1978, p. 46) believes that "everyone's main reason for living is to love and be loved." He discusses the hopelessness that is manifested in most caregivers of SCI patients. It is an attitude that contributes to the widespread suicidal despair of many of these patients. He emphasizes the importance of the nurse as a carrier of hope to such patients. In every case where a despairing patient has "been turned around," the result was attributed to a nurse. He describes the nurse as the "vital link" between the patient and the information he needs. The rapport between the nurse and the patient is special, because, as he points out, "you spend more time with him than any other staff member" (p. 48).

For many patients, when their sexual functioning is ignored in the rehabilitation process, the exclusion further contributes to their despair. Depending on the effects of injury, some ability for the male to maintain erection may be retained. The full effects of the injury on sexual functioning may not be determined for many months, until the temporary effects of trauma to the spinal cord have subsided. The final outcome is that many men no longer have erections. Of those who do, many do not ejaculate; accordingly, they are unable to have children (Griffith, 1975).

Most female patients have a return of their menses within 6 months of injury. Regarding pregnancy, 9 paraplegic female patients were studied through 11 pregnancies that produced healthy infants. Most of them were able to deliver vaginally; the remainder required cesarean section. All the women successfully breast-fed their babies. The final conclusion of the authors was that maternal roles for the paraplegic female seem to be unlimited (Robertson and Guttman, 1963).

Woods (1979) describes the major difference in sexual functioning between normal persons and persons with complete transections of the spinal cord. The SCI person no longer experiences sexual pleasure genitally. Instead, sexual pleasure is experienced emotionally and cognitively. Woods's book contains a section on the sexual adaptation of the paraplegic patient that includes an extensive review of the literature. There are other excellent books usually available in hospital libraries that can be used as references by nurses who need more information for their patients. These books can also provide many answers to bright, highly motivated patients who are seeking more information about their conditions.

Nursing Approaches

The importance of the nurse to the SCI patient was described above by Baxter. Before caregivers can commit themselves to therapeutic long-term relationships with patients, they must examine their own feelings about helplessness and other issues that constantly confront the paralyzed patient. This introspective examination is important in developing an open, empathetic relationship. The patient's ability to trust his caregivers and to perceive their caring can support his self-esteem during many critical periods.

Helping the patient to retain a sense of control about choices in care, especially during the lengthy process of rehabilitation, is an important support to him. If depression or anxiety are noted, prompt intervention using the recommendations in the prevous chapter can help to avert a crisis.

If his emotional discomfort continues despite your efforts, recommend a psychiatric liaison or social work referral early in the crisis. Strong support of the patient at the beginning of this type of frightening episode can restore equilibrium. It helps the patient to know that his caregivers are responsive to his needs and will provide extra help when he needs it to maintain his own control.

The families of SCI patients, especially quadriplegics, are at risk for coping failure. Too often, these families abandon the patient (Baxter, 1978). The need for family members to withdraw can perhaps be understood when you think about the emotional response they experience with each visit: the dashed hopes, strained communications, and perhaps a growing resentment about the emotional and financial drain because of the irreparable injury of their family member.

Can you imagine the emotional response in the patients when their spouses or family members gradually stop coming to see them or caring about them? Extra emotional support given to families at the very beginning of the patient's hospitalization may enable them to remain more committed to their loved ones. A variety of support services can help the family. Is there a clinical nurse specialist in neurosurgical, rehabilitation, or psychiatric liaison

nursing in the hospital? Social service is important in assessing the family's emotional and financial resources for sustaining such an injury. The pastoral care department or the patient's own clergyman can provide added support. With the emotional strain on the family in this illness and the high risk of relationship failure, these services ideally can be called in as a preventive measure before crisis symptoms are observed.

Allowing family members to talk about their worries, angers, sadness, and other unpleasant emotions can help them to feel relief by expressing them and to accept them as normal under the circumstances. Referral to a family therapist is recommended when compromised or disabling family coping is evident.

Baxter gives the following recommendations as guides to nurses who are working with quadriplegics or paraplegics and have the opportunity for counseling and teaching about sexual function. First, wait until the patient is ready for such discussion. There will be clues in his conversation, behavior, or mood that can alert you that he is having concerns about his sexuality or sense of worth in relation to others.

In describing the most helpful approach to use with patients, Baxter says:

> To us, partly because of the limits placed on us by our disability, the psychological aspects are more important than the physical. Companionship, touching, shared interests, and understanding the hopes and cares of our partners are the most important things to us. If counselors spent as much time and energy on this as they do on the mechanics of sex, SCI patients would be better off. [Baxter, 1978, p. 49].

He recommends telling patients that there are no right or wrong rules about having sex. Generally, audiovisual or graphic teaching aids are not well received by SCI patients.

Conclusion

Chronic illness presents untold and unpredictable numbers of challenges to patients and their families. Nurses often identify with patients who have cancer, chronic obstructive pulmonary disease, or other chronic conditions. They ask themselves, "How can they do it? I don't think I could cope with such an illness." The human mind and spirit have remarkable resiliency when a major challenge presents itself. There is no question, however, that nursing intervention in the psychosocial adaptation process can make a difference in the final outcome. Nurses spend more time with chronically ill patients than do any other caregivers. During the long hours of care, patients' perceptions of their illnesses, themselves, and the responses of others to their illnesses and themselves can be adaptively formed or revised with the assistance of an astute and caring nurse.

19

The Dying Patient and the Family

The process of dying is indeed a *process*. It usually happens over time and involves the dying person, his family, friends, co-workers, and the caregiving team of physicians, nurses, social workers, and all others who come in contact with him. There are many subsystems involved in the process. Each person is a complex being with his own intra-psychic responses to dying; these involve his beliefs about his own death or the death of another person. Another subsystem is his own body, which is changing both internally and externally. The awareness of these changes feeds back into his psyche. They are constantly adding stress to his ability to maintain his self-esteem and body image.

Another subsystem is the family unit. It is made up of two or more people, all of whom are accustomed to filling certain roles and relating with other members in specific ways; these constitute the normal dynamics of the family. The threat of death to one of the family members can cause major shifts in family functioning. It is one of the most critical events that can happen to a family (Bowen, 1976).

The fourth major subsystem is the caregiving subsystem, which is made up of many parts: the people who constitute it, the technical capacity of the institution to give quality care, and the philosophy of the institution. Although the last category may seem nebulous and inconsequential, the philosophy of an institution about the dying process can be one of the most important factors in the quality of a patient's death. "Philosophy" is an abstraction, but it is made up of the beliefs of the administrative personnel in management, medicine, and nursing, which can promote or avoid a policy of support to the dying person and his family.

Because of the multiple factors affecting the dying person, we can call the dying process dynamic. Elisabeth Kübler-Ross (1975, p. 1) has said that "the key to the question of death unlocks the door of life. . . . For those who seek to understand it, death is a highly creative force."

This chapter deals primarily with theory about the effects of dying on the patient and his family. The next chapter presents intervention recommendations for the nurse to use in caring for dying patients and discusses the effects caring for dying patients has on the nurse. The nurse's needs during this time must be recognized as well.

Death has been described by Imara as follows:

> The one journey, the one labor few of us look forward to. Fear of that final separation, death, is natural. The thought of sleep without

dreams, timelessness without concern and conversation with others is the most difficult thing we humans face [Kübler-Ross, 1975, p. 149].

Many authors have identified the nurse as the person in the hospital environment who is best able to give emotional support to the dying patient (Eisendrath and Dunkel, 1979; Houpt, 1979; Schwab, 1969; Shusterman and associates, 1973). Indeed, the nurse may be the only person in the dying patient's environment who does not abandon him emotionally.

What Does Death Mean to a Dying Person?

In order to understand how a dying person feels about dying, it is important to be aware that death has different meanings depending on the person's age. This difference in the way that death is conceptualized extends also to family members.

Nagy (1959) theorizes that there are three different stages in the way that children perceive death. These stages are the same whether the child is dying or is losing a loved one.

Under 5 Years

The child believes that death is reversible. It is as if the dying person were asleep. He will not be able to communicate, but in many respects he will still be alive. The child believes that the dead are still able to eat, sleep, feel, and so on but are no longer able to be present in relationships. He has active fantasies regarding the dying or dead person. These fantasies often result in increased feelings of guilt and fear (Nagy, 1959; Castles and Murray, 1979).

Five to 9 Years

Because of changes in cognitive development, the child in this age range views death concretely and realistically. This stage demonstrates the overlap of the stage of concrete operations identified by Piaget (Piaget and Inhelder, 1969). He is aware of the permanent nature of death. It is frightening to him, particularly if he has been raised in an environment that included threats of punishment or one in which he has experienced traumatic events (Piaget and Inhelder, 1969). Because of his developing body image, the child conceptualizes his own death (if he is the dying person) as an external assault to his body (Nagy, 1959; Castles and Murray, 1979; Spinetta, 1973; Waechter, 1971).

Over 10 Years

At this age the child is able to think in a more formal and abstract manner (Piaget and Inhelder, 1969). He reasons with conceptual thinking and begins to be aware that death is inevitable for all human beings because of internal causes (Nagy, 1959; Castles and Murray, 1979).

Adolescence

The adolescent is able to intellectualize his awareness of death but, because of his emotional immaturity, may isolate and repress his feelings about dying. Emotional awareness of the possibility of his own death is blocked because his ego is in most cases unable to acknowledge the finality of his own life. As is customary with the young, he experiences emotion intensely. During the grieving process he is likely to experience acute sadness, anger, hopelessness, and the other emotions associated with a major loss (Nagy, 1959; Castles and Murray, 1979; Evans, 1971; Kastenbaum, 1972).

Adulthood

The person in young and middle adulthood thinks of, and has concerns about, the dying process. The actual death is not as great a concern as *how* he dies. The fears associated with dying are related to pain, fear of loss of control, abandonment, and fear of the unknown. Adults are not as certain as they were in adolescence about whether there is life after death (Schneidman, 1971; Greenberg, 1965; Castles and Murray, 1979).

Old Age

Many elderly persons approach their inevitable deaths with a tranquility that is unusual in younger persons. This can be due to their desire to avoid a long, painful, and gradually helpless physical condition. They may welcome death rather then being useless and unwanted members of society (Jeffers and Verwoerdt, 1969; Castles and Murray, 1979).

Fears of the Dying

Pattison (1978) has described the period between the patient's awareness that death is inevitable and his actual death as the living-dying interval. During this time, the patient may experience many or all of the Kübler-Ross stages and may experience the following specific fears:

Fears of the Dying

1. Fear of the unknown
2. Fear of loneliness
3. Fear of sorrow
4. Fear of loss of body
5. Fear of loss of self-control
6. Fear of suffering and pain
7. Fear of loss of identity
8. Fear of regression

(Pattison E: The living-dying process. In Garfield C (ed): Psychosocial Care of the Dying Patient, p 146. New York, McGraw-Hill, 1978)

The Process of Resolution of Loss

Anticipatory Grief

A concept that has received minimal recognition, yet is very helpful in understanding the responses we see in terminally ill patients and families, is called *anticipatory grief*. It is the deep sadness experienced when a major loss is expected in the near future "as distinguished from the grief which occurs at or after the loss" (Aldrich, 1974, p. 4). Lindemann (1944, p. 147) described the stages of anticipatory grief as "depression; a heightened preoccupation with the departed; a review of all the forms of death that might befall him; and anticipation of all the modes of readjustment which might be necessitated by it." Lindemann described anticipatory grief in relation to the experiences of family members whose loved one entered the armed services and went to a dangerous battle zone. The anticipatory grief that operates with terminally ill patients is a more concrete experience because death is certain. There is a period during which all involved persons have an opportunity to "work through" the eventual death. This helps to buffer the shock of the death when it occurs. It allows the person to prepare to cope with grief.

Conventional grief is differentiated from anticipatory grief by Aldrich (1974, p. 4), who states that "anticipatory grief is usually experienced (or denied) simultaneously by both the patient and his

family, while conventional grief is experienced only by the family." *Conventional grief* is the grief occurring after a major loss. Switzer (1970) defined this type of grief as the emotional and physiological pain that is experienced as a response to a major loss. The following case example illustrates the importance of anticipatory grieving:

Case Example

Ann and Henry are in their early 70s. Henry's health has been poor. Their only son and daughter-in-law live several hundred miles away. In order to be available to help his parents, the son moved his parents to a small apartment near his home. The parents missed their old friends and became increasingly dependent on one another. Henry experienced a severe myocardial infarct (MI) and was not expected to live 24 hours. His wife's anxiety level was intense. Her ability to cope was failing. She depended on him and cared about him too much to be able to lose him.

Henry surprised his caregivers by living almost 2 more weeks. During that time, Ann and Henry sat for hours, holding hands. They talked of their years together. They laughed and cried together. Ann was strongly loved and supported by her son and his family during this time. The nursing staff talked with her as her husband slept. By the time Henry died, Ann had already begun the bereavement process. She was coping adaptively. The 2-week period had allowed her a long enough interval to integrate her anticipated loss. She and her husband had also had a special time to review their life together.

The Reaction of the Family to Anticipated Loss of a Loved One

Family members experience the same stages of grief as those outlined by Kübler-Ross and Bowlby. The patient and his family may not experience these stages simultaneously, however. For example, a spouse or family member may be at the anger stage and be very hostile while the patient is in the bargaining or depressed stage. Similarly, the patient may have slowly and painfully traversed the preliminary stages of coping and have reached the final acceptance stage after long months of introspection. His spouse may still be fixated at the stage of denial. Because of her rigid denial, there may be no communication between them about his impending death. This is frequently so when the subject of death raises the anxiety level of the patient or family or both to a point where totally avoiding discussion of death is the only way to relieve anxiety. It also occurs when each spouse tries to protect the other and avoids bringing up the subject.

Aldrich (1974) suggests that one of the reasons why denial may be more prolonged in family members than in patients is because of the family's feelings of ambivalence toward their family member. *Ambivalence* is the presence of conflicting feelings about the same object. This is caused in part by the element of hope that is present in anticipatory grief. In conventional grief, the family member has already died; there is no hope for him. The ambivalence in anticipatory grief is there because the patient is still alive. Because he is alive, the family member believes that he must take action to help him: spend more time with him, change physicians, seek a miracle cure, protect him, and so on. If these tasks are not carried out, guilt may result.

The dynamics of guilt as the cause of ambivalence can be present in both anticipatory and conventional grief: it seems wrong to accept the death of someone dear; there also may be feelings of anger toward the dying person. These feelings are intolerable. There is also guilt about being a survivor. The survivor asks himself, "Why is he dying and not me?" Ambivalence, then, may be one of the most important reasons why family members become fixated at the denial stage. The result is a failure to work through and accept the coming death of their loved one. The tragedy is especially poignant if the patient has been able to accept his own death, *but there is no one in his final social system, neither family member nor health professional, with whom he can share it.*

The ideal situation is for the patient and his spouse or family member to arrive at the stage of acceptance at the same time. When this occurs, Parkes (1972, p. 131) has found the following in his work with terminal patients:

It is sometimes possible for a husband and wife to work together towards an acceptance of the approaching death of one of them. If the circumstances are right they can share some of the anticipatory grief which each needs to feel. The striking thing about such cases is that, despite the sadness which is an inevitable component of anticipatory grieving, couples who choose to face the future in this way often seem to win through to a period of calm and contentment which persists to the end. After bereavement has occurred, the surviving spouse is likely to look back on this period with a satisfaction that contrasts with the dissatisfaction expressed by many who have chosen to hide the truth.

Families and their dying members do not always choose to hide the truth, but the conscious or unconscious denial of the intolerable truth engendered by the anxiety of the patient, his family, and professional caretakers may prevent this sharing of the process of final acceptance. The medical and nursing staffs can unintentionally join with the patient and his family in the denial process and compound it.

Stages of Bereavement

Bereavement is the actual state of experiencing a major loss, as contrasted with grief, which is the emotion experienced during the bereavement process. An important theory about the way that people react to loss has been proposed by John Bowlby (1961). He describes three stages of bereavement:

1. Beginning stage of protest: characterized by denial, weeping, clinging to the lost object, and hostility
2. Middle stage of disorganization: characterized by despair, apathy, and aimlessness
3. Termination stage of reorganization: characterized by acceptance of the image of the lost object (the bereaved person "lets go" of the painful emotional attachment) and acceptance of new objects

Bowlby's theory contains the same elements as that of Kübler-Ross; it differs only by using more emotional-sounding words to describe the process through which a bereaved person must pass in order for peaceful acceptance and resolution of a major loss to occur.

First Stage of Bereavement: Beginning State of Protest

In Bowlby's first stage, the grieving person is not able to tolerate the loss of a valued object and still clings to the memory of it. His emotional energy is still invested in the person whom he either anticipates losing or has already lost. He has not let go of the lost person; he continues to long for the memory of him or her. In psychiatric terms, this memory is called an *internal representation*.

As described above, an important phenomenon that occurs during the first stage of the bereavement process is ambivalence about the lost object;

the bereaved will first feel love and yearning for the family member and then be shocked to feel anger toward him.

Bowlby believes that the anger that a person feels toward a dying or departed loved one is part of the normal response that a person experiences during separation. He says that most separations that a person experiences in life are temporary. For example, if a beloved pet "escapes" from its home, it usually is found. Similarly, when you misplace your car keys, you probably will find them soon. Think of your normal response to these two events. Do you say peacefully, "Oh, well, I must go look for my dog now?" Or is there usually an anxious response followed by anger toward him for getting away? In fact, the anger usually results in increased energy and is the motivator behind the increased physical activity involved in retrieving the lost object.

Think also of a parent in a large department store looking for a missing 4-year-old child. Do most parents in such a situation feel anger toward the child mixed with their fear? Anger in each of these situations is a *normal* response, according to Bowlby. Anger serves the following functions: "first, it may assist in overcoming such obstacles as there may be to reunion; second, it may discourage the loved one from going away again" (1973, p. 247).

God may be another cause of anger for dying persons and their family members and friends. The bereaved may think, "*Why* did He do this?" In fact, he may feel deep rage toward God. This type of anger is frightening to most people who have a normally strong religious faith; they experience a high level of guilt about it. One of their underlying fears is that because of their anger toward Him, God may "strike" them again. The reaction of anger toward God happens to many patients and their families. Because it seems abnormal, people keep these feelings to themselves and suffer silently. In working with bereaved or dying persons, you can mention that these feelings are common in many people. If the person seems particularly troubled by them, he should be referred to an understanding hospital chaplain who may be able to relieve some of the guilt he is experiencing.

Another phenomenon of ambivalence occurs in anticipatory grief. Before the ill person dies, the family member may find himself alternately wishing for the death of the person as well as for the survival. These feelings cause high levels of guilt and are rarely shared with others because they are so disturbing. When the course of a terminal illness is examined for its effect on remaining family members, we discover many factors that contribute toward these mixed feelings. A terminal illness creates heavy emotional demands on the family system. The ill person may be hospitalized frequently for long periods. The cost of these hospitalizations, even with insurance, can seriously undermine the family's financial stability.

Visits to the hospital by family members are time consuming, and the amount of time invested in the sick person may then create extra burdens on others. For example, a middle-aged woman who visits her dying husband daily for several hours may be unavailable to her adolescent children who continue to need her support. She may not be able to keep up her normal household responsibilities. Ideally, caregivers can say that her children should take over these responsibilities out of their concern and love for her and their father. This may not be the case, however. They may be experiencing anger about the impending loss of their father and may displace some of this anger onto their mother. She, in turn, may be repressing her anger toward her husband for leaving her and may displace it onto her children because of their lack of support.

These extra pressures have an effect on all the spheres of a person's functioning: his relationships with others outside of the family system; his normal functioning at work, home, or school; his normal intrapsychic functioning, and so on. Accordingly, it is not uncommon, especially during times of fatigue, to wish that the difficult period caused by the terminal illness of the loved one could finally be over. In addition, the hope that the terminally ill person will die soon may be motivated by a genuine wish to end the loved one's suffering and pain.

Middle Stage of Bereavement: Stage of Disorganization

The middle stage is marked by disorganization. During this phase the emotional energy attached to the lost object is released; however, it has not been reinvested in another object. As a result, the emotion at times seems all encompassing and overwhelming. The emotion that is being withdrawn from the lost object is not focused because the person's grief is not resolved enough for him to reinvest it in another object. This is a time of disequilibrium intrapsychically and within the family system. Everything may seem out of control. It is not unusual for persons in this stage of bereavement to feel as though they may be losing their sanity. Indeed, rather than experiencing the unpleasant emotional and cognitive reactions of this stage, many persons remain "stuck" in the first stage of bereavement. The loss is never resolved.

Final Stage of Bereavement: Termination Stage of Reorganization

In the last stage, the grieving person's ego allows his feelings to be attached once again to a new object. The new object never replaces the old; instead, the emotional energy that was invested in the original object is refocused and invested in a new object. In many instances, the acceptance of a new object begins before the letting go of the lost object is complete. In fact, it may facilitate the final acceptance of the loss. If a person is widowed, for example, there is a longing for the spouse. Ideally, a person should eventually begin to be with other people, both men and women friends. Sometimes this occurs before the person has totally resolved the loss. By meeting and enjoying new people and eventually focusing on one of them, or by engaging in work or recreational pursuits which bring pleasure, the final acceptance of the loss of the original partner may be resolved. The most important aspect of this last stage of bereavement and the one that indicates that the grief process is complete is that the bereaved is able to invest his feelings in a replacement object. He is able to feel emotional gratification from his new situation.

Keep in mind the various types of grief reactions that can be present in a general hospital when dying patients are involved. The patient himself experiences grief in accepting the loss of himself through death. His is an anticipatory grief. The final stage of acceptance for him occurs when he lets go of the emotional energy invested in his own life and accepts that he will no longer live. Many times, belief in some type of afterlife, or perhaps reunion with previously departed family members or God, becomes the new focus.

Family members may have many months to prepare for the death. Accordingly, they may be able to work through some of the initial stages. Because of this process, by the time death occurs, some of the grief work may already have been completed. On the other hand, the loss of a family member through accidental death has a greater potential for coping failure because of its suddenness. Being able to prepare for the death of a loved one, if only for a few days, allows more coping mechanisms to develop in the family. For example, if an accident or coronary victim lives even a few days in an intensive care unit, it prevents the members of the family from having to cope suddenly with the shock of death with no warning.

The Effect of the Social Environment on the Grieving Person

Western culture rarely tolerates a grieving person's expressions of feelings for more than a few weeks after the death of a loved one. He or she is expected to adjust and cease talking about the feelings about the loss very soon. Friends and family members usually do not object to a bereaved person's mentioning his or her loss, but repeated descriptions of sadness, hopelessness, inability to sleep, and so on eventually meet with cues from the listener that he does not want to hear any more. In fact, U.S. society usually commends the bereaved person who "holds up well" and shows little or no emotion or distress during the dying process, funeral, and the weeks after the loss. Actually, this person may experience much more painful distress later due to a maladaptive grief response.

In order to eliminate some of the problems in the hospital care system, it may help for caregivers to understand the normal reactions experienced during the various stages of bereavement. It is frequently the caregiver's discomfort in listening to patients' and family members' anticipatory grief that causes distancing and avoidance to occur. By understanding the *normal* feelings of a grieving person, nurses may be able to encourage and validate these emotions.

The Normal Emotional Response to Loss

The responses to loss will vary with each person. The following descriptions of the feelings associated with a major loss are the same for a patient anticipating his own death and for family members who may be preparing for the loss of their loved one or who have already experienced the loss. The usual response to a major loss is disbelief. The ego will not accept this sudden terrible information. In an emergency room, for example, if parents are told that their child did not survive a school bus accident, they will react with cries of, "No, no, no," "I can't believe it," or "Are you sure?" The other reaction may be one of shock; the news does not seem to penetrate.

When a patient or bereaved person "holds up well," it may be because he is in denial or has repressed the news. Family members and friends usually are relieved. They compliment him on his stoicism, courage, and so on. This behavior of the patient or bereaved is positively reinforced. In a few weeks, when the repression disappears and he has full awareness, his true feelings may emerge. He may be afraid to express them, despite the fact that he may feel that he is bursting with grief. The social system of the patient or bereaved person, in effect, tells him: we cannot tolerate these feelings in you. After all, he has been complimented for being so courageous.

A normal feeling that emerges after a loss is an overwhelming sadness accompanied by crying and sobbing. The grieving person feels unable to control when the waves of sadness will occur. Seeing an item that belonged to the loved person, or thinking of him, will bring on greater depths of sadness (Loss and Grief, 1977). The effects of the social reinforcement of being stoic cause most people to fear losing control entirely. The feelings are frightening because of their intensity.

For family members in anticipatory or conventional grief, the period of awareness, when the full realization of the loss occurs, is just the beginning of grief work. This marks the beginning of the middle stage of bereavement. During this phase, the lost person is idealized. The bereaved has a great need to talk about him. He is preoccupied with thoughts of this person. Illusory phenomena are very common. For example, the bereaved may think he sees the lost person driving a car, in a crowd, or at any specific place where the two of them interacted often. These illusory phenomena, accompanied by frequent nightmares, cause the bereaved to think he is losing his sanity (Bowlby, 1980). The feeling of losing one's sanity is not unusual. This fear is so frightening that it is rarely shared with others. A very similar process can occur for the dying person, except that he experiences these thoughts and feelings about himself. He usually reviews his life, his relationships, his work, and so on. He may experience episodes of derealization. These are periods when he feels detached from the world around him.

During this time, neurovegetative signs of reactive depression may occur, including insomnia, loss of appetite, and loss of energy. The grieving person sighs frequently (Bowlby, 1980). He may feel overwhelming anxiety, which further adds to his feeling of loss of control and feelings that he is "going crazy." Another very normal emotional response in family members is one of anger toward the lost person. The anger is caused by the feeling that the dead person has abandoned them. These feelings of anger are abhorrent to

grieving persons and strong guilt is the result. Dying persons experience anger about their illness. The accompanying feelings of helplessness and hopelessness may be projected onto family and caregivers.

It is not unusual for the normal grieving process to take up to 1 year to complete (Parkes, 1972). The feelings described above may be quite intense for many months, accompanied by marked mood swings and ambivalence. The pain and the yearning for the lost person gradually diminish after that time. The bereaved begins to feel in control once again. The psyche of the dying person or the family member begins to feel more at peace as the intrapsychic conflicts created by the grief process begin to diminish.

Family System Response to a Dying Member

When a family learns that one of its members is dying, it is immediately subject to a variety of new stresses. These stresses affect all the dynamics in the family system. Whether a family is "healthy" or has many pathological coping patterns, the stress can be severe. One factor that immediately determines the severity of this stressor is the role the dying member fills in the family.

There are obvious roles that are highly valued in a family: the role of mother or father in an active family, a child of any age, a loved grandparent. Another role less recognized by many caregivers is the person who maintains equilibrium in the family. For example, this could be a single uncle who has been very involved in a family that is fatherless or in a family in which the father was weak and nonsupportive. Another example could be a very elderly woman who always encouraged her children's dependency. Accordingly, even though her children may be in their 50s or 60s, her loss may be highly threatening to one or more of them.

Family as Support System

The most important factor in a person's ability to tolerate stress is the effectiveness of his defense mechanisms. These defense mechanisms will determine if his coping is adaptive or maladaptive. The next most important factor is the way that the family system is able to manage stress. Loss of a family member is one of the most stressful events a family experiences. Accordingly, if the family's coping ability fails, it will have a definite impact on the patient's coping strength.

One of the most important factors in the way that a family responds to stress is the coping pattern of each of its members. If the members are accustomed to dealing with threatening events by using immature defenses, then the family is at greater risk for maladaptation. If a limited number of the members respond maladaptively, the more mature coping responses of the other members can help to promote the adaptation of the entire family. (More likely, however, family members respond similarly; remember, they were socialized similarly.)

Research on families in crisis has indicated that the family coping response to a very threatening event becomes formed by 1 to 4 weeks after the initial threat occurs (Parad and Caplan, 1965). During this time, it is possible to see both adaptive and maladaptive defenses working. As a reminder, the list of defense mechanisms (in order of level of maturity) that appeared in Chapter 4 is repeated below (Freedman and colleagues, 1976; Usdin and Lewis, 1979; Vaillant, 1977):

Hierarchy of Human Defenses

Narcissistic defenses
Denial
Delusional projection
Distortion

Immature defenses
Acting-out behavior
Avoidance
Hypochondriasis
Passive-aggressive behavior
Projection
Regression

Neurotic defenses
Displacement
Identification
Isolation
Reaction formation
Repression

Mature defenses
Anticipation
Sublimation
Humor
Altruism
Suppression

Many families go into crisis when they learn that a member of their family has a grave illness. The incidence is much higher than many nonpsychiatric caregivers would expect. In one study:

Eighty-seven percent of the families in the sample failed to cope adequately with the consequences of childhood leukemia and this failure created a variety of individual and interpersonal problems that were superimposed on stresses posed by the illness itself [Kaplan and colleagues, 1978, pp. 246, 247].

Another study revealed that one or more family members required psychiatric treatment at some time following the diagnosis of childhood leukemia (Binger and coauthors, 1969).

Another source of crisis in families of dying children occurs when one parent adapts and copes relatively well but the spouse does not. If the maladaptive spouse continues this pattern beyond the initial weeks, serious marital conflict can occur. Lines of communication become permanently shut down. Conflicts in discussion of the illness and grieving extend to the other children. The major cause of divorce in such families is due to the disparity in the two parents' coping levels (Binger and colleagues, 1969).

Anniversary Reaction

An *anniversary reaction* to the date of death or the date when the illness was originally diagnosed is an important phenomenon that occurs in most people. It occurs whether the grief resolution was normal or pathological. In an anniversary reaction, someone who has lost a significant person will experience an emotional or physical reaction around the time of the anniversary of the loss. He usually is at a loss to explain what is going on (Schwab, 1979). The following case example will help to clarify this concept:

Case Example

A general hospital patient was admitted for a respiratory ailment in the month of March. Her medical history revealed that she had been admitted to the hospital during February or March each year for each of the previous 6 years because of various ailments: hernia repair, cholecystectomy, abdominal pain, and so on. Questioning by the nurse revealed that one of her children had died in March 20 years earlier. Her husband's birthday was in March. She had been divorced from him in March, and he later died in March.

The month of March was highly significant to this woman. She had been unaware of the relationship between the month of March and the repressed painful memories it recalled at an unconscious level and her numerous health problems.

George Engel, one of the leading liaison psychiatrists in the United States, wrote a sensitive article about his own anniversary reactions to the deaths of his twin brother and father, with whom he had very close relationships. Engel's brother died of a heart attack in the summer of 1963. Following the death, Engel experienced most of the disquieting symptoms of grief reaction described above. He also became obsessed with the idea that he, too, would experience a heart attack. Three weeks short of the first anniversary of his brother's death his prediction was fulfilled.

Immediately after the death of his brother and on significant anniversaries, he had dreams that gave him remarkable insights about his relationship with his brother and his reaction to the deaths of his brother and father. His father died at age 58. In his own 58th year he had unusual psychological and physical experiences that were strongly associated with his brother and father (Engel, 1975).

It is easy to understand that people can be aware of upcoming anniversaries of losses of significant persons. It is more difficult to understand that the anniversary reactions described in the examples above were unconscious. People repress their awareness of these anniversaries, yet the unconscious mourning process is an active one. To the unaware person, the outward manifestations may take many forms that are never connected to the original loss.

Maladaptive Grieving Process

If a person does not proceed through the stages of grief outlined above, it is possible for a *maladaptive grieving process* to occur. A maladaptive grieving process, also known as pathological bereavement, is characterized by maladaptive coping in response to a significant loss. There is either excessive repression of grief or an excessive and prolonged emotional response that extends beyond 1 year. This can be manifested in many ways. Some persons become fixated in denial. Although there is intellectual awareness of the death of the person, there is little or no affective or feeling response. This is caused by the defense mechanism called isolation (see Chap. 4). The feelings of grief are

repressed or are delayed indefinitely. Sometimes, years later, another loss will trigger the emotional response that was denied during the first loss (Parkes, 1972). Or, the feelings of grief may never occur but the person may become socially guarded and isolated.

Such persons may never feel sadness or display the range of emotions usually associated with a major loss. Their feelings are deeply repressed. Some of the ways maladaptive grief may be demonstrated are by prolonged immobility and withdrawn states; hyperactivity, a flurry of activity that helps the bereaved to avoid the pain; excessive spending of money and pleasure seeking; and alcohol or tranquilizer abuse. Depression may also occur many months or years after the original loss. When it occurs years later, it may even be misdiagnosed as endogenous depression. Another outcome of maladaptive grieving is that the bereaved may display excessive and inappropriate anger toward some person in his social system. This person becomes the focus of his rage. This anger can also be turned inward and be expressed by a physical symptom (Schwab, 1979).

The Consequences of Unresolved Grief for Family Members

Most families have periods of several weeks to several years to begin to accept the impending loss of a family member. If the opportunity to work through the death of a person is not developed before the loss occurs, it is possible that the coping strategies developed by family members during the conventional grief stage may become more maladaptive and prolong the bereavement process (Aldrich, 1974).

The unresolved grief may lead to abnormal psychopathology. Studies have found that unresolved grief led to a larger incidence of physical and mental illness in bereaved family members (Maddison and colleagues, 1969; Maddison, 1968; Rees and Lutkins, 1967).

Engel (1961) theorized that the experience of grief imposes psychological stress that disturbs the total adjustment of the person left behind—the biochemical, physiological, and psychological spheres all can be involved in the normal as well as the abnormal bereavement response. Engel's theories are compatible with Selye's stress theory, presented in Chapter 9.

In a major study of widowed persons, Rees and Lutkins (1967) found that their mortality was 15 times higher during the 2-year period following the loss of their spouses. It has also been suggested that unresolved loss is a significant finding in a majority of cancer patients (Horne and Picard, 1979; Bahnson, 1981).

Another type of unresolved grief reaction is one in which the lost person preoccupies the grieving person's mind more than a year later. Some of the causes of a delayed grief resolution are an inability to express rage or cry about the loss, lack of supportive persons, overidentification with the dead person, anger and ambivalence toward him, an earlier unresolved grief reaction, and prolonged encouragement by a social system of the bereaved's grief reaction (secondary gain) (Parkes, 1972). It is not unusual for a delayed grief reaction to occur at or near the time of the first or a subsequent anniversary of the death.

In order to emphasize the effects of unresolved grief, the following research findings are of interest. Rosenbaum (1981), in a study of medication use of widows and widowers, discovered many significant facts about the ways in which they maladaptively coped with their spouses' deaths. A partial list of findings is as follows:

1. There is an increase in the use of psychotropic medication (tranquilizers, antidepressants, hypnotics) following the loss of their spouse. Although a slight leveling off occurred, the amount of medication used remained higher than it was before the loss.
2. The most common reasons given for taking the medication(s) was "to help relax" and "to help with sleep."
3. These people continued using psychotropic drugs, some of them for many years.
4. Most subjects reported that refills for these medications were obtained by calling the physician's office and talking to the nurse or receptionist. They were given either "no instructions" or "unsatisfactory instructions" regarding their use.
5. Of those subjects who knew their spouse was dying, only 4 of 26 had free and open discussion about death. Of those who had free discussions, none of the spouses was taking medication after the death.*

*No. 5 above is a very significant finding, which helps us to understand the dynamics of unresolved and maladaptive grief. It points out how essential it is for the nurse or *some* caregiver to promote an open environment where spouses can be honest with one another.

These and other studies reported in this chapter poignantly illustrate the great need for caregivers to be able to identify the maladaptive coping responses of dying persons and their families. Too often, caregivers assume that these responses are temporary and that after discharge these problems will decrease. *This is not usually so.* The long-term consequences of unresolved grief are of major significance.

Unless some perceptive person recognizes the problem, these people will experience a changed existence because of maladaptive coping. Their quality of life can be diminished for years, both during the terminal illness and after the death of their loved one. This maladaptation can persist through the rest of their lives.

Visiting nurses and nurses in primary and outpatient care settings are more likely to see persons with unresolved and maladaptive grief than nurses in inpatient settings; their clients should be referred for psychotherapy.

Nursing Diagnosis of Maladaptive Coping in Family Members

In general, hospital nurses usually are the first to notice the distress of families. The Fifth National Conference on Nursing Diagnosis, held in 1982, identified several categories of coping failure that are within the nurse's capability to diagnose and begin intervention. They are all applicable to the dying patient and his family members (Kim and Moritz, 1982):

> Coping, ineffective individual
>
> Family member's disabling coping response to the client's health challenge
>
> Family member's compromised coping response to the client's health challenge
>
> Family member's potential for expanded response to the client's health challenge
>
> Grieving: dysfunctional
>
> Grieving: potential dysfunctional

It is important for nurses to be able to recognize maladaptive coping patterns in families during the early part of the patient's admission. When it is obvious that the family is not coping effectively and that this ineffective coping continues to occur, then intervention should begin with the family. Intervention theory is outlined in Chapter 15: Crisis Intervention With the Maladapting Patient. Unless the problem is severe, intervention can be appropriately carried out by the nurse, using the chapters on counseling and crisis intervention as a guide. If nursing intervention does not result in evidence of adaptation, psychiatric consultation is recommended. There are a few important points to keep in mind when working with family members who are experiencing anticipatory grief or bereavement. One is that the most helpful approach for *some* persons is talking. Talking can allow the acceptance process to occur and unconscious blocks to be worked through. Chapter 12: Counseling Techniques for Nurses, can be helpful in knowing how to approach these family members. The subsection in the next chapter on what to say to a dying patient can also be applied to family members.

Another important point is that some persons do not want to talk. When your attempts to open the subject are resisted, the person is giving you the message that he is not ready or willing to talk. If you persist, you will only increase his anxiety. Do continue to test his resistance gently every day or so. Some of the reasons why people are unable to talk are denial, as described earlier in the chapter, and certain personality styles that cannot tolerate interpersonal intimacy. These personality styles are the aloof and uninvolved, suspicious, controlling, and superior (see Chap. 5: Personality Styles Seen in General Hospital Patients).

The nurse should also include the attending physician in her care plan for the family. When the nurse articulates the problems he or she has observed and outlines the intervention approach that will be used, the physician will be more aware of the maladaptive process and may be able to provide extra support to the family. House officers too are usually receptive to such discussion.

Conclusion

This chapter has presented information about the responses that can be observed when working with dying patients and their families. This theory can also be generalized and used when caring for any patient who is experiencing a major loss as the result of illness that will have an ongoing effect on his life. The patient may have undergone coronary artery bypass surgery or amputation of a limb or have been diagnosed with a chronic, degenerative, and ultimately terminal illness. Nonetheless, he and his family will respond with the same emotions and process as the dying patient and his family, but to a lesser degree in most cases. The interventions recommended in this chapter and the next one can be helpful with him and his loved ones.

Care of the dying patient and his family can be one of the greatest challenges in nursing. Sometimes it is difficult to know the "right" way to talk with these patients and their families. Many nurses worry that they will say or do something that will add even more distress. This chapter will present various concepts that I hope can be useful to you in your work. It is important to remember one thing: there is no "right" way to work with a dying person.

Because the personality of *every* human is unique, there are a vast variety of interpersonal responses that are right. What you would do with a dying person might be quite different than another nurse, yet both approaches can be equally therapeutic. In addition to the sections on specific aspects of care of the dying person, the latter part of this chapter examines the stress that nurses themselves experience in caring for the dying.

Specific Issues of Caring for Dying Patients

Should the Patient Be Told He Is Dying?

Although it may be difficult to acknowledge, the question about whether it is upsetting to a patient to talk about his own death may actually be a projection of the upset that *we* feel in talking to a dying patient about his death. A study by Kübler-Ross (1975) reported that only 2% of dying patients did not want to talk about their deaths. Murray Bowen (1976), in his work with physically ill patients who were dying as well as psychiatric patients who wanted to die, found that they were relieved to find someone they could talk with about dying; they felt better afterward.

The patient should be told he is dying in most cases. The patient's physician is responsible for telling the patient and the family. It is not uncommon for the patient to deny the original discussion with the physician in which he learns that he is dying. On occasion, nurses become angry with physicians who they believe are not being honest with dying patients. Before making such a judgment, it is important to talk with the physician about what he or she has told the patient. Remember that a person's ego is on constant guard to protect him from disturbing awarenesses. The dying patient's ego will maintain denial of unpleasant reality until its more mature defenses are able to cope with troubling thoughts and feelings.

20

The Nurse and the Dying Patient

It can be helpful for the nurse to be present when the physician is actually telling the patient his prognosis. Telling a patient that he has a terminal illness is difficult, and the physician may understandably choose to do this alone with the patient. If he or she is willing to have the nurse present, the following advantages to the patient can occur:

1. The nurse will be able to support the patient when he is being told the threatening prognosis.
2. The nurse will be able to reinforce the information given to the patient by the physician.
3. The nurse knows exactly what the patient was told and will be in a position to assess the patient's response and plan appropriate interventions to promote adaptation.

Intervention (Not Confrontation) With Denying Patients

If the patient's denial continues beyond a few days, it is important to begin to intervene gently to determine the strength of the denial. It is essential *never* to confront a denying patient directly with the reality that he is struggling to avoid. The persistence of strong denial of more than a day or two should indicate that the awareness of impending death is *terrifying*. The anxiety that the denial is masking could overwhelm the patient.

In order to understand how direct and forceful confrontation will cause further emotional difficulties, think of the following analogies. The denial of such a patient can be compared to an egg shell. It appears hard, *but it is brittle.* A direct blow will cause it to fracture and the contents to spill out with no control; direct confrontation could crack the patient's denial. His inability to keep out the unbearable awareness could cause his anxiety to overwhelm him.

Earlier in the book an analogy was used in which a patient who is in denial is compared to a person who is frightened and goes into a room to seek refuge. He shuts the door to keep out the environment he fears (comparable to a moderate level of denial). Can you understand how caregivers' or family members' direct confrontation of such a patient only results in a more disabling type of denial?

Because of the amount of time nurses spend with patients, they are in a better position than the physician, who makes a brief, daily visit, to test denial gradually and gently in order to know how strong it is. The answers that patients formulate to nurses' questions can help them to accept the reality of their illness gradually, *at their own pace.*

In thinking of the frightened person in the room mentioned above, you are allowing the patient to open the door rather than breaking it down yourself. Remember, too, that the patient's "door" is closed to you because of his level of anxiety. You can still talk to the patient through the "door" of his denial, however, by asking him how he is feeling, whether he is comfortable, how he thinks he is doing, and so on. The following list includes questions that can be used with dying patients who are denying their illnesses.

Questions to Test the Strength of Denial in Dying Patients

How are you feeling today?

How do you think you are doing?

How does your physician think you are doing?

How does your family feel about your being in the hospital?

What does your family think about your illness?

How much longer do you think you will be in the hospital?

These questions should never be asked in a series; rather, they should be interspersed in your normal conversation with the patient as you are caring for him. Similar questions can be asked each day so that you can compare his level of denial to previous days. If the answers you receive indicate that he is continuing to rigidly deny awareness of his terminal status beyond a few days, it is strongly recommended that you talk to the attending physician. Present specific examples of this strong denial. Ask the physician if he or she should talk to the patient again.

If there is a clinical specialist (oncology, pulmonary, gerontology, or some other specialty) working with the dying patient, make certain that he or she is aware of your concerns. Find out if the specialist has observed denial in the patient and whether he or she thinks it is at an adaptive or maladaptive level. Ask for specific recommendations of what you can do, or not do, to help the patient. If, despite the assistance of these caregivers, the patient's denial persists, psychiatric liaison consultation should be considered. This should be discussed with the clinical specialist, who may or may not believe that the patient's emotional complexity requires psychiatric intervention.

If it is decided that psychiatric intervention is necessary, approach the physician, using clinical examples and the charted documentation by you and the clinical specialist showing that the patient's level of denial is placing him at strong risk for maladaptation and potentially severe psychiatric problems.

One of the important reasons why a continuation of strong denial is maladaptive is that the psychic energy required to maintain the defense is both an emotional and physical drain. It causes the patient's openness as a person to be diminished. His guardedness has a serious effect on the quality of his relationships with others. His family, especially his spouse, may need to be able to talk to him, but he holds them away. Eventually, his unyielding denial can undermine the effectiveness of the family system in coping with his impending death. Another negative effect of this strong denial is due to general system effects. The level of stress that results from constant psychic strain eventually causes the sympathetic nervous system to respond. This triggers a stress response in all of the other body systems (cardiovascular, pulmonary, gastrointestinal, and so on).

Withholding Information From the Dying Patient

Often, caregivers and family members withhold information from the patient about his condition. They believe they are helping him. May (1974) argues that such withholding places the patient in a dependent position. He is treated like a child and has no control or choice in the care he receives. The patient is done a gross disservice. Actually, this "protectiveness" can provoke a level of anxiety and distrust in the patient that undermines his emotional well-being through the remainder of his illness.

If families and physicians do choose to keep patients' prognoses from them, patients frequently are able to deduce the actual situation. The tragedy in these cases is that the patient too must keep up the charade. He believes that he must shield his family and caregivers from the pain of his own death. He withholds his feelings of anger, grief, and so on in order to protect them. He also fears their rejection and abandonment if he is too honest with them and they are frightened away. No one is being honest with anyone. What potential for loneliness for all concerned! Pattison has listed the ways in which a patient picks up clues from those around him that he is dying:

1. Direct statements from the physician
2. Overheard comments of the physician to others

3. Direct comments from other personnel, including aides, nurses, technologists
4. Overheard comments by staff to each other
5. Direct statements from family, friends, clergy, lawyer
6. Changes in the behavior of others toward the patient
7. Changes in the medical care routines, procedures, medications
8. Changes in physical location
9. Self-diagnosis, including reading of medical books, records, and charts
10. Signals from the body and changes in physical status
11. Altered responses by others toward the future

(Pattison E: The living-dying process. In Garfield C [eds]: Psychosocial Care of the Dying Patient, p. 144. New York, McGraw-Hill, 1978)

Importance of Control in the Dying Process

Kastenbaum (1978) reminds us that the anxiety-provoking aspects of working with dying patients frequently cause caregivers to need to control many aspects of the dying process:

Their own feelings about the patient's death.

The patient's feelings about his own death. (If the patient becomes out of control, they possibly would feel inadequate in helping him.)

Caregivers, in their desire to give care, may indeed give good technical care but may become unaware of the way that they remove the patient's control of his own dying process. This poignant case example may give you a better understanding of how this happens:

Case Example

Amos is a 53-year-old man with an 8-year history of chronic obstructive pulmonary disease. His condition is terminal. He is not expected to live more than a few days. He has been a patient in the respiratory intensive care unit for 6 weeks. He is intubated by permanent tracheostomy. He is fully alert and very anxious. When his anxiety becomes acute, he has an order for a low dose of morphine. (Sedation of patients with advanced lung disease is usually avoided becuase it would compromise respiratory status.)

During his hospitalization, when he experienced respiratory distress despite the intubation, he asked for frequent "bagging." (Bagging is the extra breath of oxygen that can be given by attaching the oxygen to a semisolid plastic ball or bag, as it is called.) He asked for extra bagging three or four times an hour. He was very anxious before the bagging began and relaxed markedly when he received the extra oxygen. Eventually, he wanted to be bagged almost every 5 to 8 minutes. Recent x-ray studies, however, demonstrated that Amos's lung tissue was becoming dangerously dilated. There was danger that rupture of a segment of lung could occur with the extra pressure of bagging. Death would be the certain result.

His physicians abruptly ordered the cessation of all bagging. The patient was told of the decision. The nurses, who were at the patient's bedside almost constantly, cried because of their concern about the patient's emotional response to the loss of his only security in the unit. They also were crying because they had lost the only means *they* had to decrease his anxiety level and give him at least a small level of comfort.

What about the patient in this situation? Did *he* have any choice? Was he given any choice about the amount of medication that could have given him a more comfortable emotional state and helped him to die more peacefully? Was he given any choice in the bagging decision? What would you have wanted for yourself if you were the patient in this situation? If the patient were someone whom you loved?

The ultimate question of whether the care of this patient was the most supportive and allowed him any control of his own death is complicated by ethical questions. The ability to maintain life in sophisticated intensive care units often removes the chance to die naturally.

It is important to remember, however, that patients and families should be informed by physicians so that these decisions are not made by the physicians alone with no input from the patient or family. Most patients and families follow physicians' recommendations, but certain intelligent and thoughtful people may want to make the final decision after being informed of the alternatives. Certainly, a patient who has always been independent and in control of his life (see Chap. 5) will respond with high levels of anxiety and distrust if all control of his own dying process is removed by his caregivers or family members.

These are difficult questions. There continue to be many physicians who maintain complete control over the patient's dying process. They believe it is *their* responsibility to make these choices.

Neither a passive nor aggressive approach by a nurse will ever cause a change in such a physician's beliefs. Perhaps a gentle yet assertive approach by the nurse to such a physician on the behalf of the patient or family will be able to effect gradual change. The process can be slow, however, especially if the physician has been dealing with patients in this manner for many years. Intelligent study of these issues by hospital ethics committees made up of well-informed representatives of the various caregiving professions can potentially reduce the emotional distress caused by cases such as the one described above.

Maintaining the Patient's Choices

On some occasions, medical and nursing caregivers make choices for dying patients about treatment plans, use of analgesics, or decisions regarding resuscitation in case of death. It is important to remember that *this is the patient's life*. He or she, if mentally competent, can be presented the various choices of his or her options. For example, it may be a dying person's very important but unexpressed wish to be fully awake and alert as long as possible before death in order to interact with his family.

Well-meaning caregivers may decide that the patient's pain would be well controlled by a morphine drip that would maintain a constant analgesia and *decrease alertness*. They may have received approval from the family for this measure. Before caregivers assume that they know what is best for the patient, however, it is the alert patient's right to be a part of this decision-making process; the advantages and disadvantages of the possible alternatives can be described. Caregivers can strongly encourage particular approaches; usually the patient agrees. This patient, even when he agrees with his caregivers' recommendations, will develop a deeper trust in his caregivers for having been given the opportunity to make the final decision. The lack of this approach may cause some caregivers to carry burdens of responsibility that they have taken on themselves.

Where to Die?

The staffing patterns and wards of general hospitals generally are not designed to provide the supportive and comfort-promoting measures that can contribute to a peaceful death. The main goal of general hospitals and caregivers is to save or maintain lives; death is not easily accepted there. Caregivers frequently consider the death of a patient to be a reflection on themselves and their care (Eisendrath and Dunkel, 1979; Schwab, 1969).

Another alternative to care in the general hospital is a hospice. A *hospice* is a special institution for the dying that provides strong support to all persons involved in the dying process: the patient, his family, and his caregivers. The hospice concept was begun in England and is being introduced in other countries in hospice institutions as well as in hospice home care programs run by visiting nurse agencies. In a hospice, the following occurs:

> [Care is] given by nurses who are able to accept their own feelings about death in order that they are able to listen compassionately and constructively to the fears of others. They provide physical and psychological support that enables the patient to make the transition from life to death peacefully [Castles and Murray, 1979, p. 319].

A third alternative in providing care to a dying person is allowing him to remain at home. Before advocating one type of care over another, there are some important considerations. How is the patient coping with his impending death? How is the family coping with the patient's dying? The patient and a majority of his family members may cope by maintaining high levels of denial. There may be virtually no openness in family communication. If these factors are present, this patient would not do well at home until, and unless, the denial level is lowered in both. If a patient is discharged into a home where either he or his family is maintaining a high level of denial, there inevitably will be potential for high anxiety and maladaptation because of the strained communications in the family system.

Accordingly, the patient and family who are grieving about the upcoming loss and have a very low level of defense and are not coping well will be at further risk if they attempt to have the patient die at home. They will need the extra support available in an institution as well as the chance to be away from the patient for extended hours. Support is essential to the patient and family if the grieving is to proceed in an adaptive manner. A hospice environment would be ideal in helping them to work through these uncomfortable and overwhelming feelings.

Remember that persons cannot will defense mechanisms into use. They are unconsciously set into action by a well-functioning ego. The external supportive environment provided by caring nurses in a hospice can avert a crisis until the temporarily overwhelmed egos resume their adaptive capabilities.

The home can be an ideal environment for a dying patient if the patient *and* most of his family members are coping well. They may be experiencing the emotional upheaval of dying, but their emotional responses are not stagnant. It is essential that the caregivers in the home receive support from others outside of the home. A prolonged illness in the home can result in family caregivers' emotional and physical exhaustion by the time their loved one dies. Home nursing services should be used in order to provide support. If a hospice approach to home nursing services is available, this can provide needed psychological support to the patient and family.

Pain Management

One day, while working with a staff who was feeling great concern and caring about a dying patient who was experiencing severe pain, I suggested that nurses are in a prime position to monitor patients' pain and make recommendations for pain management. When I asked if the nurses thought this might be so, they agreed unanimously. When I asked them why, they said, "Because we see how they suffer, and the physicians don't." Indeed, nurses do watch patients suffer, sometimes for many days. Many nurses experience anger at physicians for allowing this to happen.

This is an important instance of nurses being able to serve patients as advocates. *Unless* the physician is given specific examples of the patient's response to pain, he or she cannot make a decision regarding changes in pain management. In addition, nurses can and should make specific recommendations for medication management that they believe would help the patient. These include types of medication, doses, and time intervals.

The nurse who has cared for many dying patients has had an opportunity to observe patients' responses to particular types of medications, doses, and so on. If the physician chooses not to follow the nurse's recommendations, that is his or her choice. (Usually, most physicians are receptive to these recommendations and frequently are willing to adopt all or part of nurses' recommendations for pain management in complex patients.) If the physician chooses not to follow the nurse's suggestion, it frequently is because of an underlying reason why the change could further complicate the patient's physical condition. Without an opportunity for the physician to explain his or her rationale, the nurse may mistakenly believe the physician is insensitive and uncaring.

The advantage of nurses being honest with physicians in these types of cases is that honesty promotes communication within the caregiving team at a time when the patient needs *all* members of the team to be working in his behalf. If conflict is present because nurses are angry at physicians' management of the patient, the patient's care becomes less than optimum.

Margo McCaffery is a nurse who works with nurses and physicians in order to help them better understand and care for the patient who is in pain. After working closely with patients in pain for many years, she has formed the following beliefs:

I believe pain relief is a legitimate therapeutic goal.

I believe pain relief contributes significantly to the patient's physical and emotional well-being.

I believe pain relief should rank high in the list of priorities in patient care.

I believe the patient has a *right* to pain relief unless it endangers another person.* Within this context, I believe the patient has a right to decide the duration and intensity of pain he is willing to tolerate, to be informed of all possible methods of pain relief along with the favorable and unfavorable consequences, as well as the controversial aspects, to choose which methods he wishes to try, and to choose to live without pain.

High and Low Pain Thresholds

High and low pain thresholds are concepts that should be understood in caring for dying patients. Pain threshold is sometimes misunderstood as a specific neurological point at which *any* person experiences pain. In the past, this inaccurate concept held that all humans experienced pain at the same point and that the point was unchangeable (Hardy and colleagues, 1940). Continued research has proved that pain is a perceived

---

*For example, the mother's right to take certain medications strictly for her own comfort during pregnancy or labor and delivery may be questioned if these medications endanger the health or life of the infant. Similarly, one may question the right of an individual to take an analgesic that also sedates him while he is driving a vehicle or operating any other machinery that could injure someone else if it is managed improperly. (McCaffery M: Nursing Management of the Patient With Pain, 2d ed, p. 3. Philadelphia, JB Lippincott, 1979)

---

experience that can vary among people. It can also vary with time and setting in the same person. McCaffery, in her original book on pain, defined it as "whatever the experiencing person says it is, existing whenever he says it does" (1968, p. 95). The capacity to tolerate great pain reflects the patient's willingness to tolerate severe pain; conversely, low pain tolerance reflects the patient's lack of willingness to endure pain (McCaffery, 1979).

In addition, I believe that another important factor in the patient's ability to tolerate pain is his ego defensive structure. A stoic patient is, in most cases, a person who has an internal locus of control (see p. 67) and usually uses a moderate level of denial in dealing with unpleasant external or internal stimuli. He frequently also is a person with a high level of differentiation between his intellect and emotion (see Chap. 8), so that his intellect is able to maintain control over the unpleasant feeling state associated with pain. This patient frequently may choose to remain "in control" of his pain. He may choose not to feel drugged. His perception of pain may indeed be at a level that is more tolerable for him than it would be for another patient with a similar disease.

Accordingly, there can be another type of patient who has always been highly dependent on others, has an external locus of control, and has a low level of denial in dealing with threatening perceptions. This patient may choose to be medicated as often and as much as possible, because otherwise he would feel out of control. His feelings often are at a low level of differentiation from his intellect; accordingly, the sensation of pain may quickly overwhelm him. The issue of the nurse's concern regarding patients' possible addiction to narcotic analgesia can be found in Chapter 16.

The final analysis of what nurses should do for dying patients in pain is to present the alternatives the patient has open to him for the control of pain and then let the patient decide what *he* needs. The nurse then becomes the liaison, if necessary, between patient and physician, so that the physician has the information necessary to order appropriate pain relief for the patient. Your ongoing assessment and evaluation of the patient's response to pain medication are essential if revisions in the physician's orders are necessary.

In pediatric, geriatric, and intensive care settings, it is not uncommon for nurses to be asked by family members to medicate their loved ones. The nurse may assess that the patient is not in pain. In these instances it is helpful to sit with the family member, who often is feeling helpless and guilty about his or her inability to do something to assist the loved one. With the opportunity to talk about these feelings, family members may become less insistent in their requests for pain medication that actually may not be necessary.

Religion and the Dying Patient

Most large hospitals employ chaplains. Hospital chaplains have prepared for their role with special counseling courses. In many instances thay have completed pastoral counseling programs. They are aware of the effects of loss on the human spirit and are prepared to intervene with patients or family members. In many cases the patients and families have relationships with the clergy of the houses of worship to which they belong. From them they receive extra support during their time of crisis.

Nurses are usually the care coordinators of dying patients. They know what resources are available to them. It is important to offer the services of pastoral care to the dying patient and the family. During this difficult period it can be comforting for family members to speak with a clergyman. The number of emotions that people experience at such a time may cause them concern and guilt. Frequently, it is only by talking with an understanding clergyman that feelings of guilt can be relieved. Medical and nursing caregivers may be able to discuss these issues with them, but often they need to have their guilt relieved by talking with a religious professional.

A frequent cause for concern in many dying patients and family members is their anger toward God for allowing the terminal illness to occur. These feelings arouse strong guilt. Only when they are assured of the normality of these feelings, and their usually temporary status, does the feeling of guilt begin to diminish. Patients and family members also worry about their sins of omission and commission toward one another. Family members' feelings of ambivalence toward their dying member also arouse strong guilt feelings. If you offer to call a chaplain and are refused, remember that later the patient or family member may be relieved by talking with a religious person. At appropriate intervals continue to offer the availability of the hospital chaplain to the patient.

What Can You Say?

In the physical care of patients, we carry out treatments with somewhat rigid guidelines about how to carry out each step of the procedure. Many nurses experience self-expectations of, "I should be able to do something to help." Usually these self-expectations can be carried out in the physical care of the patient in the general hospital setting. There seems to be a never-ending list of medications to be given, treatments to be done, nursing care plans to be written, and so on. When caring for patients, nurses usually have a predetermined list of things to do. Their talking with patients usually falls into three categories:

1. Discussing the patient's physical and emotional response to his illness.
2. Formal teaching regarding hospital or home care protocols.
3. Superficial conversation about weather, news events, and so on.

When working with a long-term patient whose condition is terminal and who will be hospitalized until death, think of what happens to the categories mentioned above:

1. Discussing the patient's responses to his illness may become taboo. Nurses may be afraid of patients' feelings and fear that they won't know how to respond to them.
2. Formal teaching is no longer needed by this patient because his care has become supportive and palliative rather than restorative.
3. Superficial conversation may not be appropriate because the patient may be depressed, in pain, or both.

The consequence of nurses' loss of these normal communications usually causes some anxiety. It is important to recognize that this is a normal response. When we are not sure how to act in a situation, we usually feel anxiety and, whenever possible, avoid the situation as a way of eliminating it.

Rather than being a situation to be avoided, it is possible that working with dying patients can be one of the most rewarding aspects of nursing. In order to work comfortably with dying patients, caregivers must be able to be aware of some major philosophical questions and factors that influence their comfort or discomfort with the dying patient. They are as follows:

How do you feel about your own death?

What do you think happens after death?

To what emotional or physical degree should life be maintained?

These are questions that touch people at their core. The cannot be superficially answered; rather, they are pondered, sometimes for a lifetime.

When nurses are able to work through their own feelings and fears about their own deaths, they frequently find themselves more at ease with dying patients. Sometimes it is by working with and learning from the dignity and peace of dying persons that nurses' fears of death are decreased. Nurses who have thought about and resolved some of their concerns about death are able to be more open with dying patients. They are able to perceive accurately the emotional state of a dying person at a given time. By commenting to a patient, "You seem worried today" or "You seemed sad after your son left tonight," you are telling the patient you understand. This is not an invasion of his privacy.

If you are wrong in your perception, or if the patient does not want to talk about his feelings at that time, he will tell you. Remember, the dying person is responsible for his feelings; the chance that you will suddenly trigger a strong emotional response is much less than triggering relief in allowing his bottled-up feelings to come out. If he should begin to cry, this can be a relief for him. Your concern can be very supportive; stay with the patient, sit with him, or hold his hand. His tears will subside. He may need to talk, or he may need you to sit quietly. Take your clues from the patient.

Many nurses worry that they will say something "wrong" to a dying patient. If a nurse genuinely cares about a patient, it is far more likely that his or her comments will tell the patient that he is understood. An important point to remember is that your presence and touch may be far more comforting to the patient than your conversation. Do not feel compelled to speak comforting words. Do what *you* feel comfortable with.

Can Nurses Show Emotion When Working With Dying Patients?

An issue that is rarely discussed is whether it is all right for nurses to show emotion when working with dying persons and their families. A general feeling among many nurses is that it is not professional to be emotional with patients. They report that this belief came from their nursing education process. Accordingly, they judge themselves unprofessional if they are moved to tears by the tragedy of a stillbirth or the courage of a young dying father.

Stop and think for a moment. When you experienced a major disappointment or personal tragedy, was there someone you talked with whom you found very caring and supportive? Did that person stare at you without expression? Did that person rapidly shift the conversation to another "safer" topic? Did that person occupy herself with busywork as a way of avoiding further awareness of your problem?

The answer is probably no. If she had done any of the things mentioned above, it is doubtful you would have considered her caring and supportive. Instead, she probably sat quietly and listened; she probably asked a few questions that let you know she understood. She most likely had an expression of caring and concern on her face. Her own eyes may have contained tears in response to your emotional pain. Which type of person described above is more aware of the feelings of others? Which type of person described above is more aware of his or her *own* feelings?

A common fear of all people is that they may become emotionally overwhelmed in a difficult circumstance. They really are not sure what is "OK" or "not OK" to feel. Because of this fear, they block their own emotional responses to some experiences. If you are moved to tears with a patient, there is no need to apologize to anyone. (Remember, there is a difference between having your eyes fill with tears and crying uncontrollably.) The patient will know that you care. Your nursing peers will be able to understand; if not, it is their loss—and their patients'—that they have never felt such emotion. It also may help them to be able to allow such emotion in themselves.

You may have spent 1½ or 2 months caring for certain patients on a daily basis, several hours a day. Is it really "unprofessional" to find that you care deeply about some of these patients? Is it possible that by continually having to deny, repress, suppress, and avoid such feelings, we may be diminishing our own humanity as well as that of our patients and their family members?

As the death of a patient approaches, particularly a tragic death, you may occasionally find yourself crying on your way home from work or when at home. You may talk about the patient with a spouse or nonnursing colleague and be moved to tears. All these responses are normal. They are part of the grief response. You are, after all, losing someone who is special. You may know the person more intimately than anyone else during his dying process. It is possible that his family members, because of a maladaptative response to his death, may have been unable to support him.

If you are concerned about whether you are

overinvolved emotionally with a dying patient, seek out a senior staff member or a clinical specialist who works with the dying. He or she can help you to explore the possible causes of your feelings. Understanding the dynamics that cause you to feel attached to a particular patient can help re-establish an objective, empathic posture. As described above, an existential type of relationship with a patient does not occur frequently or with the majority of patients. After the patient dies, most nurses experience the normal bereavement process but for a briefer period than one would experience with a family member or good friend. Again, it is important for nurses to acknowledge their sadness rather than try to stifle it or judge themselves "unprofessional" because of it. Many nurses, after this type of loss, find that they become more emotionally distant from their new patients for a time. Eventually, they are able to resume normal relationships with patients.

Nurse's Role as Patient Advocate

An important aspect of care of the dying person is the nurse's ability to assess the patient's needs for supportive care. On occasion, the physician's awareness of those needs may be different than that of nurses. As discussed above, physicians may concentrate on the patient's biological rather than psychosocial and comfort needs. Many nurses express anger about what they consider to be physicians' insensitivity with dying patients. We must remember, however, that their orientation to patient care is different than nurses'. Rather than being angry toward physicians and lamenting the plight of the patient, there are ways in which the nurse can promote a holistic approach to the care of the dying patient.

The following is a case example of the powerful role that a nurse can play as the dying patient's advocate in a complex hospital care system:

Case Example

Jennifer was a bright, sophisticated 22-year-old woman. At age 17 she attended a professional school in a South American city away from her family. She became fatigued, listless, and ill. Despite the persistence of symptoms, no laboratory work was done, and she was told that she had mononucleosis. When she returned to the United States 7 months later, she had several disquieting physical symptoms. A diagnostic medical workup revealed that her liver was permanently damaged from an undiagnosed and untreated case of hepatitis.

Despite aggressive medical treatment, her liver status continued to deteriorate. Her college education was consistently interrupted by her frequent illnesses and hospitalizations over several years; it ultimately had to be abandoned. Her 22nd year was punctuated by acute medical emergencies and several episodes of organic brain syndrome (OBS) caused by buildup of toxic wastes that the liver could not metabolize.

During her last admission, Jennifer was admitted to a medical teaching unit where her care was supervised by a large medical team who did not know her from previous admissions. At that time, Jennifer was hemorrhaging into all her body tissues because of the failure of two liver-produced clotting factors. She had severe ascites.

Her abdomen was swollen larger than the abdomen of a full-term pregnant woman. Her body was emaciated from metabolic wasting. On admission she was semicomatose because of liver-related encephalopathy (OBS). She became fully alert within 2 days. The chief medical resident and staff physicians were concerned about maintaining whatever liver function she had. They refused to order pain medication because they did not want to stress the liver further with metabolism of complex analgesics.

Her kidneys began to fail. It was obvious to nursing staff members who had cared for her on earlier admissions that death was near. The physicians remained committed to aggressive treatment. They refused to consider a no-resuscitation order in case of death because of her age. The nurses were upset because they believed that the patient had been through enough and should not have to experience the assault of a medical "rush" emergency.

The staff nurse caring for Jennifer approached the chief resident and gave him specific examples of Jennifer's excruciating pain in her abdomen, back, and legs. Jennifer whimpered when any part of her body was touched. Even when she temporarily lapsed into semiconsciousness, she cried out with pain when moved. With the nurses' examples, the chief resident quickly reversed the no-analgesic orders of the intern and other residents. The next day the head nurse approached him about reconsidering his order for an all-out resuscitation attempt in case of death. She emphasized that all the physical systems were in failure, that resuscitation, if effective, could not be maintained by Jennifer's body, that the patient had been through enough pain, and that both the patient and family had been through enough heartache and were prepared for her death. He then ordered that there be no resuscitation attempt and ordered that the patient's comfort level be maintained by adequate analgesics. Jennifer died peacefully 3 days later.

In this case the nurses did not aggressively confront the physicians, nor did they angrily or passively withdraw from their advocacy role. Instead, they continued to bring forward the aspects of the patient's care that they believed were important for consideration in order to ensure the patient the most peaceful and comfortable death possible.

Reasonable Limits of the Nurse's Emotional Involvement With the Dying Patient

Working with dying patients and their families is not easy. When done therapeutically, the emotional investment of the caregiver can cause a drain on his or her emotions. Therapeutic involvement cannot occur unless the caregiver *cares* and *gives*. There are no shortcuts or ways to avoid it.

When you care very much about a dying patient, you may find yourself crying with him, laughing with him, and loving him and his humanity. You feel committed to his well-being and may be the only person who is able to stay with him in his final days. Sister Madeleine Clemence Vaillot (1966, p. 504) advanced an existentialist explanation of commitment, in which she states:

Commitment is the full, willing, and open-eyed acceptance of one's full share of life . . . . It is the acceptance of full responsibility for one's actions . . . . Lack of commitment, on the other hand, is a refusal: a refusal to use one's freedom to choose, to involve one's self with life's difficulties.

Feeling such attachment to a patient is a rare gift for both the patient and the nurse. It goes beyond the normal nurse-patient relationship. In it there is an existential experience. *Existential* refers to the existence, the living process, of a human being. In an existential relationship the two people share an encounter that is unique. There is full understanding and acceptance of the other. Both lives are permanently touched to their emotional

depths, and sometimes to depths never before experienced (Clemence Vaillot, 1966; May and colleagues, 1976). Some nurses may never experience such a relationship. Others experience this closeness at infrequent intervals during their professional lives, perhaps only once a year, once every 2 or 3 years, or once in a working lifetime.

The reason why such an intense relationship does not happen routinely for a nurse with all dying patients is because of the protective functioning of the nurse's defense mechanisms. Even a healthy, mature ego would have difficulty resolving repetitive grief reactions to losses of innumerable patients in whom so much of the nurse's self was invested. Accordingly, the ego unconsciously uses the mechanisms of denial, repression, avoidance, and isolation as a way of coping with the stress of working with dying patients. A chart of those defense mechanisms is presented below.

Whether nurses experience an emotional commitment or maintain a mildly detached, yet still involved, relationship with dying patients, it is important that they accept their own emotional reactions as normal. Some nurses experience anxiety about working with dying patients. Much of this anxiety appears to be caused by the nurse's discomfort with dying. In fact, in a study of staff nurses on general hospital units, nurses were asked to rank the most common stressors they experienced in their everyday work. The list of stressors included 25 items, such as too frequent rotation of shifts, poor relationship with supervisors, lack of respect from subordinates, being overworked, inadequate staffing, and so on. The highest ranking stressor that staff nurses reported was working with dying patients. The second highest stressor reported by many nurses was having to deal with physicians who avoided discussions with dying patients or family members (Barry, 1981).

Maladaptive Grief in Caregivers

One of the reasons why working with dying patients is stressful for staff nurses is that they are reminded of their own eventual death and the eventual deaths of their loved ones. Another reason may be the unresolved loss of a loved person. A third reason is not described in the literature but appears to be an important factor in nurses with whom I have worked; it is the unresolved loss of a significant patient or patients during the formal training period.

Most nurses are able to recall quickly many of the specific details about a special patient they cared for during their student experiences. In fact,

Defense Mechanisms Normally Observed in Caregivers of Dying Patients

Denial	When the nurse cares for the dying patient, he or she engages in light banter, with no emphathetic awareness of the patient's emotional reaction to dying.
Repression	The nurse performs technical nursing care in an acceptable way. When unpleasant feelings such as sadness or hopelessness about the patient are initially experienced, they are excluded from conscious awareness by the ego.
Avoidance (also called withdrawal or professional distancing)	When the dying process is coming to an end, the nurse may feel helpless and hopeless about the patient's condition. Rather than checking on him periodically, the nurse has many other tasks that keep her busy and away from the patient. He or she responds to call lights of dying patients more slowly than to those of other patients.
Isolation (also called rationalization or intellectualization)	The nurse is aware on an intellectual or superficial level of what the dying patient and his family are experiencing. There is little or no affective or emotional component to this awareness, however. The nurse's discussion of the patient's response to dying has a cold, professional-sounding tone. He or she is able to identify the patient's current response to his own death and is able to accurately describe the particular "stage" the patient is in.

frequently they cry as they describe how they felt as they cared for their special patients during their terminal care and ultimate deaths. This is so even though many years have elapsed and they had not thought of the patients during the intervening time.

When asked if they shared this sadness with their instructors or student peers, they often reply that they did not dare. They feared disapproval from others because they had been socialized that such expression of feelings would be considered unprofessional; they could be accused of being too emotional or of being overinvolved with the patient. In addition to disapproval, they also expected that their attitude would affect their clinical nursing grade. Because of their deep sadness about the death of a patient, many of them felt inadequate as nurses. They had been taught that excessive emotion was unacceptable. Can you remember the first dying patient you cared for whose death was a very sad event for you? Can you bring back those feelings? Would you have been comfortable sharing them with your instructor at that time? With your classmates? Why? Remember that nursing faculty members experienced the same socializing process in their student days as you did. Many of them may have been taught that grief about the loss of a patient is unprofessional behavior for a nurse.

When nurses experience such feelings, and I suspect that most nurses do, these feelings are too uncomfortable if there is no place to vent them.

Accordingly, the ego protects the person by repressing them. Remember that repressing feelings does not eliminate them; they are not destroyed. Rather, they are held in the unconscious. This is why, years later, when nurses recall a patient about whom they cared very much, the sadness returns as though the patient had just died.

I believe that it is the result of this type of early unresolved loss that contributes to the anxiety of many caregivers as they work with dying patients. After one or two of these special, but unsupported, encounters with dying patients, the nurse eventually may begin to defend against similar unpleasant feelings about future dying patients. Rather than allowing themselves to get close to other patients, nurses who have not been "allowed" to grieve by their nursing social system unconsciously protect themselves by using avoidance and other mechanisms.

What Can Be Done To Support Nurses Caring for Dying Patients

The most commonly recommended approach is to provide nurses with a group in which they can discuss their reactions to working with dying patients (Eaton, 1976). Such groups are usually led by psychiatrists, social workers, psychiatric nurse specialists, or psychiatric liaison nurse specialists. Whenever possible, I think that the most appropriate leaders for this type of nurse group are psychiatric liaison nurse specialists. Their theoretical and clinical training is related to the stressful aspects of physical illness of all concerned: patients, families, and nurses. They are familiar with the interaction effects of these people within a complex hospital caregiving system. Psychiatric or psychiatric liaison nurse group leaders are able to understand the specific issues of nurses that can contribute to the stress of working with dying patients. Some of these issues are the socialization process of the nursing student, which may have encouraged repression of unpleasant affects such as sadness, anger, and guilt about dying patients; the type of stress involved in long, unbroken hours of nursing care, as opposed to the much briefer contacts of nonnursing caregivers; and, most important, the philosophy of nursing, which is strongly psychosocially oriented when compared to the more predominant interest of medical caregivers in the patients' biological processes.

An essential aspect of working with dying patients is for nurses to be aware of their own feelings about their patients. Without an opportunity to vent this emotion, it remains trapped within.

Support of the Student Nurse Working With Dying Patients

In addition to such a group for graduate nurses, it is important that nursing educators review the philosophy of their curricula, as well as their own convictions about what types of responses of students to dying patients are acceptable. One of the strongly contributing factors in nursing students' repression of unpleasant emotion can be caused by the clinical grade administered by their clinical instructor. Students frequently fear that these grades will be affected if they display more than a mild emotional response to the death of a patient.

One way of avoiding this problem is to consider an ongoing group experience for students. The group should be led by a member of the faculty who is a psychiatric liaison or psychiatric clinical specialist. Such a group can have a positive outcome with an every-other-week meeting. The focus of the group could be discussion of the students' feelings about specific patients and of psychosocial care problems of specific patients. There should be no grading involved in this group experience and confidentiality of the group should be maintained.

The healthy ego will not allow an intolerable amount of emotion to accumulate. In its adaptation attempt, it will either repress the painful emotion or not allow it to be experienced. Remember that repression can be a very adaptive response in nurses in the care of acutely ill patients. However, repeated episodes of unpleasant emotion or deep continued repression that occurs with patient encounters are not conducive to positive adaptation; rather, they may cause nurses to "shut down." They may no longer be able to be as open or responsive to their patients.

Conclusion

This chapter has been written in order to help you work with dying persons and their families. I hope you will find that some of the concerns that you have had or may someday have about your own emotional responses as well as those of the patient, his family, and other caregivers will be more understandable.

Part Three

Adaptation to Nursing

The final chapter in this book is for the nurse himself or herself. There is stress in caring for chronically or critically ill human beings who are reacting to some of the most frightening experiences they will ever know. Nurses are expected to adapt constantly in their care of others. This chapter is written for nurses everywhere in the hope that it will provide for them some of the care they so readily give to others.

This chapter is written especially for nurses. In my work with nurses in many hospitals, I have found them to be givers. Rarely do they place their own needs on an equal plane with those of patients. Rather, they set high standards of patient care and struggle constantly to perform to these expectations.

Many thoughts and concepts will be presented in this chapter that can potentially decrease the levels of stress that many nurses experience in today's health care settings. Just as maintaining patients' quality of life is a high priority of nurses, so should it be an essential goal in our own lives. It is widely recognized that nursing is one of the most stressful of all occupations. Our ability to recognize our own stress responses and to reduce them will have a significant effect on our capacity to enjoy life and experience full development as human beings.

Stress: What's It All About?

Stress and its implications in the lives of all persons was discussed in Chapter 9. The main theme of this book has been to teach nurses how to assess and intervene with the patient or family who is not able to adapt to the stress of illness and is at risk for maladaptation. Before beginning to write the book, I decided that the last chapter would be devoted to nurses themselves in order to help them to be more aware of the particular stresses that are inherent in nursing and some of the underlying dynamics. I believe that if we are better able to tolerate the level of stress in our working environment, we will have more emotional reserves to support our patients and ourselves. Frequently, if we are able to understand intellectually what is happening to us, it helps us to cope, adapt, and manage the stressful feelings we experience more effectively.

Can We Change the Way We Respond to Stress?

Stress Management

By the time we reach late childhood and adolescence, the way that we respond to stress is already a part of our personality. Most of the time we respond unconsciously to stressors. For example, a 13-year-old girl may suspect that two other girls

21

Stress in Nursing Practice

who are giggling and looking in her direction are talking about her. This is a stressor for her. She may respond in various ways, depending on her normal personality style and the way that her ego uses defense mechanisms:

Walk up to them, smiling, and say hello (no defense, because she was unthreatened, denial, or reaction formation)

Walk by them with her head down, embarrassed (threatened, but no defenses are operating; self-esteem is decreased)

Turn around and walk the other way (avoidance)

Immediately look for another friend and begin to gossip about the other two (acting-out behavior or projection)

Go to her basketball practice and consistently slam the ball against the backboard (displacement onto inanimate object)

Go home and be angry with her innocent young brother (displacement onto other person)

The way we respond to stress depends on our basic personality styles and our own unique defensive style (the defense mechanisms that we customarily use, unconsciously, when under stress).

The next time you are under stress, tune in to the way you are responding. Think back to times of severe stress in your life. If you can be objective about yourself, you will discover what your normal defensive or coping style is. This will be the coping style you will continue to use during your lifetime, unless a major personality reorganization occurs. Understandably, this type of major change is quite rare. A person's coping style is used automatically and *unconsciously* to varying degrees, depending on the level of stress encountered.

What Is the Difference Between Stress Management and a Coping Style?

Stress management is a different concept from coping style. The difference is that defense/coping mechanisms are, for the most part, unconscious and based on a person's normal personality style. Stress management is the *conscious* use of mental or physical maneuvers that reduce feelings of tension. These maneuvers are a shift in personal tactics and are used when a person begins to

detect an uncomfortable level of stress in himself. They can be learned.

Basic Principles of Stress That Relate to Nursing

A stressor can be a psychological or physiological threat. If a person wakes up to find his house on fire, his awareness of the threat causes a series of psychological and physiological responses that should help him to think and act rapidly. If the person is burned, the body responds immediately with a vast variety of physiological mechanisms designed to promote homeostasis.

In hospital environments, nurses are frequently working in stressful conditions. Imagine yourself in the following situation:

Case Example

On the night shift you have 22 surgical patients directly under your care; there are heavier medications and treatments tonight than normal; two of the fresh postoperative patients are bleeding; the vital signs of one of them are not stable. The son of one of your patients was in an automobile accident yesterday and is in critical condition in another hospital. The evening charge nurse told you that the patient is upset and needs to talk.

Your staff is one RN and one LPN. At 2 AM the night supervisor calls. Because of an emergency elsewhere, she is pulling the LPN to another unit.

At 3 AM the surgical resident decides that the unstable postoperative patient should be returned to the operating room. The other patients are restless. There are more requests for pain medication than normal.

At 5:50 AM as you are preparing your 6 AM medications, the surgical patient is returned to the floor with an order for every-15-minute signs, changes in intravenous fluid, medication and treatment orders, and an order for shock blocks.

At 6:45 AM you are running to complete your treatment list. All night your treatments were behind schedule because of the unexpected events.

At 7 AM the day staff arrives. Before you begin report, the head nurse takes you aside to tell you that she is not pleased with the condition of the unit and that the treatment room was not straightened up after your shift yesterday.

Sound familiar? Unfortunately, too familiar, right? No matter what shift you work, you will be able to identify with the nurse above. Nursing is not easy work. The time pressures alone are very stressful. Add to that the unexpected emergencies in which you must act very quickly and with a level head. Add also the interpersonal stress of working closely with the same group of nurses and patients for extended periods. Perhaps then you can acknowledge that there are legitimate reasons why you go home some days feeling as if you had been put through a wringer. Is it any wonder that at times you are less than pleasant company when you arrive home? This unrelieved stress can take its toll on your personal life and relationships with others as well.

Realistically, the hospital environment and the functions that nurses perform in hospitals cannot be dramatically altered. Stress *is* a part of nursing. There can be positive and negative types of stress, however. The negative stress of a conflict or problem within the system *can* be examined, and resolution may indeed be possible. An example of positive stress is a well-staffed intensive care unit in which an experienced nurse is challenged by the unpredictability of the environment and feels good that his or her responses are essential to patients' well-being.

The Stress Response

This section has been written to present suggestions about what to do when you are negatively stressed. Stop and think how you feel when you are stressed. Recall how you felt during a recent time when you were very stressed. What sensations did you experience? The following chart presents the common physiological, emotional, and intellectual responses to stress.

For many people, the effect is an unpleasant physical feeling in addition to the emotional and intellectual responses described. When people are asked what stress feels like, they reply:

> I get pressure in the back of my neck that moves up into my head and becomes a massive headache.
>
> My head feels as if it were popping.
>
> My stomach feels as if it were turning inside out.
>
> My chest feels tight.
>
> My whole body feels exhausted. I feel as if I can't do anything.
>
> My bursitis flares up.
>
> All my joints ache.

What causes these unpleasant effects of stress? Essentially, the body of early man was designed to respond to a threatening event by "fight or flight" (Cannon, 1929). Either way, a whole series of physiological responses were set into motion by the flood of increased adrenaline and norepinephrine into the body. Some of the physiological effects of these catecholamines are as follows:

1. Stimulation of the sympathetic nerves that supply the involuntary muscle in the walls of the arterioles, causing these muscles to contract and the blood pressure to rise accordingly
2. Conversion of the glycogen of the liver into sugar, which is poured into the blood and brought to the voluntary muscles, permitting them to do an extraordinary amount of work
3. Increased heart beat
4. Dilation of the bronchioles through relaxation of the smooth muscle of their walls

The body needed extra energy to maintain the extra physical effort to escape from the dinosaur or

Responses to Stress

Physiological

Increased heart rate	Diarrhea
Elevated blood pressure	Nausea, vomiting, or both
Tightness of chest	Sleep disturbance
Difficulty in breathing	Anorexia
Sweaty palms	Sneezing
Trembling, tics, or twitching	Constant state of fatigue
Tightness of neck or back muscles	Accident proneness
Headache	Susceptibility to minor illness
Urinary frequency	Slumped posture

(continued)

Responses to Stress
(*continued*)

Emotional

Irritability
Angry outbursts
Feeling of worthlessness
Depression
Suspiciousness
Jealousy
Restlessness
Anxiousness
Withdrawal

Lack of interest
Diminished initiative
Tendency to cry
Sobbing without tears
Reduction of personal involvement with others
Tendency to blame others
Critical to self and others
Self-deprecating

Intellectual

Forgetfulness
Preoccupation
Rumination
Mathematical and grammatical errors
Errors in judging distance
Blocking
Diminished fantasy life
Lack of concentration

Reduction in interest
Lack of attention to details
Past oriented rather than present or future oriented
Lack of awareness of external stimuli
Reduction in creativity
Diminished productivity

(After Reres M: Editorial: coping with stress in nursing. The American Nurse 9:4, 1977)

to fight off the bigger caveman. The brain needed to think clearly of the options: where to run or how to hit the other man. By the time the fight or flight was over, the body had "burned up" the extra adrenaline, norepinephrine, blood sugar, and other biochemicals released during the original alarm. Homeostasis returned. The caveman felt no aftereffects except perhaps normal fatigue, which can be a pleasant, comfortable sensation. There were no lingering mental or physical effects of stress.

Let us compare the effects of stress on prehistoric man to man of the 20th century. Does 20th-century man usually have the opportunity to fight or flee when under stress? (Remember that fighting as described above is a physical exchange, not an intellectual argument.) How about the night nurse in the example above?

- Could she start a fight with the supervisor when she pulled the LPN from the unit?
- Could she run away when she realized by 1 AM that it was going to be a bad night?
- Could she run the other way when a fresh postoperative patient was returned to the unit with a pageful of new orders?
- Could she start a fight with her head nurse who lectured her about the treatment room?

No. She could not. Her body, however, responded with the hormones and subsequent physiological changes necessary for fighting and fleeing. Where does all of this available energy go? Nowhere. It remains in the body as unreleased tension. It dissipates very gradually. When she finished work and went home to go to bed, she wondered why she could not sleep!

Stress has become a big word in our culture. People everywhere are experiencing more stress in their lives than did their fathers and grandfathers. It is partially the result of the exponential rate of change in our society (Toffler, 1970).

Because of the increased numbers of stressors in our everyday world, it is possible that we are continually operating with increased levels of adrenaline and tension in our bodies. There is not time for them to wear off before another stressor comes along and triggers more adrenaline. Is there any way that this effect can be brought down to a more comfortable level and the constant feeling of tenseness relieved?

An active physical exercise program has been found to contribute to an increase in a person's sense of well-being and a decrease in depression. In research on college students, Hochberg (1980) divided 21 of them into two groups. Before her intervention with them, the rate of depression determined by a validated depression index scale in the two groups was equal. The students in the experimental group then participated in an 8-week jogging program, which involved running three times a week. At the end of that time the two groups were again measured for levels of depression. The experimental group had a significantly decreased rate of depression compared to the control group. Similar findings of decreased depression in people who participated in active exercise programs compared to depression rates in persons who did not exercise regularly have also been reported by Morgan and colleagues (1970), Greist and colleagues (1979), and Brown and colleagues (1978). Although Hochberg could not give a specific reason for this change, one of her theories was that running released the aggressive drive that had previously been repressed and caused a depressive process. I believe that another reason why people experience relief is that the exertion of physical exercise "uses up" the extra neurotransmitters, such as adrenaline, that contribute to a feeling of stress.

Setting up an exercise program for yourself is an important way of managing stress. If you feel fatigued and believe that you do not have the energy for extra activity, schedule a physical examination in order to relieve your mind that there is no physical reason for the fatigue. If there are no problems, then plan to begin.

Most people find that they lack the discipline to keep on with an exercise program of their own design. Some popular alternatives are to exercise at an exercise or health club. These clubs are very popular with many nurses. They are usually open from very early to very late, and you may schedule your time at your own convenience. The personnel design exercise programs specifically to meet your needs. These clubs also offer the advantage of meeting other people. A similar type of exercise program is usually available at lower cost through the recreation departments of many communities. Some progressive hospitals have established exercise facilities for their personnel. For beneficial stress reduction to occur, the exercise session should be an hour long and be done two or three times a week. Intellectual pursuits, such as classes or reading, are sometimes suggested as diversions for nurses' stress, but they lack the advantage of releasing physical tension and the related elevated levels of neurotransmitters.

Recommendations for Reducing Stress

In addition to physical exercise, the following suggestions are recommended as ways of reducing stress:

1. *Be good to yourself.* Nurses always seem to be in a giving role—to patients, family, friends. How often do you take time just for yourself? At least once a week pamper yourself. Go out to lunch with a friend. Have a long, quiet, luxurious bath. Buy yourself something you think you shouldn't. You *are* special.

2. *Budget your energy and time.* Nurses frequently give themselves away. Others will continue to ask things of you as long as you say yes. Begin to value yourself more. Learn to say no. Restrict your professional time so that you have more time for your family and friends out of the hospital. Learn to say no, on occasion, to your family so that you have *some* time to yourself. As you value your own time, so will you find others valuing you.

3. *Understand the role you play.* Know what the *reasonable* expectations are for your various roles. You are a nurse, daughter, son, mother, father, wife, husband, and so on. Determine what people can fairly expect of you. Pay close attention to the expectations *you impose on yourself.* Sometimes our self-expectations are motivated by trying to avoid guilt feelings. Others may not expect as much of us as we think they do.

4. *Learn to communicate.* Learn to express your real feelings, rather than using avoidance or passivity or suppressing anger. Bottled-up feelings can lead to burnout at work, depression, or physical ailments such as headaches, stomach problems, high blood pressure, and so on.

5. *Make decisions.* When you vacillate between choices, you burn up more energy. Once you make up your mind, you can move on with your decision. Being indecisive is similar to a car caught in mud. Its wheels are spinning. It uses up a lot of energy but gets nowhere.

6. *Let your emotions out.* When you are alone, allow yourself to feel emotions that you do not feel comfortable allowing others to see. Although you may not be able to release some work-related emotions at work, on the way home when you remember your dying patient and feel sad, it's OK to cry. Or, it is all right to blast the tennis ball extra hard after work when you remember the rudeness of a family member earlier in the day. Burying these feelings can result in a general feeling of tenseness.

7. *Train yourself to let your intellect rule, not your emotions.* Emotions, when unchecked, can make a person feel miserable. Nurses, for

example, find that guilt about all the things they think they *should* be doing can drive them to a near frenzy of activity. Instead, when a difficult situation is caused by events beyond your control—understaffing, unusually sick patients, and so on—train your intellect to take charge. In such a case the intellect can reason, "I'm doing the best I can." Rather than allowing emotion to flood the intellect, you will be able to prioritize objectively the many jobs that need doing. You *can* gain a sense of control over the situation.

These suggestions can make a difference in your life and the way that you value yourself as a person.

Ten Basic Rights for Women in the Health Professions

Speaking of valuing yourself as a person, you may find that the following "basic rights" proposed by Chenevert (1978) can help you to assess your views about yourself and your profession. Although addressed to women, they pertain to all nurses, male and female.

Ten Basic Rights for Women in the Health Care Professions

1. You have the right to be treated with respect.
2. You have the right to a reasonable workload.
3. You have the right to an equitable wage.
4. You have the right to determine your own priorities.
5. You have the right to ask for what you want.
6. You have the right to refuse without making excuses or feeling guilty.
7. You have the right to make mistakes and be responsible for them.
8. You have the right to give and receive information as a professional.
9. You have the right to act in the best interest of the patient.
10. You have the right to be human.

(Chenevert M: Special Techniques in Assertiveness Training for Women in the Health Professions, p 39. St. Louis, CV Mosby, 1978)

Assertiveness vs. Aggressiveness

All this consciousness raising sometimes leaves nurses feeling uncertain about whether it is "OK" to stand up for themselves. Frequently, the cause of this discomfort for female nurses is that they do not want to become unfeminine. It *is* possible to value yourself and be honest with others and retain their respect without being pushy and unfeminine.

The problem is that many nurses confuse assertiveness with aggressiveness.

There are major differences between being assertive and being aggressive. Study the following chart carefully; it will clarify some of the differences. It also includes the characteristics of passivity, which have frequently been applied to women as part of their traditional role (Miller, 1976). By implication, because nursing is a woman-dominated profession, passivity is a common characteristic of many nurses. The chart to the right lists several characteristics of each of the three major styles in which people relate with others.

Professional Stress in Nursing

Several years ago I was asked by a visiting nurse agency to come in and do psychiatric consultation with staff nurses about their complex patients. I entered the room to meet 24 tired- and hostile-looking nurses. I introduced myself and asked them to tell me how they had used the consultation time with their former consultant, a psychiatrist. They told me "formal case presentations." I asked how that had gone, and they said that they had not liked it. I asked if they had any suggestions about how they would like to change the format. There was silence. I briefly presented some possible ways in which we could examine patient care issues. I asked them what they thought about the possibilities. There was more silence. The assistant director of the agency was sitting in the group, and I thought how impressed she must be! After a very long silence I said, "What would *you* like to do with this time?" The nurses sat slouching, looking at the floor and occasionally at each other, with a "what a waste of time" look. Finally, one of them said, "I'm sick of talking about patients. All we do is put out and put out, I want to talk about me and what *I'm* going through taking care of *them*."

Suddenly, everyone in the room sat up. It was as if they were thinking, "Who is this bold person who dares to say these words out loud!" One by one, other nurses began to pour out the pressures they felt in their work, their discouragement and fatigue at never being able to catch up, never feeling that they were doing a whole job anywhere.

These feelings had been present in them for a long time. Other than occasional comments of frustration to colleagues or expressions of anger or resentment about their jobs to family members, they had never fully expressed these feelings, which, for many, had reached a helpless and

Interpersonal Styles of Nurses

	Characteristics	Feelings in Self	Reactions of Others
Assertive	Open	At peace inside	Respect
	Honest	Good self-esteem	
	Does not impinge on others' beliefs	Respects other's rights	
Passive	Weak	Uncertainty	Pity
	Yielding	Tries to please	Uncertainty
	Self-denying	others	Unconcern
	Hidden bargaining	Resentfulness	Annoyance
	Deceptive about real feelings		
Aggressive	Quarrelsome	Anger	Indignation
	Bold	Contempt for others	Displeasure
	Degrades others	Extreme self-pride	Hurt
	Bulldozes over others' opinions, beliefs, and feelings with no respect for others	Anxiety when aggressiveness is out of control	Disgust

hopeless point. They seemed relieved to express them. They found that they were not alone. All of them discovered that they felt the same way, but they had never realized it. Within the first group meeting, support from each member to all other members was expressed. As the group time ended, the air in the room was lighter, people were smiling, and there were many voices chattering as the nurses went off to their daily patient rounds. I wondered if the quality of care they gave that day was different from the care they gave the day before.

After the nurses left, I spoke to the assistant director and asked, "What do we do now?" She said, "Let's go with it." She had known that the staff was going through a difficult time but had not been aware of the depth of their discouragement. In subsequent meetings with that group and another group that formed as the result of staff members' talks with nurses from another field location within the agency, I formed some preliminary conclusions about the value of support groups for nurses to deal with work-related stress.

Nurse Support Groups in the Work Setting

Support groups provide nurses with a place to ventilate bottled-up feelings. Nurses carry many emotions that are a direct result of patient care.

They feel grief about dying patients or patients with multiple tragedies in their lives. They feel frustration in wanting to do more for their patients but being limited by time constraints. In addition, there are difficult, noncompliant patients who severely test the patience of the best nurses. These diverse situations often result in nurses feeling inadequate. The usual outcome is guilt, which is the most common unpleasant emotion nurses report.

Another set of unpleasant emotions is the result of working in an institution. Working with multiple caregiving disciplines can result in conflict between them that seems unresolvable. Anger, followed by hopelessness, is the result. Seemingly unchangeable institutional policies can also result in negative and hopeless feelings in nurses.

Support groups provide a place for nurses to look intellectually at the conflicts that are undermining their work satisfaction. Frequently, nurses do not have an intellectual awareness of the dynamics of these problems. Instead, they react with feelings. Their emotions dominate their intellects (see Chap. 8) and their ability to resolve the problem. When emotions are in control, the opportunity to use a step-by-step problem-solving approach is lost. With proper leadership, an intellectual approach to problem identification and resolution can be achieved.

Traditionally, staff nurses have not been a part of the problem-solving process in resolving *their own problems*. Instead, they have passively asked nursing or hospital administrators to solve their problems for them. When staff nurses do not articulate their problems or present sufficient objective data, nursing leaders have solved the problems from their own perspectives. The solutions designed by nursing administrators frequently result in more staff anger because the solution was not what staff members wanted. More standoffs occur.

Nurses *can* solve their own problems. It is rare that a person or group that is having a problem cannot think of solutions to the problem. Only those who *live* with a problem fully understand the dynamics. By understanding all the contributing factors of a problem, the process of looking at the solutions becomes easier. It is essential, when problems become acute and emotions, rather than intellect, are in control, that an objective, unbiased outsider be brought into the problem-solving process. This can be a sensitive nursing service supervisor if he or she can effectively lead a group of emotional people. Another recommendation is a psychiatric liaison clinical specialist whose training involves assessment of intrapsychic and social system functioning. It is preferable for this problem solver to be a nurse rather than a member of some other professional group. In most instances I believe that someone with a nursing background can best understand the specific issues that are of concern to nurses.

Support groups can provide a place for nurses to regain a sense of hope. Nurses find that seemingly unresolvable problems or conflicts are indeed not hopeless. In addition, such a group can provide a vehicle for support of the person. This type of feedback can have a positive effect on self-esteem and job satisfaction in the professional setting. Discussion of the formation of such a group appears later in this chapter.

Burnout

One of the most popular words in our society today is burnout. *Burnout* is the perceived accumulation of stressful events over time and the belief that nothing can be done about them. *Perceived* and *accumulation* are two important words. Remember, that what one person considers to be a stressor may be a challenge and joy for another. (Think of the example of parachute jumping in Chap. 9.) An important dynamic in the development of burnout in some people is unrealistically high expectations of their own performance.

The second part of the definition provides the key to what burnout feels like: belief that nothing can be done about these stressors. This belief results in feelings of hopelessness, resignation, resentment, and sometimes depression. It is usually preceded by a stage of anger. It is during the stage of anger that the nurse has the potential to *do* something to make the situation better for himself or herself.

Remember that feelings of anger come from the aggressive drive. This is one of the two main drives in every human being. Both these drives, the libidinal and the aggressive, provide motivation in our daily lives. These drives, simply stated, help us to feel good in our relationships and to go about our routine activities. With the energy of the aggressive drive sparked by anger, there is potential for people to work on problem solving. This can be a necessary component in the desire to resolve a problem. It is important to differentiate, however, between anger that is emotional and volatile and usually destructive in a conflict situation and a reasonable level of anger that can be channeled into an intellectual problem-solving approach.

Once the anger has worn out or burned out, the result is a void of hopelessness or helplessness. Even worse, if the anger is repressed, it can result in depression. Burnout occurs everywhere, not just in nursing. It occurs in any job situation, in school settings, relationships with others, and in a person's general feelings about life.

A very important part of preventing burnout is being able to recognize the warning signs. Being able to recognize your own legitimate anger is one of the most important indicators. Once you become aware of negative feelings about one or more situations, rather than continually stifling these feelings, ask yourself if this is a problem for other people as well. If it is, then it is probably a problem that can potentially contribute to the burnout of others. While the energy-producing effects of anger are still present, it can be worthwhile to see what you can do about it.

In surveying staff nurses from over 30 institutions, I found these descriptions of the factors that are contributing to discouragement in their positions:

- Lack of challenge because of lack of respect for nurses' judgment from other professionals
- Understaffed—consequently overworked emotionally and physically

- Too little gratitude from patients and superiors
- Tension with physicians
- Understaffing
- Disorganization
- Lack of staff
- Low morale
- Stress
- Self-expectations that are too high
- Lack of attainable goals
- Low wages
- Emotional and physical fatigue
- Frustration over being unable to change those areas that require change
- Stress in coping with poor quality of physician
- Frustration with self—incapability to cope with job situation
- Trying to do too much in a given time
- Too many years of ideas and enthusiasm being totally ignored
- Frustration at the inability to care for patient adequately because of lack of staff; feeling personally responsible for patients not happy with treatment
- Frustration in dealing with administration in trying to promote change in patient care—difficult to get change when needed.

It does sound depressing, doesn't it? *It is not hopeless, however.* In some of these comments you can hear hopelessness. That is due to nurses' going beyond the anger stage. They have lost their energy to work toward solutions.

Changing the Climate in Hospitals

Many nurses working at the staff nurse level are not aware that hospitals and nursing administrators are genuinely and seriously concerned about the well-being of their nurses; the distress and dissatisfaction of their nursing staffs troubles them. Before you chuckle at this comment, remember that staff nurses are *essential* if hospitals are to remain open. How many of you work in hospitals in which beds have had to be closed because of lack of nursing staff? The current state of nursing will not change in the immediate future. Decreases in federal funding for nursing students, other job opportunities opening for women, the negative impact of the media's attention to the nursing shortage on young women considering nursing as a career, more demand for nurses in nonhospital settings as

well as in hospital positions, and so on are all contributing factors to this prediction.

Accordingly, if hospitals are going to continue to care for patients, an adequate nursing staff is essential. When available nurses existed in large numbers in our society, they were expendable. Astonishingly high turnover rates were of little concern to hospital administrators because there were always more nurses available. That attitude is now changing. Nurses *are* needed. Their value is unquestioned. Progressive hospitals have begun to realize that they must listen to their nurses or they will lose them; replacing them is costly.

Nurses *Can* Help Themselves

There are many ways that overworked nurses can reexamine their working style and educate hospital administrators about the realities of continuing policies that existed during previous eras with markedly different staffing patterns. Nurses themselves know which elements of their work are essential and which elements can be restructured, eliminated, or shifted to paraprofessionals.

For example, old policies cause increased stress in nurses. It may be hospital policy that *every* patient on a unit must receive a backrub before bedtime, including ambulatory patients. Finding the time to give backrubs to eight ambulatory patients who do not need them might result in a frequently incontinent patient being turned less often than is necessary to avoid skin breakdown. The nurse knows that the consequence of lack of turning could be a decubitus ulcer that takes 6 weeks to heal, but hospital policy has been so ingrained into him or her that priorities become confused and the work pace is frantic. The incontinent patient may be turned only twice in a shift, but the backrubs all get done.

Stress Reduction by Conflict Resolution

If you review the list of nurses' statements of frustration listed above, you will see that if nurses could come together in a group to solve problems, some problems could be resolved and a more supportive and realistic working environment could result.

In order to assist nurses in resolving conflicts that are contributing to their burnout, I will present a general format that can be useful to nurses who want to try a problem-solving approach. Remember that the alternative to a problem-solving approach is a helpless and hopeless feeling that can ultimately cause a nurse to leave his or her job. Some of you who are reading this chapter may be in your second or third position, and you may be beginning to get this helpless feeling again. Here is an approach that can help you to create a working environment where you can meet not only the needs of the patient and the institution, *but your own as well*. This problem-solving concept can be useful in *every* nursing setting, institutional or academic. Nursing students have found it helpful in approaching their teachers about situations that they felt were "hopeless."

In order to address a problem, it is important to identify the source of the problem. The main types of problems that result in burnout in nursing service and education are frustration, overload, and deprivation. They are described in the following chart:

Causes of Conflict That Lead to Burnout

Frustration: person is in situation where he is blocked from accomplishing something he wants to do

Overload: more is demanded of person than he can give because of lack of available time or lack of ability

Deprivation: the environment is withholding and denying a person something he needs

The Problem-Solving Approach

If you are experiencing stress as the result of a long-standing problem and find that you are experiencing unpleasant physical, intellectual, or emotional symptoms as a result of that stress, you do have options open to you:

1. *Leave your place of employment or your school of nursing.* Before you do, however, think of the consequences. Will it *really* solve your problem? It is possible that you might experience quick relief but eventually regret leaving a job or giving up a goal that essentially was very meaningful to you. If so, then the other options, although they will involve more time, more work, and more self-control, may be better choices.

2. *Use the stress-reduction suggestions that appeared earlier in this chapter.* After a few weeks of using these recommendations, do you feel any different? If not, then it is indeed possible that other people are experiencing the same problems you are. Rather than it being a problem of personal inadequacy, it is very possible that it is a systems problem. Rather than continuing to personalize the problem and finding yourself inadequate, realize that the problem may be the result of an inadequacy somewhere in the overall nursing service or education system. It is not impossible to solve problems in a system.

In order to initiate a problem-solving process, informally discuss your thoughts with some co-workers or fellow students. Learn if they feel as you do. If you find your thoughts validated by them, then informally poll a larger circle of persons *within* the group that is having the problem. If you violate boundaries and discuss it with other nurses from other units or other classes, you may escalate the problem. If the other members of your group also believe that the problem is a significant one, schedule a meeting that will include all persons who are immediately involved, including the head nurse or faculty member in direct authority.

An objective group leader is necessary to help you to maintain reality testing about both the problem and the solutions you decide on. If your hospital employs a psychiatric liaison clinical specialist, he or she is an ideal person to help in this process. Lacking a psychiatric liaison nurse, a clinical specialist in psychiatric nursing can assist in the process. Administrative personnel who have responsibility to your unit are in a difficult position to lead such a group because of their required administrative involvement and need to report and act on the problem; their objectivity is nearly impossible to maintain in such a situation. As discussed earlier, it is usually unwise to bring in a nonnursing person to lead such a group. They do not understand basic nursing dynamics. Interdisciplinary misunderstandings can also occur. *The leader should not be judgmental or be involved in bringing the results of the meeting to a decision-making authority person.* His or her position after the meeting is to maintain the confidentiality of the group. It is, after all, not his or her problem. You do not want that person speaking on your behalf, or you may find that the solution is one that is acceptable to him or her but not to you.

If the problem affects an entire nursing unit, a time convenient to all should be arranged. The meeting should be scheduled for one full hour. Less time prevents full discussion and problem-solving potential. More time can result in idle discussion or discussion of more than one problem. Proceed as follows:

A. Identify the problem:
   1. Allow adequate time to talk about the problem. Allow emotions about the problem to come forth for approximately one third of the meeting time. People think more clearly after unpleasant emotion is released. *Make sure you identify the source of the problem:*
      a. Present several examples of the problem so that the group is in agreement about the basic problem.
      b. Temporarily discard any problems that are different than the basic problem the group identifies. They can confuse the issue and should be addressed at a different time.

B. Brainstorm ways of solving the problem. Put together a list of several solutions:
   1. Include all solutions presented:
      a. If a few impractical but amusing solutions are presented, include them. A sense of humor during such a meeting can be valuable.
   2. Stop and review the course of action involved in each solution and, most important, think of the possible outcome of each solution:
      a. Many times nurses do not look at the possible outcome of their actions:
         (1) Without this step, you may either complicate the problem or may prematurely inhibit your actions when no negative outcomes are possible.

C. Decide on the best solution that is agreeable to all. The group's choice of a solution should be unanimous. Unanimity usually is not difficult to achieve when the steps described above are worked through. Otherwise, splintering and divisiveness can undermine the later effectiveness of the solution.

D. Bring the problem to the attention of the one person who has decision-making authority about the problem:
   1. Above all, do not violate boundaries in this process. For example, if you are having

problems with a group of new *medical* house officers who are disrespectful to nurses, do not "sound out" the director of *surgical* residents to find out how you should best approach the director of medical residents. Go directly to the person involved.
   2. The choice of who brings the solution to the decision maker is up to the group. It can be the entire group, part of the group, or a spokesperson chosen by the group. The person(s) presenting the solution should make it clear to the decision maker that the solution is the unanimous choice of the group and that it was arrived at by a consensual process.

E. Present the problem with your recommended solution to the authority person. Allow no more or no less than 1 hour for this meeting:
   1. Allow time to adequately explain the problem. Maintain intellectual control of yourself in your discussion.
   2. Do not allow emotions to dominate.
   3. *Be articulate.*
   4. Give the person time to ask questions so that you know he or she understands the problem.
   5. Allow the person time to talk about your solution:
      a. There may be circumstances that prevent your solution from being fully implemented:
         (1) Listen well. Be open to new ideas.
         (2) Be prepared to compromise.

F. Ask for a follow-up appointment of 30 minutes in 1 week for evaluation and for mutual feedback:
   1. Be open and honest in this meeting.
   2. If there has been no change in the problem, be prepared to implement your second-choice solution.

Frequently, in these situations both the group with the problem and the final decision maker are surprised to discover that neither understood all the factors involved in the others' viewpoint. Once the lines of communication are open, the potential for conflict resolution can be very real indeed. Nurses who have been prepared to leave their positions have found, to their surprise, that their level of optimism and hopefulness about their work returns after this type of approach to their problem. Surprisingly, only one or two such meetings may be necessary to resolve the problem to the satisfaction of both parties.

Desiderata

Go placidly amid the noise & haste, & remember what peace there may be in silence. As far as possible without surrender be on good terms with all persons. Speak your truth quietly & clearly; and listen to others, even the dull & ignorant; they too have their story. Avoid loud & aggressive persons, they are vexations to the spirit. If you compare yourself with others, you may become vain & bitter; for always there will be greater & lesser persons than yourself. Enjoy your achievements as well as your plans. Keep interested in your own career, however humble; it is a real possession in the changing fortunes of time. Exercise caution in your business affairs; for the world is full of trickery. But let this not blind you to what virtue there is; many persons strive for high ideals; and everywhere life is full of heroism. Be yourself. Especially, do not feign affection. Neither be cynical about love; for in the face of all aridity & disenchantment it is perennial as the grass. Take kindly the counsel of the years, gracefully surrendering the things of youth. Nurture strength of spirit to shield you in sudden misfortune. But do not distress yourself with imaginings. Many fears are born of fatigue & loneliness. Beyond a wholesome discipline, be gentle with yourself. You are a child of the universe, no less than the trees & the stars; you have a right to be here. And whether or not it is clear to you, no doubt the universe is unfolding as it should. Therefore be at peace with God, whatever you conceive Him to be, and whatever your labors & aspirations, in the noisy confusion of life keep peace with your soul. With all its sham, drudgery & broken dreams, it is still a beautiful world. Be careful. Strive to be happy.

Conclusion

This chapter includes many concepts that can improve the quality of your professional and personal life. They are presented so that you can better understand yourself and the choices open to you.

There is a final message that I want to leave with you. You may find it helpful. It is an inspirational message called Desiderata that is inscribed at Old St. Paul's Church, Baltimore, and dated 1692.

Appendix

Approved Nursing Diagnoses (1980 and 1982)

Airway Clearance, Ineffective

Etiology	Defining characteristics
Decreased energy/fatigue	Abnormal breath sounds (rales [crackles], rhonchi [wheezes])

Tracheobronchial
  Infection
  Obstruction
  Secretion
	Changes in rate or depth of respiration
	Tachypnea
	Cough, effective or ineffective, with or without sputum

Perceptual/cognitive impairment	
Trauma	Cyanosis
	Dyspnea

Comments: New diagnosis. This is a component of the previous nursing diagnosis, respiratory dysfunction.

Bowel Elimination, Alteration in: Constipation

Etiology	Defining characteristics	Other possible defining characteristics
To be developed	Decreased activity level	Abdominal pain
	Frequency less than usual pattern	Appetite impairment
	Hard formed stool	Back pain
	Palpable mass	Headache
	Reported feeling of pressure in rectum	Interference with daily living
	Reported feeling of rectal fullness	Use of laxatives
	Straining at stool	

Comments: This is an updated and refined diagnosis.

Bowel Elimination, Alteration in: Diarrhea

Etiology	Defining characteristics	Other possible defining characteristics
To be developed	Abdominal pain	Changes in color
	Cramping	
	Increased frequency	
	Increased frequency of bowel sounds	
	Loose, liquid stools	
	Urgency	

Comments: This is an updated and refined diagnosis.

(After Kim M, Moritz D [eds]: Classification of Nursing Diagnoses: Proceedings of the Third and Fourth National Conferences, pp 283-319. New York, McGraw-Hill, 1982. By permission of North American Nursing Diagnosis Association)

Bowel Elimination, Alteration in: Incontinence

Etiology	Defining characteristics
To be developed	Involuntary passage of stool

Comments: More specific signs and symptoms still are needed.

Breathing Pattern, Ineffective

Etiology	Defining characteristics
Neuromuscular impairment	Dyspnea
Pain	Shortness of breath
Musculoskeletal impairment	Tachypnea
Perception/cognitive impairment	Fremitus
Anxiety	Abnormal arterial blood gas
Decreased energy or fatigue	Cyanosis
	Cough
	Nasal flaring
	Repiratory depth changes
	Assumption of three-point position
	Pursed-lip breathing/prolonged expiratory phase
	Increased anteroposterior diameter
	Use of accessory muscles
	Altered chest excursion

Comments: New diagnosis. This is a component of the previous nursing diagnosis, respiratory dysfunction.

Cardiac Output, Alteration in: Decreased

Etiology	Defining characteristics	Other possible defining characteristics
To be developed	Variations in blood pressure readings	Change in mental status
	Arrhythmias	Shortness of breath
	Fatigue	Syncope
	Jugular vein distension	Vertigo
	Color changes in skin and mucous membranes	Edema
	Oliguria	Cough
	Decreased peripheral pulses	Frothy sputum
	Cold, clammy skin	Gallop rhythm
	Rales	Weakness
	Dyspnea	
	Orthopnea	
	Restlessness	

Comments: Further development of this diagnosis in the framework of nursing practice is recommended. Debate continues on whether this problem can be independently treated by nurses or whether it falls more into the collaborative realm.

Comfort, Alteration in: Pain

	Defining characteristics	
Etiology	*Subjective*	*Objective*
Injuring agents Biological Chemical Physical Psychological	Communication (verbal or coded) of pain descriptors	Guarding behavior, protective Self-focusing Narrowed focus (altered time perception, withdrawal from social contact, impaired thought process) Distraction behavior (moaning, crying, pacing, seeking out other people or activities, restlessness) Facial mask of pain (eyes lackluster, "beaten look," fixed or scattered movement, grimace) Alteration in muscle tone (may span from listless to rigid) Autonomic responses not seen in chronic stable pain (diaphoresis, blood pressure and pulse rate change, pupillary dilatation, increased or decreased respiratory rate)

Communication, Impaired Verbal

Etiology	Defining characteristics
Decrease in circulation to the brain	Unable to speak dominant language*
Physical barrier, brain tumor, tracheostomy, intubation	Speaks or verbalizes with difficulty*
	Does not or cannot speak*
Anatomical deficit, cleft palate	Stuttering
Psychological barriers, psychosis, lack of stimuli	Slurring
	Difficulty forming words or sentences
Cultural difference	Difficulty expressing thought verbally
Developmental or age related	Inappropriate verbalization
	Dyspnea
	Disorientation

Comments: Needs further development

*Critical defining characteristic. Degree of independent nursing therapy: high.

Coping, Ineffective Individual

Definition: Ineffective coping is the impairment of adaptive behaviors and problem-solving abilities of a person in meeting life's demands and roles.

Etiology	Defining characteristics
Situational crises Maturational crises Personal vulnerability	Verbalization of inability to cope or inability to ask for help* Inability to meet role expectations Inability to meet basic needs Inability to problem solve* Alteration in societal participation Destructive behavior toward self or others Inappropriate use of defense mechanisms Change in usual communication patterns Verbal manipulation High illness rate High rate of accidents

Comments: Further development is needed in the defining characteristics and critical characteristics. Changed and refined from previous nursing diagnosis, coping patterns; individual, maladaptive.

*Critical defining characteristic.

Coping, Ineffective Family: Compromised

Definition: A usually supportive primary person (family member or close friend) is providing insufficient, ineffective, or compromised support, comfort, assistance, or encouragement which may be needed by the client to manage or master adaptive tasks related to his or her health challenge.

Etiology	Defining characteristics Subjective	Objective
Inadequate or incorrect information or understanding by a primary person Temporary preoccupation by a significant person who is trying to manage emotional conflicts and personal suffering and is unable to perceive or act effectively in regard to client's needs Temporary family disorganization and role changes Other situational or developmental crises or situations the significant person may be facing The client providing little support in turn for the primary person Prolonged disease or disability progression that exhausts the supportive capacity of significant people	Client expresses or confirms a concern or complaint about significant other response to his or her health problem Significant person describes preoccuption with personal reactions, e.g., fear, anticipatory grief, guilt, anxiety, to client's illness, disability, or to other situational or developmental crises Significant person describes or confirms an inadequate understanding or knowledge base that interferes with effective assistive or supportive behaviors.	Significant person attempts assistive or supportive behaviors with less than satisfactory results Significant person withdraws or enters into limited or temporary personal communication with the client at time of need Significant person displays protective behavior disproportionate (too little or too much) to the client's abilities or need for autonomy

Comments: Differential diagnosing: the coping strategies of family members addressed in this diagnosis are basically constructive in nature. The constructive but compromised response and intent fall short of their realistic potential for effective situation or crisis management. Changed and refined from previous nursing diagnosis, coping patterns, ineffective family.

Degree of independent nursing therapy: high.

Coping, Ineffective Family: Disabling

Definition: The behavior of a significant person (family member or other primary person) disables his or her own capacities and the client's capacities to effectively address tasks essential to either person's adaptation to the health challenge.

Etiology	Defining characteristics
Significant person with chronically unexpressed feelings of guilt, anxiety, hostility, despair, and so on	Neglectful care of the client in regard to basic human needs or illness treatment
Dissonant discrepancy of coping styles being used to deal with the adaptive tasks by the significant person and client or among significant people	Distortion of reality regarding the client's health problem, including extreme denial about its existence or severity
Highly ambivalent family relationships	Intolerance
Arbitrary handling of a family's resistance to treatment that tends to solidify defensiveness as it fails to deal adequately with underlying anxiety	Rejection
	Abandonment
	Desertion
	Carrying on usual routines, disregarding client's needs
	Psychosomaticism
	Taking on illness signs of client
	Decisions and actions by family that are detrimental to economic or social well-being
	Agitation, depression, aggression, hostility
	Impaired restructuring of a meaningful life for self, impaired individualization, prolonged overconcern for client
	Neglectful relationships with other family members
	Client's development of helpless, inactive dependence

Comments: Regarding the family member's disabling coping response to the client's health challenge, one can describe a family member's response as disabling if it involves short-term coping behaviors that are highly detrimental to the welfare of the client or the significant person. In addition, chronically disabling patterns by a primary person are described as continued use of selected coping skills that have interrupted the person's longer-term capacity to receive, store, or organize information or to react in regard to it. This diagnosis is changed and refined from the previous nursing diagnosis, coping patterns, ineffective family.

Degree of independent nursing therapy: moderate to high.

Coping, Family: Potential for Growth

Definition: The family member has effectively managed adaptive tasks involved with the client's health challenge and is exhibiting desire and readiness for enhanced health and growth in regard to self and in relation to the client.

Etiology	Defining characteristics
The person's basic needs are sufficiently gratified and adaptive tasks effectively addressed to enable goals of self-actualization to surface	The family member attempts to describe growth impact of crisis on his or her own values, priorities, goals, or relationships
	Family member is moving in direction of health-promoting and enriching life style that supports and monitors maturational processes, audits and negotiates treatment programs, and generally chooses experiences that optimize wellness
	Individual expresses interest in making contact on a one-to-one basis or on a mutual-aid group basis with another person who has experienced a similar situation

Comments: New diagnosis

Degree of independent nursing therapy: high.

Diversional Activity, Deficit

Etiology	Defining characteristics
Environmental lack of diversional activity	Patient's statements regarding
Long-term hospitalization	Boredom
Frequent, lengthy treatments	Wish there were something to do, to read, and so on
	Usual hobbies cannot be undertaken in hospital

Comments: New nursing diagnosis.

Fear

Definition: Fear is a feeling of dread related to an identifiable source that the person validates.

Etiology	Defining characteristics
To be developed	Ability to identify object of fear

Comments: In extensive discussion, the group agreed to accept the diagnosis of fear as a nursing diagnosis. Some group members expressed concern over the fact that fear may be a symptom of ineffective coping and others. The defining characteristics and etiologies of fear require further development and refining. As the diagnosis is further developed, it may be discovered that fear is not an appropriate nursing diagnosis and is a symptom analogous to the symptom of anxiety.

The following nursing diagnoses related to fear developed in 1973 were deleted: functional fear, mild; functional fear, moderate; functional fear, severe; functional fear, panic; nonfunctional fear, mild; nonfunctional fear, moderate; nonfunctional fear, severe; nonfunctional fear, panic. The nursing diagnosis of anxiety was also subsumed under fear in 1980.

Fluid Volume Deficit, Actual (1)

Etiology	Defining characteristics	Other possible defining characteristics
Failure of regulatory mechanisms	Dilute urine	Possible weight gain
	Increased urine output	Hypotension
	Sudden weight loss	Decreased venous filling
		Increased pulse rate
		Decreased skin turgor
		Decreased pulse volume and pressure
		Increased body temperature
		Dry skin
		Dry mucous membranes
		Hemoconcentration
		Weakness
		Edema
		Thirst

Comments: Consider further development as subcategories of alterations in nutrition.

Fluid Volume Deficit, Actual (2)

Etiology	Defining characteristics	Other possible defining characteristics
Active loss	Decreased urine output	Hypotension
	Concentrated urine	Thirst
	Output greater than intake	Increased pulse rate
	Sudden weight loss	Decreased skin turgor
	Decreased venous filling	Decreased pulse volume and pressure
	Hemoconcentration	Change in mental state
	Increased serum sodium	Increased body temperature
		Dry skin
		Dry mucous membranes
		Weakness

Comments: Consider further development as subcategories of alteration in nutrition.

Fluid Volume Deficit, Potential

Etiology	Defining characteristics
Extremes of age	Increased output
Extremes of weight	Urinary frequency
Excessive losses through normal routes, *e.g.*, diarrhea	Thirst
Loss of fluid through abnormal routes, *e.g.*, indwelling tubes	Altered intake
Deviations affecting access to, intake of, or absorption of fluids, *e.g.*, physical immobility	
Factors influencing fluid needs, *e.g.*, hypermetabolic states	
Knowledge deficiency related to fluid volume	
Medications, *e.g.*, diuretics	

Comments: Etiologies listed are high risk that could lead to the diagnosis.

Gas Exchange, Impaired

Etiology	Defining characteristics
Ventilation, perfusion imbalance	Confusion
	Somnolence
	Restlessness
	Irritability
	Inability to move secretions
	Hypercapnea
	Hypoxia

Comments: This is a new diagnosis, a component of the previous nursing diagnosis, respiratory dysfunction.

Grieving, Anticipatory

Etiology	Defining characteristics	
To be developed	Potential loss of significant object	Choked feelings
	Expression of distress at potential loss	Changes in eating habits
	Denial of potential loss	Alterations in sleep patterns
	Guilt	Alterations in activity level
	Anger	Altered libido
	Sorrow	Altered communication patterns

Grieving, Dysfunctional

Etiology	Defining characteristics
Actual or perceived object loss (object loss is used in the broadest sense); objects include people, possessions, a job, status, home, ideals, parts and processes of the body	Verbal expression of distress at loss
	Denial of loss
	Expression of guilt
	Expression of unresolved issues
	Anger
	Sadness
	Crying
	Difficulty in expressing loss

	Alterations in
	    Eating habits
	    Sleep patterns
	    Dream patterns
	    Activity level
	    Libido

	Idealization of lost object
	Reliving of past experiences
	Interference with life functioning
	Developmental regression
	Labile affect
	Alterations in concentration or pursuits of tasks

Comments: Changed and refined from previous nursing diagnosis, grieving.

Home Maintenance Management, Impaired

Definition: The client is unable to independently maintain a safe, growth-promoting immediate environment.

	Defining characteristics	
Etiology	Subjective	Objective
Individual/family member disease or injury	Household members express difficulty in maintaining their home in a comfortable fashion*	Disorderly surroundings
Insufficient family organization or planning	Household requests assistance with home maintenance*	Unwashed or unavailable cooking equipment, clothes, or linens*
Insufficient finances	Household members describe outstanding debts or financial crises*	Accumulation of dirt, food wastes, or hygienic wastes*
Unfamiliarity with neighborhood resources		Offensive odors
Impaired cognitive or emotion functioning		Inappropriate household temperature
Lack of knowledge		Overtaxes family members, e.g., exhausted anxious family members*
Lack of role modeling		Lack of necessary equipment or aids
Inadequate support systems		Presence of vermin or rodents
		Repeated hygienic disorders, infestations, or infections*

Comments: Changed and refined from previous diagnosis, functional performance, variations in home maintenance management.

*Critical defining characteristic.

Injury: Potential for

Etiology

Definition: Interactive conditions between individual environment that impose a risk to the defensive and adaptive resources of the individual.

Internal factors, host	External environment
Biological	Biological
Chemical	Chemical
Physiological	Physiological
Psychological perception	Psychological
Developmental	People or Provider

Defining characteristics

Internal	*External*
Biochemical	Biological
Regulatory function	Immunization level of community
Sensory dysfunction	Microorganism
Integrative dysfunction	Chemical
Effector dysfunction	Pollutants
Tissue hypoxia	Poisons
Malnutrition	Drugs
Immune-autoimmune	Pharmaceutical agents
Abnormal blood profile	Alcohol
Leukocytosis or leukopenia	Caffeine
Altered clotting factors	Nicotine
Thrombocytopenia	Preservatives
Sickle cell	Cosmetics and dyes
Thalassemia	Nutrients (vitamins, food types)
Decreased hemoglobin	Physical
Physical	Design, structure, and arrangement of
Broken skin	community, building, or equipment
Altered mobility	Mode of transport or transportation
Developmental	Nosocomial agents
Age	People or Provider
Physiological	Nosocomial agent
Psychosocial	Staffing patterns
Psychological	Cognitive, affective, and psychomotor factors
Affective	
Orientation	

Comments: Etiological factors depend on the epidemiological model. The outline of characteristics is provided as a framework for future task work; it is not considered to be all inclusive. Further development is needed. This diagnosis has three subcomponents, A, B, and C.*

A. Poisoning, Potential for

Definition: The client has accentuated risk of accidental exposure to or ingestion of drugs or dangerous products in doses sufficient to cause poisoning.

B. Suffocation, Potential for

Definition: The client has accentuated risk of accidental suffocation (inadequate air available for inhalation).

C. Trauma, Potential for

Definition: The client has accentuated risk of accidental tissue injury, *e.g.*, wounds, burns, fractures.
Comments: Major work needed; changed and refined from previous diagnosis, injury: susceptibility to hazard.

*For further description of defining characteristics see Kim M, Moritz D (eds): Classification of Nursing Diagnoses: Proceedings of the Third and Fourth National Conferences. New York, McGraw-Hill, 1982.

Knowledge Deficit

Etiology*	Defining characteristics
Lack of exposure	Verbalization of the problem
Lack of recall	Inaccurate follow through or instruction
Information misinterpretation	Inadequate performance of test
Cognitive limitation	Inappropriate or exaggerated behaviors, *e.g.*, hysterical, hostile, agitated, apathetic
Lack of interest in learning	
Unfamiliarity with information resources	

Comments: Changed from previous nursing diagnosis, knowledge, lack of (1978).

Degree of independent nursing therapy: high.
*From the survey done by Ann Reilly and Claire Bennett, during the fourth national conference, on the interpretation of etiological statements regarding the diagnosis of knowledge deficit.

Mobility, Impaired Physical

Etiology	Defining characteristics
Intolerance to activity and decreased strength and endurance	Inability to move purposefully within the physical environment, including bed mobility, transfer, and ambulation
Pain and discomfort	
Perceptual and cognitive impairment	Reluctance to attempt movement
Musculoskeletal impairment	Limited range of motion
Depression and severe anxiety	Decreased muscle strength, control, or mass
Neuromuscular impairment	Imposed restrictions of movement, including mechanical, medical protocol
	Impaired coordination

Comments: Use of a scale when patients are rated from dependence to independence is suggested. The diagnosis has been changed and expanded from the previous diagnosis, mobility, impaired physical.

Suggested Code for Functional Level Classification

0   Completely independent
1   Requires use of equipment or device
2   Requires help from another person for assistance, supervision, or teaching
3   Requires help from another person and equipment or device
4   Is dependent, does not participate in activity

(After Jones, E, et al: Patient Classification for Long-Term Care: Users' Manual, DHEW pub. no. HRA-74-3107. Washington, DC, U.S. Government Printing Office, 1974)

Noncompliance (Specify)

Definition: Noncompliance is a person's informed decision not to adhere to a therapeutic recommendation.

Etiology	Defining characteristics

Patient value system
  Health beliefs
  Cultural influences
  Spiritual values
Client-provider relationships
	Behavior indicative of failure to adhere by direct observation, statements by patient or significant others*
	Objective tests (physiological measures, detection of markers)
	Evidence of development of complications
	Evidence of exacerbation of symptoms
	Failure to keep appointments
	Failure to progress

Comments: Further development and refinement of all areas are needed.

*Critical defining characteristic.

Nutrition, Alterations in: Less Than Body Requirements

Etiology	Defining characteristics	
Inability to ingest or digest food or absorb nutrients due to biological, psychological, or economic factors	Loss of weight with adequate food intake 20% or more under ideal body weight Reported inadequate food intake less than recommended daily allowance (RDA)* Weakness of muscles required for swallowing or mastication Reported or evident lack of food Lack of interest in food Perceived inability to ingest food Aversion to eating Reported altered taste sensation Satiety immediately after ingesting food	Abdominal pain with or without pathology Sore, inflamed buccal cavity Capillary fragility Abdominal cramping Diarrhea or steatorrhea Hyperactive bowel sounds Pale conjunctive and mucous membranes Poor muscle tone Excessive loss of hair Lack of information, misinformation Misconceptions

*Critical defining characteristics.

Nutrition, Alterations in: Potential for More Than Body Requirements

Etiology	Defining characteristics
Hereditary predisposition	Reported or observed obesity in one or both parents*
Excessive energy intake during late gestational life, early infancy and adolescence	Rapid transition across growth percentiles in infants or children*
	Reported use of solid food as major food source before 5 months of age
Frequent, closely spaced pregnancies	Observed use of food as reward or comfort measure
Dysfunctional psychological conditioning in relationship to food	Reported or observed higher baseline weight at beginning of each pregnancy

Membership in lower socioeconomic group	Dysfunctional eating patterns
	  Pairing food with other activities
	  Concentrating food intake at end of day
	  Eating in response to external cues such as time of day, social situation
	  Eating in response to internal cues other than hunger, e.g., anxiety

*Critical defining characteristic.

Nutrition, Alterations in: More Than Body Requirements

Etiology	Defining characteristics
Excessive intake in relationship to metabolic need	Weight 10% over ideal for height and frame
	Weight 20% over ideal for height and frame*
	Triceps skin fold greater than 15 mm in men and 25 mm in women*
	Sedentary activity level

	Reported or observed dysfunctional eating patterns
	  Pairing food with other activities
	  Concentrating food intake at end of day
	  Eating in response to external cues, e.g., time of day, social situation
	  Eating in response to internal cues other than hunger, e.g., anxiety

*Critical defining characteristic.

Parenting, Alterations in: Actual or Potential

Defintion: Parenting is the ability of a nurturing figure(s) to create an environment that promotes the optimum growth and development of another human being. It is important to state as a preface to this diagnosis that adjustment to parenting in general is a normal maturational process that elicits nursing behaviors for prevention of potential problems and health problems.

Etiology	Defining characteristics
Lack of available role model	For actual and potential lack of parental attachment behaviors†
Ineffective role model	Inappropriate visual, tactile, auditory stimulation
Physical and psychosocial abuse of nurturing figure	Negative identification of infant or child's characteristics
Lack of support between or from significant other(s)	Negative attachment of meanings to infant or child's characteristics
Unmet social or emotional maturation needs of parenting figures	Constant verbalization if disappointed in gender or physical characteristics of the infant or child
Interruption in bonding process, *i.e.*, maternal, paternal, other	Verbalization of resentment toward the infant or child
Unrealistic expectation for self, infant, partner	Verbalization of role inadequacy
Perceived threat to own survival, physical and emotional	Inattentive to infant or child's needs*
	Verbal disgust at body functions of infant or child
Mental or physical illness	Noncompliance with health appointments for self, infant, or child
Presence of stress: financial, legal, recent crisis, cultural move	Inappropriate caretaking behaviors (toilet training, sleep or rest, feeding)*
Lack of knowledge	Inappropriate or inconsistent discipline practices
Limited cognitive functioning	Frequent accidents
Lack of role identity	Frequent illness
Lack of or inappropriate response of child to relationship	Growth and development lag in the child
Multiple pregnancies	History of child abuse or abandonment by primary caretaker*
	Verbalizes desire to have child call himself/ herself by first name versus traditional cultural tendencies
	Child receives care from multiple caretakers without consideration for his or her needs
	Compulsively seeking role approval from others
	For actual
	Abandonment†
	Runaway†
	Verbalization cannot control child†
	Evidence of physical and psychological trauma†

Comments: These diagnoses were not acted on in 1980 except for the recommendation that they be developed further. There is a need to differentiate actual and potential. Further research is needed to identify critical data.

*Critical factors.
†Highly critical factors.

Rape-Trauma Syndrome

Definition: Rape is forced, violent sexual penetration against the victim's will and without the victim's will and consent. The trauma syndrome that develops from this attack or attempted attack includes an acute phase of disorganization of the victim's life style and a long-term process of reorganization of life style. This syndrome includes the following three subcomponents: A, B, and C

A. Rape, Trauma

Defining characteristics	
Acute phase	*Long-term phase*

Emotional reactions
  Anger
  Embarrassment
  Fear of physical violence and death
  Humiliation
  Revenge
  Self-blame
 	
Multiple physical symptoms
  Gastrointestinal irritability
  Genitourinary discomfort
  Muscle tension
  Sleep pattern disturbance
	Changes in life style (changes in residence, dealing with repetitive nightmares and phobias, seeking family support, seeking social network support)

B. Compound Reaction

Defining characteristics

All defining characteristics listed under rape-trauma

Reactivated symptoms of such previous conditions, *i.e.*, physical illness, psychiatric illness

Reliance on alcohol or drugs

C. Silent Reaction

Abrupt changes in relationships with men

Increase in nightmares

Increasing anxiety during interview, *i.e.*, blocking of associations, long periods of silence, minor stuttering, physical distress

Marked changes in sexual behavior

No verbalization of the occurrence of rape

Sudden onset of phobic reactions

Self-Care Deficit: Feeding, Bathing/Hygiene, Dressing/Grooming, Toileting

Etiology

Intolerance to activity, decreased strength and endurance

Pain, discomfort

Perceptual or cognitive impairment

Neuromuscular impairment

Musculoskeletal impairment

Depression, severe anxiety

A. Self-Feeding Deficit (level 0 to 4)†

Defining characteristics

Inability to bring food from a receptacle to the mouth

B. Self-Bathing and Hygiene Deficit (level 0 to 4)†

Defining characteristics

Inability to wash body or body parts*

Inability to obtain or get to water source

Inability to regulate temperature or flow

C. Self-Dressing and Grooming Deficits (Level 0 to 4)†

Defining characteristics

Impaired ability to put on or take off necessary items of clothing*

Impaired ability to obtain or replace articles of clothing

Impaired ability to fasten clothing

Inability to maintain appearance at a satisfactory level

D. Self-Toileting Deficit (Level 0 to 4)†

Etiology (broad categories)	Defining characteristics
Impaired transfer ability	Unable to get to toilet or commode*
Impaired mobility status	Unable to manipulate clothing for toileting*
Intolerance to activity, decreased strength	
Pain, discomfort	Unable to carry out proper toilet hygiene*
Perceptual or cognitive impairment	
Neuromuscular impairment	Unable to flush toilet or empty commode
Musculoskeletal impairment	Unable to sit on or rise from toilet or commode*
Depression, severe anxiety	

*Critical defining characteristic.
†For definition of code see mobility, impaired physical.

Self-Concepts, Disturbance in: Body Image, Self-Esteem, Role Performance, Personal Identity

Definition: A disturbance in self-concept is a disruption in the way one perceives one's body image, self-esteem, role performance, and/or personal identity. These four subcomponents, in turn, have their own etiologies and defining characteristics (Figure 1).

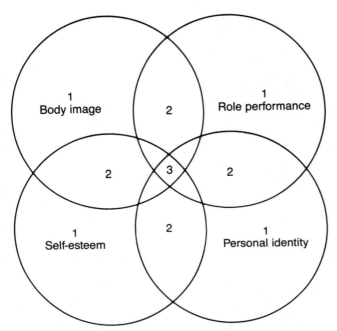

Defining characteristics of a disturbance in self-concepts are (1) critical characteristic or cluster of characteristics specific to the subcategory, (2) characteristic or cluster of characteristics shared by subcategories but not common to all subcategories, (3) characteristic or cluster of characteristics common to all subcategories.

A. Body Image, Disturbance in

Etiology	Defining characteristics
Biophysical	Either A or B must be present to justify the diagnosis of body image, alteration in:
Cognitive perceptual	A. Verbal response to actual or perceived change in structure or function*
Psychosocial	
Cultural or spiritual	B. Nonverbal response to actual or perceived change in structure or function*
	The following clinical manifestations may be used to validate the presence of A or B

Objective	Subjective
Missing body part	Verbalization of
Actual change in structure or function	Change in life styles
	Fear of rejection or of reaction by others

*Critical defining characteristics.

(continued)

A. Body Image, Disturbance in
(continued)

Objective	Subjective
Not looking at body part	Focus on past strength, function, or appearance
Hiding or over-exposing body part (intentional or unintentional)	Negative feelings about body
	Feelings of helplessness, hopelessness, or powerlessness
Trauma to nonfunctioning part	Preoccupation with change or loss
Change in social involvement	
Change in ability to estimate spatial relationship of body to environment	Emphasis on remaining strengths, heightened achievement
	Extension of body boundary to incorporate environmental objects
	Personalization of part or loss by name
	Depersonalization of part or loss by impersonal pronouns
	Refusal to verify actual change

Degree of independent nursing therapy. This may be related to etiology:
Biophysical: low degree of nursing independence
Psychosocial: medium to high degree of nursing independence
Cognitive perceptual: high degree of nursing independence
Cultural spiritual: medium to high degree of nursing independence

It may be possible to identify high-risk populations, e.g.,
Missing parts
Dependence on machine
Significance of body part or functioning with regard to age, sex, developmental level, or basic human needs
Physical change due to biochemical agents (drugs)
Physical trauma or mutilation
Pregnancy or maturational changes

B. Self-Esteem, Disturbance in

Etiology	Defining characteristics
To be developed	Inability to accept positive reinforcement
	Lack of follow through
	Nonparticipation in therapy
	Not taking responsibility for self-care (self-neglect)
	Self-destructive behavior
	Lack of eye contact

C. Role Performance, Disturbance in

Etiology	Defining characteristics
To be developed	Change in self-perception of role
	Denial of role
	Change in others' perception of role
	Conflict in roles
	Change in physical capacity to resume role
	Lack of knowledge of role
	Change in usual patterns or responsibility

(continued)

D. Personal Identity, Disturbance in

Definition: Inability to distinguish between self and nonself.

Etiology	Defining characteristics
To be developed	To be developed

Comments: Change from the previous diagnosis, self-concept, alteration in. Further development in the following areas is recommended:

1. Define and develop each of the four subsets of self-esteem, body image, role performance, and personal identity.

2. Develop etiologies and characteristics for the four subset areas.

3. Identify most commonly shared characteristics of the four subset areas.

4. Use previously documented work (as included in this section) as a basis for further development.

5. Consider including such components as "group relations, noneffective" and "sexuality."

Sensory-Perceptual Alterations: Visual, Auditory, Kinesthetic, Gustatory, Tactile, Olfactory Perception

Etiology	Defining characteristics	Other possible defining characteristics
Altered environmental stimuli, excessive or insufficient	Disoriented in time, in place, or with persons	Complaints of fatigue
Altered sensory reception, transmission or integration	Altered abstraction	Alteration in posture
	Altered conceptualization	Change in muscular tension
Chemical alterations, endogenous (electrolyte), exogenous (drugs)	Change in problem-solving abilities	Inappropriate responses
Psychological stress	Reported or measured change in sensory acuity	Hallucinations
	Change in behavior pattern	
	Anxiety	
	Apathy	
	Change in usual response to stimuli	
	Indication of body-image alteration	
	Restlessness	
	Irritability	
	Altered communication patterns	

Comments: Etiologies and defining characteristics are too broad and general, since they relate to the diagnosis, sensory-perceptual alterations. These must be differentiated and further developed to be specific for each of six subcomponents.

Sexual Dysfunction

Etiology	Defining characteristics

Biopsychosocial alteration of sexuality
  Ineffectual or absent role models
  Physical abuse
  Psychosocial abuse, *e.g.,* harmful
  relationships
  Vulnerability
  Misinformation or lack of
  knowledge
  Values conflict
  Lack of privacy
  Lack of significant other
  Altered body structure or function:
  pregnancy, recent childbirth,
  drugs, surgery, anomalies,
  disease process, trauma,
  radiation
	Verbalization of problem
	Alterations in achieving perceived sex role
	Actual or perceived limitation imposed by disease or therapy
	Conflicts involving values
	Alteration in achieving sexual satisfaction
	Inability to achieve desired satisfaction
	Seeking confirmation of desirability
	Alteration in relationship with significant other
	Change of interest in self and others

Comments: Changed from previous diagnosis, sexuality, alterations in pattern of. Further development and refinement are required in keeping with the change of the diagnostic terminology. Etiology and defining characteristics of the previous diagnosis are presented for this task.

Skin Integrity, Impairment of: Actual

Etiology		Defining characteristics
External (environmental)	*Internal (somatic)*	
Hyperthermia or hypothermia	Medication	Disruption of skin surface
Chemical substance	Altered nutritional state, *e.g.,* obesity, emaciation	Destruction of skin layers

Mechanical factors
  Shearing forces
  Pressure
  Restraint
	Altered metabolic state
	Altered circulation
	Altered sensation
		Invasion of body structures

Radiation	Altered pigmentation	
Physical immobilization	Skeletal prominence	
Humidity	Developmental factors	
	Immunological deficit	
	Alterations in turgor (change in elasticity)	

Comments: Group recommended consideration of a universal grading system for impaired skin integrity (1978). There were no changes made in 1980; further development was recommended.

Skin Integrity, Impairment of: Potential

Etiology	Defining characteristics*	
	External (environmental)	Internal (somatic)
Not applicable	Hypothermia or hyperthermia	Medication
	Chemical substance	Alterations in nutritional state, e.g., obesity, emaciation
	Mechanical factors	
	Shearing forces	Altered metabolic state
	Pressure	Altered circulation
	Restraint	Altered sensation
	Radiation	Altered pigmentation
	Physical immobilization	Skeletal prominence
	Excretions or secretions	Developmental factors
	Humidity	Alterations in skin turgor (change in elasticity)
		Psychogenic
		Immunologic

Comments: This diagnosis remains the same as that of 1978, but the group recommended further development.

*Presence of one or more risk factors (something that increases the possibility of a condition's occurring).

Sleep Pattern Disturbance

Definition: Disruption of sleep time that causes a patient discomfort or interferes with the patient's desired life style.

Etiology	Defining characteristics
Sensory alterations	Verbal complaints of difficulty falling asleep*
Internal factors	Awakening earlier or later than desired*
Illness	
Psychological stress	Interrupted sleep*
External factors	Verbal complaints of not feeling well rested*
Environmental changes	Changes in behavior and performance
Social cues	Increased irritability
	Restlessness
	Disorientation
	Lethargy
	Listlessness
	Physical signs
	Mild, fleeting nystagmus
	Slight hand tremor
	Ptosis of eyelid
	Expressionless face
	Thick speech with mispronunciation and incorrect words
	Dark circles under eyes
	Frequent yawning
	Changes in posture

Comments: Changed from previous diagnosis, sleep-rest activity, dysrhythm of.

*Critical defining characteristics.

Spiritual Distress (Distress of the Human Spirit)

Definition: Distress of the human spirit is a disruption in the life principle that pervades a person's entire being and that integrates and transcends his or her biological and psychosocial nature.

Etiology	Defining characteristics
Separation from religious or cultural ties Challenged belief and value system, e.g., due to moral or ethical implications of therapy because of intense suffering	Expresses concern with meaning of life or death or belief systems*
	Anger toward God
	Questions meaning of suffering
	Verbalizes inner conflict about beliefs
	Verbalizes concern about relationship with deity
	Questions meaning for own existence
	Unable to participate in usual religious practices
	Seeks spiritual assistance
	Questions moral and ethical implication of therapeutic regimen
	Gallows humor
	Displacement of anger toward religious representatives
	Description of nightmares and sleep disturbances
	Alteration in behavior or mood evidenced by anger, crying, withdrawal, preoccupation, anxiety, hostility, apathy

Comments: Changed from previous diagnoses of spirituality: spiritual concern; spirituality: spiritual distress; spirituality: spiritual despair. Further refinement and development of the defining and critical characteristics are needed.

*Critical defining characteristic.

Thought Processes, Alteration in

Etiology	Defining characteristics	Other possible defining characteristics
To be determined	Inaccurate interpretation of environment	Inappropriate or nonreality-based thinking
	Cognitive dissonance	
	Distractibility	
	Memory deficit or problems	
	Egocentricity	
	Hypervigilance or hypovigilance	

Comments: Previous diagnosis, consciousness, altered level of, is subsumed under this diagnosis. This diagnosis needs further development.

(After Fish S, Shelly JA: Spiritual Care: The Nurse's Role. Downers Grove, IL, InterVarsity Press, 1978)

Tissue Perfusion, Alteration in: Cerebral, Cardiopulmonary, Renal, Gastrointestinal, Peripheral

Etiology

Interruption of flow, arterial

Interruption of flow, venous

Exchange problems

Hypervolemia

Hypovolemia

Defining characteristics with estimated sensitivities and specificities

Characteristic	Chances defining characteristic will be present given diagnosis	Chances defining characteristic not explained by any other diagnosis
Skin temperature: cold extremities	High	Low
Skin color		
Dependent, blue or purple	Moderate	Low
Pale on elevation, and color does not return on lowering leg*	High	High
Diminished arterial pulsations*	High	High
Skin quality: shining	High	Low
Lack of lanugo	High	Moderate
Round scars covered with atrophied skin		
Gangrene	Low	High
Slow-growing, dry, thick, brittle nails	High	Moderate
Claudication	Moderate	High
Blood pressure changes in extremities		
Bruits	Moderate	Moderate
Slow healing of lesions	High	Low

Comments: Further work and development are required for the cerebral, renal, and gastrointestinal subcomponents.

*Critical defining characteristic.

Urinary Elimination, Alteration in Patterns

Etiology	Defining characteristics

Multiple casualty
  Anatomical obstruction
  Sensory motor impairment
  Urinary tract infection
	Dysuria
	Frequency
	Hesitancy
	Incontinence
	Nocturia
	Retention
	Urgency

Comments: This category pertains only to urine elimination, not urine formation. Polyuria, oliguria, and anuria are indicative of kidney function, and the nurse may not be able to alter this with nursing intervention. The nurse may also need to add "alterations in pattern not otherwise specified." This diagnosis has been changed and refined from the previous diagnosis, urinary elimination, impairment of: alteration in patterns.

Violence, Potential for (Self-Directed or Directed at Others)

Etiology	Defining characteristics	Other defining characteristics*
Antisocial character	Body language Clenched fists, facial expressions, rigid posture, tautness indicating intense effort to control	Increasing anxiety levels
Battered women		Fear of self or others
Catatonic excitement		Inability to verbalize feelings
Child abuse	Hostile threatening verbalizations; boasting of prior abuse to others	Repetition of verbalizations: continued complaints, requests, and demands
Manic excitement		
Organic brain syndrome	Increased motor activity, pacing, excitement, irritability, agitation	Anger
Panic states		Provocative behavior, e.g., argumentative, dissatisfied, overreactive, hypersensitive
Rape reactions	Overt and aggressive acts; goal-directed destruction of objects in environment	
Suicidal behavior		Vulnerable self-esteem
Temporal lobe epilepsy	Possession of destructive means, e.g., gun, knife, weapon	Depression (specifically, active, aggressive, suicidal acts)
Toxic reactions to medication	Rage	
	Self-destructive behavior or active aggressive suicidal acts	
	Substance abuse or withdrawal	
	Suspicion of others, paranoid ideation, delusions, hallucinations	

*From doctoral dissertation of Patricia Clunn.

New Diagnoses Accepted for Clinical Testing at 1982 Conference

Activity Intolerance

Etiology	Defining characteristics
Bedrest and immobility	1. Verbal report of fatigue or weakness*
Generalized weakness	2. Abnormal heart rate or blood pressure response to activity
Sedentary life style	3. Exertional discomfort or dyspnea
Imbalance between oxygen supply/demand	4. Electrocardiographic changes reflecting arrythmias or ischemia

*Critical defining characteristic.

Anxiety

Definition: A vague, uneasy feeling, the source of which is often nonspecific or unknown to the individual.

Etiology	Defining characteristics
Unconscious conflict about essential values and goals of life	I. *Subjective*
	1. Increased tension
Threat to self-concept	2. Apprehension
Threat of death	3. Painful and persistent increased helplessness
Threat to or change in health status	
Threat to or change in socio-economic status	4. Uncertainty
	5. Fearful
Threat to or change in role functioning	6. Scared
Threat to or change in environment	7. Regretful
Threat to or change in interaction patterns	8. Overexcited
Situational/maturational crises	9. Rattled
Interpersonal transmission/contagion of unmet needs	10. Distressed
	11. Jittery
	12. Feelings of inadequacy
	13. Shakiness
	14. Fear of unspecific consequences
	15. Expressed concerns about change in life events
	16. Worried
	17. Anxious
	II. *Objective*
	1. Sympathetic stimulation, such as cardiovascular excitation, superficial vasoconstriction, pupil dilatation*
	2. Restlessness

*Critical defining characteristic.
(*continued*)

(After Kim M, McFarland G, McLane A [eds]: Classification of Nursing Diagnoses: Proceedings of the Fifth National Conference. New York, CV Mosby, [in press]. By permission of North American Nursing Diagnosis Association)

Anxiety
(continued)

Etiology	Defining characteristics
	3. Insomnia
	4. Glancing about
	5. Poor eye contact
	6. Trembling or hand tremors
	7. Extraneous movement (foot shuffling, hand or arm movements)
	8. Facial tension
	9. Voice quivering
	10. Focus "self"
	11. Increased wariness
	12. Increased perspiration

Family Processes, Alteration in

Etiology	Defining characteristics
Situation transition or crises	1. Family system unable to meet physical needs for its members
Development transition or crisis	2. Family system unable to meet emotional needs of its members
	3. Family system unable to meet spiritual needs of its members
	4. Parents do not demonstrate respect for each other's views on child rearing practices
	5. Inability to express or accept wide range of feelings
	6. Inability to express or accept feelings of members
	7. Family unable to meet security needs of its members
	8. Inability of the family members to relate to each other for mutual growth and maturation
	9. Family uninvolved in community activities
	10. Inability to accept or receive help appropriately
	11. Rigidity in function and roles
	12. Family does not demonstrate respect for individuality and autonomy of its members
	13. Family inability to adapt to change or deal with traumatic experience constructively
	14. Family fails to accomplish current or past developmental task
	15. Unhealthy family decision-making process
	16. Failure to send and receive clear messages
	17. Inappropriate boundary maintenance
	18. Inappropriate or poorly communicated family rules, rituals, symbols
	19. Unexamined family myths
	20. Inappropriate level and direction of energy

Fluid Volume, Alteration in: Excess

Etiology	Defining characteristics
Compromised regulatory mechanism	1. Edema
Excess fluid intake	2. Effusion
Excess sodium intake	3. Anasarca
	4. Weight gain
	5. Shortness of breath, orthopnea
	6. Intake greater than output
	7. S_3 heart sound
	8. Pulmonary congestion: chest x-ray film
	9. Abnormal breath sounds: crackles (rales)
	10. Change in respiratory pattern
	11. Change in mental status
	12. Decreased hemoglobin and hematocrit
	13. Blood pressure changes
	14. Central venous pressure changes
	15. Pulmonary artery pressure changes
	16. Jugular vein distention
	17. Positive hepatojugular reflex
	18. Oliguria
	19. Specific gravity changes
	20. Azotemia
	21. Altered electrolytes
	22. Restlessness and anxiety

Health Maintenance Alteration

Definition: Inability to identify, manage, and/or seek out help to maintain health.

Etiology	Defining characteristics
Lack of, or significant alteration in, communication skills (written, verbal, or gestural)	1. Demonstrated lack of knowledge regarding basic health practices
Lack of ability to make deliberate and thoughtful judgments; perceptual or cognitive impairment; complete or partial lack of gross or fine motor skills	2. Demonstrated lack of adaptive behaviors to internal or external environmental changes
Ineffective individual coping/dysfunctional grieving	3. Reported or observed inability to take responsibility for meeting basic health practices in any or all functional pattern areas
Unachieved developmental tasks	4. History of lack of health seeking behavior
Ineffective family coping: disabling spiritual distress	5. Expressed client interest in improving health behaviors
Lack of material resources	6. Reported or observed lack of equipment or financial or other resources
	7. Reported or observed impairment of personal support system

Oral Mucous Membrane, Alterations in

Etiology	Defining characteristics
Pathological conditions, such as oral cavity radiation to head or neck dehydration	1. Oral pain or discomfort
	2. Coated tongue
Trauma	3. Xerostomia (dry mouth)
Chemical (*e.g.,* acidic foods, drugs, noxious agents, alcohol)	4. Stomatitis
Mechanical (*e.g.,* endotracheal or nasogastric, ill-fitting dentures, braces, tubes, surgery in the oral cavity)	5. Oral lesions or ulcers
	6. Lack of or decreased salivation
	7. Leukoplakia
Nothing by mouth for more than 24 hours	8. Edema
Ineffective oral hygiene	9. Hyperemia
Mouth breathing	10. Oral plaque
Malnutrition	11. Desquamation
Infections	12. Vesicles
Lack of or decreased salivation	13. Hemorrhagic gingivitis
Medication	14. Carious teeth
	15. Halitosis

Powerlessness

Definition: The perception of the individual that one's own action will not significantly affect an outcome. Powerlessness is a perceived lack of control over a current situation or immediate happening.

Etiology	Defining characteristics
Health care environment	I. *Severe*
Interpersonal interaction	1. Verbal expressions of having no control or influence over situation
Illness-related regime	2. Verbal expressions of having no control or influence over outcome
Life style of helplessness	3. Verbal expressions of having no control over self-care
	4. Depression over physical deterioration that occurs despite patient compliance with regimens
	5. Apathy
	II. *Moderate*
	1. Nonparticipation in care or decision making when opportunities are provided
	2. Expressions of dissatisfaction and frustration over inability to perform previous tasks or activities
	3. Does not monitor progress
	4. Expression of doubt regarding role performance
	5. Reluctance to express true feelings, fearing alienation from caregivers
	6. Passivity
	7. Inability to seek information regarding care
	8. Dependence on others that may result in irritability, resentment, anger, and guilt
	9. Does not defend self-care practices when challenged
	III. *Low-Passivity*
	1. Expressions of uncertainty about fluctuating energy levels

Social Isolation

Definition: Condition of aloneness experienced by the individual and perceived as imposed by others and as a negative or threatened state.

Etiology	Defining characteristics

Factors contributing to the absence of satisfying personal relationships, such as:
1. Delay in accomplishing developmental tasks
2. Immature interests
3. Alterations in physical appearance
4. Alterations in mental status
5. Unaccepted social behavior
6. Unaccepted social values
7. Altered state of wellness
8. Inadequate personal resources
9. Inability to engage in satisfying personal relationships
	I. *Objective*
	  1. Absence of supportive significant other(s): family, friends, group
	  2. Sad, dull affect
	  3. Inappropriate or immature interests or activities for developmental age or stage
	  4. Uncommunicative, withdrawn, no eye contact
	  5. Preoccupation with own thoughts; repetitive, meaningless actions
	  6. Projects hostility in voice, behavior
	  7. Seeks to be alone or exists in a subculture
	  8. Evidence of physical or mental handicap or altered state of wellness
	  9. Shows behavior unaccepted by dominant cultural group
	
	II. *Subjective*
	  1. Expresses feelings of aloneness imposed by others
	  2. Expresses feelings of rejection
	  3. Experiences feelings of difference from others
	  4. Inadequacy in or absence of significant purpose in life
	  5. Inability to meet expectations of others
	  6. Insecurity in public
	  7. Expresses values acceptable to the subculture but unacceptable to the dominant cultural group
	  8. Expresses interests inappropriate to developmental age or stage

Glossary

abstract thinking. The ability to derive a conclusion from a logical reasoning process.

acrophobia. Fear of high places.

acting-out behavior. An immature defense mechanism by which an inner tension is not dealt with but is acted out behaviorally in an impulsive way. It is the outward manifestation of an inner need.

adaptation. A positive psychosocial adjustment to stress: the person's or family's quality of life after the event returns to normal or is improved.

advising relationship. A process in which a helper works with a client who is trying to make a decision and makes a strong recommendation for action. Advice giving is almost always contraindicated in a counseling situation.

affect. The external signs of a person's feelings. It can be the visible sign of a drive, the feeling side of a thought or idea, or the emotional reaction to a person or object. The word is often used interchangeably with *mood.*

aggression. Rage, anger, or hostility that is excessive or seems unrelated to a person's current situation.

aggressive drive. The motivating force of all activity and thus of life itself: this drive is not limited to hostility.

aggressiveness. A personality characteristic marked by boldness, lack of concern for others' feelings, and conflictual responses to others.

agitation. Anxiety associated with severe motor restlessness.

agnosia. A loss of ability to interpret sensory perceptions of vision, hearing, and so on.

agoraphobia. Fear of being in an open place.

akathisia. Extreme restlessness.

akinesia. The complete or partial loss of muscle movement.

alexithymia. The inability to describe feelings.

altruism. A mature defense mechanism that replaces the desire to satisfy one's own narcissistic needs with a desire to satisfy the needs of others. The result is constructive and gratifying service to others.

ambivalence. The presence of conflicting and opposite feelings about the same object.

amnesia. Complete or partial inability to recall past experiences.

anticipation. A mature defense mechanism by which the ego acknowledges both intellectually and emotionally an upcoming situation that is expected to provoke anxiety. Some of the anxiety is thereby worked through and resolved in advance.

anticipatory grief. The deep sadness experienced when a major loss is expected in the near future.

antisocial personality style. Traits of this personality style include unreliability, manipulativeness, lack of guilt, lack of responsibility in interpersonal relations, and superficial charm.

anxiety. An unpleasant feeling experienced in the ego. It occurs when id drives and the superego are in conflict. The person is unable to describe the cause of this unpleasant feeling.

apraxia. The loss of motor control of all or specific parts of the body.

assertiveness. A personality characteristic marked by openness, honesty, and respect for others' beliefs and feelings.

attending behavior. The way the counselor acts during the time he or she is with the person being helped. These behaviors or kinesics are eye contact, posture, gesture, and verbal behavior.

authenticity. (Also called transparency and genuineness.) The ability to share one's self, to be human and real in a relationship.

autonomic nervous system. The part of the nervous system that is concerned with control of involuntary bodily functions such as heart rate, blood pressure, and pupil dilation. Contains the sympathetic and parasympathetic nervous systems.

aversive stimulus. Any event that results in an unpleasant feeling.

avoidance. An immature defense mechanism by which the ego does not have any level of awareness of the situation, object, or activity that would be anxiety producing and is therefore bypassed. The person is never aware of the reason for the change in his motivation.

behavior modification. A type of behavioral treatment in which patterns of undesired responses are changed to more desirable responses by rewarding the desired behavior and not rewarding unwanted behavior.

bereavement. A process with several stages that a normal person goes through after the loss of a significant object. It includes all the stages involved in resolution of and adaptation to the loss.

blocking. Sudden cessation in the train of thought or in the midst of a sentence for no apparent reason.

blunted affect. See *flat affect*.

body image. The way that a person thinks about his body as a whole: the various parts of his body, the functions of his body, and the internal and external sensations associated with it. Body image development is a complex, lifelong process and is closely entwined with the development of personality.

bonding. A two-way attachment process between mother and child. The strength and character of this attachment is thought to influence the quality of the infant's relationships with other people.

boundaries. The unwritten rules within a family system that keep the role of one family member separate from another.

burnout. The perceived accumulation of stressful events over time and a feeling that nothing can be done about them.

castration anxiety. Fear of the loss of or injury to the genitals. A characteristic of the Freudian phallic stage of development in which the young boy fears that his father may remove his penis.

catastrophic reaction. A panic response that is triggered by overwhelming anxiety. It is frequently associated with organic brain syndrome.

catatonic. A fixed, immobile posture.

categories of organic brain syndrome.
1. Acute organic brain syndrome: *delirium*
2. Chronic organic brain syndrome: *dementia*

characteristics of a counseling relationship.
1. Friendship level
2. Encounter level
3. Altruistic level
4. Erotic level

circumstantiality. A flow of spoken thoughts that allows the person to reach a conclusion after many digressions to associated ideas.

clarifying. The listener not only rephrases what the client says but also takes a guess about what he thinks the person is saying.

claustrophobia. Fear of being in an enclosed place.

closed system. An assemblage of specific variables that react with a predictable outcome because of dynamics that are relatively rigid.

close-ended questioning style. A questioning style used in the counseling setting that requires only a one-word answer. This approach discourages discussion and elaboration.

clouding of consciousness. Incomplete clearmindedness with disturbance in perception and attitudes.

cognitive appraisal. Man's constant evaluation and reevaluation about the events occurring in his life. This is the cornerstone of Lazarus's theory about man's capacity to cope with threatening events.

coma. Profound degree of unconsciousness.

coma vigil. Coma in which the eyes stay open but the person is unconscious.

concrete thinking. The person interprets what he sees and hears in a rigid way and does not apply abstract judgment to decide meanings.

confabulation. The filling in of gaps in memory with untrue statements. This is done unconsciously. Frequently seen in dementia caused by chronic organic brain syndrome and in alcoholics.

confronting. A leading skill in which a direct statement is made by the counselor that challenges the client with realistic information that opposes the client's own beliefs.

confusion. Disturbance of orientation to time, place, or person.

conscious. A person's awareness of what is happening at a specific moment, including what he is thinking and feeling.

content. The actual verbatim accounting of what occurred during an interview. The factual recording of the conversation. Also see *process*.

contract. A personal relationship in which those involved have an understanding of what their responsibilities are and what the relationship means to them. These contracts may be formal or informal.

controlled personality style. A personality style characterized as "obsessive–compulsive." The person is self-disciplined and rigid and tends to be dominated by thinking rather than feeling. Sometimes used interchangeably with *type A personality style*.

conversion. An immature defense mechanism by which the ego changes emotional conflict between the instinctual pleasure-seeking–sexual drive or the aggressive drive into physical symptoms.

coping. A combination of conscious strategies that have worked successfully in the past with unconscious defense mechanisms in order to reduce the level of stress that a person is experiencing.

coping mechanism. A conscious strategy or maneuver that a person uses to reduce an unpleasant feeling of stress.

counseling. A term used broadly to describe a talking style of interpersonal relationship between a helper and a client. The definition of a formal counseling relationship appears below.

counseling relationship. A relationship in which the helper serves as a catalyst for self-exploration by the client as he strives to resolve conflicts, make decisions, and solve problems.

countertransference. The conscious or unconscious emotional response of the therapist to the patient determined by the therapist's inner needs rather than by the patient's needs.

crisis. A state of reaction within a person whose normal coping abilities are unable to adapt to a threatening event.

decompensation. Failure or breakdown of a higher level of defense mechanisms to a markedly less mature level of defense mechanisms. Frequently accompanied by panic.

defense mechanisms. Automatic, primarily unconscious devices used by the ego as a means of protecting itself against unwanted thoughts, feelings, or external reality.

déjà vu. A feeling that one has experienced a new situation on a previous occasion.

delirium. (Toxic brain syndrome.) An acute organic brain syndrome characterized by rapid changes in the patient's wakefulness, alertness, attention span, and ability to perceive the environment accurately.

delusion. A false belief, not consistent with a patient's intelligence and cultural background, that cannot be corrected by reasoning.

delusional projection. A narcissistic defense mechanism by which the ego develops a false belief that is abnormal for one's intelligence and cultural background. It has a persecutory basis and is not an adaptive mechanism in adults.

delusion of grandeur. An exaggerated belief about one's abilities or importance.

delusion of persecution. A false belief that others are seeking to hurt or damage a person either physically or by insinuation.

delusion of reference. A false belief that one is the center of others' attention and discussion.

dementia. Chronic brain syndrome that develops over an extended period. Characterized by gradual deterioration in a person's intellectual, emotional, and perceptual functioning and an exaggeration of the person's previously existing personality characteristics.

denial. A narcissistic defense mechanism that the ego uses to shut out external reality that is too frightening or threatening to tolerate; conscious awareness is blocked.

dependent personality style. A personality style that exhibits clingy, needy, and demanding behavior and has a low level of tolerance for frustration. An underlying fear of abandonment motivates much of this type of person's behavior.

depersonalization. A loss of sense of control over oneself, a feeling of detachment from one's surroundings.

depression. A hopeless feeling of sadness, grief, or mourning; prolonged and excessive sadness associated with a loss (exogenous) or not attributable to an external event (endogenous).

derealization. A sense of unreality about the environment or a distortion or frank loss of reality about the environment.

developmental crisis. A critical period that occurs as the result of poor adaptation to the emotional, physical, or social challenges of the normal processes of growth and aging.

developmental task. A challenge that a person's ego must work at and resolve during sequential stages of growth.

differentiation of self. The degree to which a person's intellect or emotions control his functioning (Bowen, 1976a).

1. *low level of differentiation.* The intellect and its ability to reason and analyze situations is dominated by feelings. The person is strongly controlled by the emotional tone of the group he is with.

2. *moderate level of differentiation.* The intellect and reasoning ability is equally dominated by feelings and capacity to retain intellectual control. The *pseudo self* dominates in this person, who is strongly relationship oriented.

3. *high level of differentiation.* The person with a high level of differentiation of self demonstrates strong evidence of *solid self.* He remains independent and is not totally dependent on relationships.

direct leading. A counseling skill in which the helper uses statements that ask for specific responses from the client.

displacement. A neurotic defense used by the ego to redirect feelings about one object toward another object. The feelings are shifted, but the instinct or motivation behind the feelings remains the same.

distorted body image. The phenomenon of perceiving one's body to be different than it actually is. This distortion occurs in the ego and is the result of the interaction of the person's intrapsychic makeup and external events.

distortion. A narcissistic defense mechanism that the ego uses to reshape external reality to suit internal needs.

dramatizing personality style. A personality style in which persons respond to events in an emotional, dramatic way. They have a captivating personality and feelings tend to dominate rather than thinking.

dreamy state. (Twilight.) Disturbed consciousness with hallucinations.

drive. The basic inborn motivating force of human behavior. There are two main drives in every person: the drive to feel pleasure and the aggressive drive. Believed to be physiologically induced.

dyad. A two-person relationship.

dynamics. A multiple and ever-changing force that causes motion. In the field of psychiatry, this term refers to the multiple intrapsychic forces that shape a person's personality and behavior.

dyskinesia. Excessive movement of mouth, protruding tongue, and facial grimacing (e.g., tardive dyskinesia, a side-effect of phenothiazine medication).

dysphoria. Unpleasant feelings of any kind.

echopraxia. The mimicking of the body movements of the interviewer.

ego. The regulator part of the psyche that acts as a buffer between the drives of the id and the judgments of the superego. It contains conscious and unconscious components. The ego has many functions, including intellect, reasoning, memory, sensing, and spatial relatedness.

egocentricity. Self-centeredness in one's interactions with others'; preoccupied with oneself and lacking interest in others.

ego-dystonic. Ideas or impulses that are not in harmony or compatible with the psyche.

ego-syntonic. Ideas or impulses that are compatible with the ego and are therefore allowed to enter into the awareness of the ego.

Electra complex. The erotic attachment of a girl to her father. A characteristic of the phallic stage of development. Corresponds to the *Oedipal complex* in boys.

empathy. The ability to be aware of the feelings of others so that one can respond to and understand their experiences on their terms. The helper is always aware of his own separateness.

encephalopathy. Any type of organic brain dysfunction.

Erikson, Erik. Described the psychosocial development of man on a continuum from birth to death in eight stages.

euphoria. Excessive and inappropriate feeling of well-being.

exaltation. Intense elation accompanied by feelings of grandeur.

extended family. The family network beyond the *family of origin*, including grandparents, uncles, aunts, and cousins.

external locus of control. A person believes that events are beyond his control. He perceives them as being the result of chance, luck, or power of others.

extinction. The complete inhibition of a conditioned reflex as a result of failure of the environment to reinforce it.

facies. Facial expressions. Different types are animated, fixed, sad, angry, color of face (pale, reddened), and so on.

family of origin. The family into which a person is born, including immediate family members and any other person who is a consistent member of the household.

fear. Fright caused by consciously recognized danger or threat.

feedback. The mechanism by which each of the units in a system communicates between and among all members of that system.
1. *positive feedback.* One member of the system reinforces a particular action or behavior of another member and promotes similar behavior in the future.
2. *negative feedback.* One member of the system discourages a particular action or behavior and potentially promotes change within the overall system.

fixations. An incomplete working through of one of the earlier stages of psychosexual development as a result of too little or too much restraint imposed on the developing child.

flat affect. (Blunted affect.) Absence of emotional range.

flight of ideas. Rapid speaking with a quick shifting from one idea to another.

focusing. A leading skill in which the helper zeroes in on a specific aspect of the client's explorations to help uncover feelings.

formal counseling. A prearranged and contractual professional relationship.

Freud, Sigmund. A psychoanalyst who developed many theories about intrapsychic functioning and personality development. Considered by many to be the "father" of psychiatry.
Stages of psychosexual development
1. Oral stage (0 to 12 months)
2. Anal stage (1 to 3 years)
3. Phallic stage (3 to 6 years)
4. Latency stage (6 to 12 years)
5. Genital stage (12 to 20 years)

functional psychiatric disorder. A psychiatric illness caused by a dysfunction in the abstract psychic structures of the id, ego, or superego. Unlike organic brain syndrome (OBS), it has no identifiable physiological etiology.

fusion. In a family system, fusion exists when two or more persons consistently relate to one another on a more emotional level than they do with other members of the same family. A similar concept is that of enmeshment.

general adaptation syndrome. (GAS.) The measurable structural and chemical changes produced in the body when stress affects the whole body (proposed by Hans Selye):

1. The alarm reaction in which the body attempts to fight off the effects of the stressor.
2. The stage of resistance in which the body maintains its resistance or fails to resist.
3. The stage of exhaustion in which the organism's energy is depleted and death ensues.

grief. The emotion experienced when a loss occurs; the affective result of a loss.

guiding relationship. A relationship in which the helper knows and presents all available options to the person being helped so that he can make his own decision.

guilt. An internal feeling that occurs when a person violates his own conscience or moral code. It represents a conflict between the id and the superego.

hallucinations. False sensory perceptions that do not exist in external reality.

    auditory hallucinations. The person hears sounds that are nonexistent.

    gustatory hallucinations. The person tastes a taste that is nonexistent.

    hypnagogic hallucinations. The person senses any type of false sensory perception during the twilight period between being awake and being asleep.

    olfactory hallucinations. The person smells a smell that is nonexistent.

    tactile hallucinations. The person feels objects or sensations that are nonexistent.

    visual hallucinations. The person sees objects that are nonexistent.

holistic health care. The approach to health care in which the person is viewed as a complex whole with physical, intellectual, emotional, social, and cultural dimensions. The focus is not on a specific disease but rather on the total health of the human being.

homeostasis: family. A balance created by the total contributing dynamics of each family member. It can be well functioning or pathological. It is *normal* for that family, however.

humanistic psychology. The view of personality development in which the driving force is seen as man's need for satisfaction, happiness, and growth. Abraham Maslow was a pioneer in this school of psychology.

humor. A mature defense mechanism used by the ego when it cannot fully acknowledge a difficult situation. It is used without expense to the self or to others.

hypochondriasis. An immature defense mechanism by which guilt caused by real or imagined aggressive or critical feelings toward others is transformed into physical complaints.

hysterical personality style. A personality style characterized by excitable, emotional, dramatic behavior. A more pathological form of the dramatizing personality style.

id. The unconscious, instinctual part of the psyche that contains the basic drives of man—the libidinal and aggressive drives.

identification. A neurotic defense mechanism by which a person accepts other's thoughts, attitudes, feelings, or particular experiences as if they were his own.

illusion. A distortion or misinterpretation of an actual stimulus by the ego.

inadequate personality style. This personality style is characterized by an unpredictable, immature, emotional response to physical, intellectual, or emotional stress.

indirect leading. A counseling skill in which the helper uses statements that are deliberately vague and general so that the client is allowed a more flexible response.

infantile sexuality. The early drive for pleasure in children; the experience of positive body sensations.

informal counseling. A less structured type of professional relationship in which meetings are not pre-arranged and no formal contracts are made.

intellectualization. See *isolation.*

internal frame of reference. The beliefs and feelings of the person being helped.

internal locus of control. A person believes that he has some ability to modify or control environmental situations and that he has some power over his own responses.

interpreting. A leading skill in which the counselor explains the meaning of events to the client so that he is able to see his problems in new ways.

interviewing relationship. A question-and-answer situation in which the focus is on obtaining factual data from the client.

intimacy. The ability to be emotionally close to another person, to be open and honest, to trust, and to take risks in a relationship.

intrapsychic. Pertaining to any functioning of the mind. See *psyche.*

intuition. The ability to gain knowledge without using conscious reasoning.

isolation. A neurotic defense mechanism by which the ego represses the feelings associated with a particular thought or idea. Also known as rationalization and intellectualization.

judgment. The ability of a person to behave in a socially appropriate manner.

Kübler-Ross, Elisabeth. A psychiatrist who developed the best-known theory of the bereavement process. The stages are denial, anger, bargaining, depression, and acceptance.

la belle indifférence. This term is used to describe an unusual lack of worry or concern in a difficult situation.

lability. Mood swings. Alternating periods of elation and depression or anxiety in the same person within a limited time.

leading skills. Types of statements that invite the person being helped to respond. The skills of the helper include focusing, questioning, summarizing, confronting, interpreting, and advice-giving. These skills are defined elsewhere in the glossary.

level of awareness. An observable aspect of brain functioning that can range from unconsciousness and frank coma through normal levels of alertness.

liaison. A connection or means of communication for promoting mutual understanding.

liaison psychiatry. A clinical science that works with the patient, the family, and all caregivers in dealing with the emotional dynamics of people in their psychosocial adaptation to the stress of illness.

libidinal drive. The motivating force to obtain and feel pleasure.

libido. The energy existing in a person that is the basis of his pursuit of pleasurable feelings.

limit setting. A nursing approach designed to reduce undesired behavior.

locus of control. The degree to which a person senses that events are under his control or are outside of his control. Also see *internal locus of control* and *external locus of control.*

long-suffering personality style. There are two variations of this personality style. In one, the person suffers silently, is selfless, and needs to sacrifice and do for others; the other type of person seems to enjoy relating the awfulness of his situation.

long-term memory. The ability to recall events from the distant past.

loss. An actual or threatened change in status of a significant object.

Mahler, Margaret. A psychoanalyst who developed the stages of psychological development of infants:
1. Autistic phase (0 to 3 or 4 weeks)
2. Symbiotic phase (1 to 4 months)
3. Separation–individuation phase:
   a. Differentiation subphase (5 to 10 months)
   b. Practicing subphase (10 to 18 months)
   c. Rapprochment subphase (18 to 22 months)
   d. Object constancy subphase (22 to 28 months)

maladaptive grieving process. See *pathological bereavement.*

Maslow, Abraham. One of the founders of humanistic psychology. Maslow believed that there are five levels of need in man:
1. Physiological needs
2. Safety needs
3. Love and belonging needs
4. Esteem needs
5. Self-actualization needs

masochism. The deriving of gratification from experiencing physical or mental pain. This pathology is linked to a childhood that is marked by harsh discipline and strong guilt instilled by the person's caregivers.

mental status examination. An evaluation that determines if there are abnormalities in the level of consciousness, thinking, feeling, perceptions, memory, or behavior of the person being examined.

mood. The internal feelings experienced by a person. The word is often used interchangeably with *affect.*

narcissism. An exaggerated form of self-love. Normal and healthy in toddlerhood, pathological if it persists strongly into adulthood.

narcissistic defense mechanisms. The earliest level of defenses used by the ego. They are commonly used by children under 5 years and include the use of denial, delusional projection, and distortion. Also used by adults with character disorders or normal adults under moderate to severe stress.

narcissistic supplies. Internal, intrapsychic sources of positive self-worth.

negative reinforcement. The rewarding of a stoppage of an undesirable event or behavior.

neologism. A new word that a person makes up.

neurosis. A mild to moderate psychopathology in which the neurotic defenses of displacement, identification, isolation, reaction formation, and repression are used heavily and affect the person's capacity to enjoy life.

neurotic defense mechanisms. (Listed above.) Levels of defense mechanisms normally operating in children between 4 and 6 years of age, persons with neuroses, and psychologically healthy adults under moderate to severe stress.

nuclear family. A family consisting of a mother and father and their child(ren).

object. A word used in psychiatry to describe a person or aspect of a person.

object relations. A term used to refer to the amount of emotional energy that a person invests in another person or an aspect of himself.

obsessive thought. An unwelcome idea, emotion, or urge that repeatedly enters a person's consciousness.

Oedipus complex. A characteristic of the phallic stage of development in which a child's sexual interest is attached chiefly to the parent of the opposite sex and the child has aggressive feelings for the parent of the same sex. It is sometimes used only to describe a boy's response to his mother. See *Electra complex,* which is the corresponding complex for girls.

open-ended questioning style. A questioning style used in the counseling setting. The helper asks questions that promote the potential for a wide range of responses. The client's responses are not pre-structured by the question; the question invites him to explore his own thoughts and feelings.

open listening. A counseling technique in which no matter what the client says or feels, the counselor accepts the client as he is. Also known as unconditional positive regard.

open system. An assemblage of smaller parts (subsystems) in which there is an unlimited number of changing dynamics.

operant conditioning. Conditioning or influencing behavior by rewarding a person for certain forms of behavior. Also called behavioral psychology.

organic brain syndrome. (OBS.) An organic psychiatric illness caused by a dysfunction in the actual anatomical structures or the biochemistry of the brain, resulting in emotional, intellectual, or perceptual changes in mental status.

organismic viewpoint. The view that all organisms are organized things and each biological system is interdependent on another. Defined by Ludwig von Bertalanffy.

organization of thought. The associations or the connections between a person's thoughts.

orientation. The person's ability to identify who he is, where he is, and the time and date.

paranoia. A form of psychopathology in which the person unconsciously projects onto the environment his own objectionable thoughts and feelings. A more pathological form of the suspicious personality style.

paraphrasing. The helper listens to what the client says and repeats and rephrases it in his own words. The helper avoids adding his own ideas.

parkinsonian movement. Fine tremor accompanied by muscular rigidity.

passive-aggressive behavior. An immature defense mechanism in which the person's anger is not expressed directly toward another but is expressed passively in ways that are frequently self-defeating and are offensive in some way to the other person.

passivity. A personality characteristic demonstrated by weakness, excessive self-denial, and uncertainty.

pathological bereavement. Also called maladaptive bereavement. A grieving process characterized by maladaptive coping in response to a significant loss. There is either excessive repression of grief or an excessive and prolonged emotional response that lasts longer than 1 year.

perception. The way that a person senses himself, the environment, and his relationships with others in his environment. Includes all senses: vision, hearing, touch, smell, and taste.

perception checking. A counselor's statement of his perceptions of the general theme of what a client has been saying.

perseveration. Repetition of the same thoughts or word in response to different questions.

personality. The accumulated characteristic behaviors, adjustment techniques, and thoughts unique to each human being.

personality trait. Characteristics unique to a person. They comprise his habitual, normal style of interacting with others as well as his coping responses to stress. They are acquired during the early childhood maturing process.

pheochromocytoma. A tumor of the adrenal medulla that releases increased levels of epinephrine. The predominant symptom is the person's high level of anxiety with episodic panic attacks.

phobia. A strong fear of a particular situation.

Piaget, Jean. A Swiss psychologist who developed and described the cognitive stages of development of children:

1. Sensorimotor stage (0 to 18 months)
2. Preoperational thought stage (1½ to 2 to 7 to 8 years)
3. Stage of concrete operations (8 to 11 years)
4. Stage of formal thought (12 years to adulthood)

placebo. Any medication used to relieve symptoms, not by pharmacological action but because of the patient's expectation of pain relief.

positive reinforcement. When a person's behavior results in a positive response from others, he experiences a feeling of acceptance and internal pleasure. He is likely to repeat the same behavior.

preconscious. That which is not present in consciousness but consists of memories that can be easily recalled. Also called subconscious.

preoccupation of thought. The person connects all occurrences and experiences to a central thought, usually one with strong emotional overtones.

presenile dementia. A term used to describe changes in mental status that occur earlier than would be expected in the normal aging process. It is caused by degenerative diseases that occur in midlife and that attack brain tissue (*e.g.*, Alzheimer's disease).

primary appraisal. The first step of Lazarus's cognitive appraisal theory about man's ability to perceive the events in his environment. During this state, man makes judgments and decisions that help him to know if an event is threatening or harmless.

process. The underlying dynamics of what happened and why in the counseling interview. Also refers to an ongoing series of events.

professional distancing. An unconscious psychological defense in which professionals deny themselves awareness of their own feelings as well as the feelings of their patients.

projection. An immature defense mechanism by which a person is unable to acknowledge thoughts or feelings in himself and attributes them to others.

pseudo self. The self that a person presents to the world. It is the result of the emotional pressure applied by a person's social system to conform to specific role expectations.

psyche. All that constitutes the mind and its processes. It contains the id, ego, and superego and their conscious and unconscious components.

psychogenic. A physical condition that has a psychological basis in its cause or etiology.

psychosis. A severe psychopathology in which the person has lost touch with reality. There is a major impairment of ego function and the defenses of denial, delusional projection, and distortion are used predominantly.

punishment. A type of reinforcement in which a negative behavior elicits a negative response from the environment. The outcome is a cessation or stopping of negative behavior.

questioning. A leading skill that includes use of queries that either encourage or discourage further discussion. *See open-ended* and *close-ended questioning style.*

rationalization. See *isolation.*

reaction formation. A neurotic defense mechanism by which the ego, because of anger and hostility, elicits the exact opposite impulse, feeling, thought, or behavior of the original impulse or feeling.

reappraisal. The third stage of Lazarus's cognitive appraisal theory. During this state the person realizes that his initial coping attempts are not working and institutes new changes in his conscious coping attempts.

recent memory. The ability to recall events in the unconscious that have occurred in the immediate past and up to 1 or 2 weeks ago. It is first to be affected in memory loss.

regression. An immature defense mechanism by which the personality returns to an earlier level of functioning in response to a severe environmental or intrapsychic stressor.

reinforcement. Increasing the likelihood of desired behavior by giving specific responses. There are three types of reinforcement: positive, negative, and punishment.

repression. A neurotic defense mechanism that the ego uses to defend itself by unconsciously excluding awareness of thoughts, feelings, urges, fantasies, and memories that would be unacceptable or threatening if they were conscious. It is the main mechanism that the ego uses to defend itself.

resistance. The conscious or unconscious opposition of the ego to the uncovering of the unconscious ego defense mechanisms that maintain their strength in order to prevent full awareness of threatening id impulses.

scapegoat. A person who is made the victim of the other members of the group.

schizoid. A type of personality characterized by withdrawal, remoteness, and detachment. These traits result from the person's early disappointments in trying to establish a loving relationship with the important persons in his life. A more pathological form of the uninvolved personality style.

secondary appraisal. The second stage of Lazarus's cognitive appraisal theory. During this stage the person realizes that there is a threatening event in his environment and applies conscious coping strategies.

secondary gain. The support, sympathy, and attention that is unconsciously and consciously sought and received by a person. It is frequently associated with illness.

self-esteem. The degree to which a person feels valued, worthwhile, or competent.

situational crisis. A critical period that is the result of a stressful event that threatens a person's physiological or social equilibrium.

social readjustment rating scale. The Holmes and Rahe stress scale. It is a list of 43 life events, each of which is assigned an item value. People report the types of changes that they have experienced in the previous year. A total point value over 300 is a positive predictor of development of illness.

solid self. The beliefs that a person has about himself and his environment resulting from his life experiences since birth.

somatization. The phenomenon of a person's reaction to psychological stressors and conflicts with bodily symptoms. The defense mechanisms involved are repression (of feelings) and displacement (of conflicts and feelings).

speech. Characteristics or aspects of speaking style that should be observed are rate, volume, modulation, flow, and production.

splitting. An unconscious defense mechanism in which the person manipulatively makes one person or group become an adversary of another. The term is also used to describe an intrapsychic mechanism that determines the way in which thoughts, feelings, or memories are repressed.

state. Temporary behaviors and reactions of a person brought on by acute stress.

stress. The internal feeling response to the demands of a stressor.

stress management. The conscious use of mental or physical maneuvers that reduce feelings of tension.

stressor. Any type of internal or external demand on a person. It results in an internal feeling that is called stress.

structural theory. Freud's description of the abstract structures of the psyche that include the id, the ego, and the superego.

stupor. Lack of reaction to and unawareness of surroundings.

sublimation. A mature defense mechanism by which a repressed urge or desire is expressed in a socially acceptable or useful way, thereby giving the original impulse a more socially acceptable outlet.

subsystem. A concrete or abstract entity that belongs to a larger system and relates in specific ways with all the parts of the larger system.

suicidal ideation. Occasional or persistent thoughts of suicide.

summarizing. A leading skill in which a statement is made at the close of a discussion that briefly describes the content and process of the interview.

sundowning. A worsening of the patient's mental status at night.

superego. The unconscious part of the psyche that includes moral judgments and establishes goals for the person. It develops as a result of internalizing the "right and wrong" teachings of parents and early authority figures.

superior personality style. The person with a superior personality style has an exaggerated sense of importance that, in actuality, is a defense against conscious and unconscious feelings of poor self-esteem.

support. A beneficial aspect of a therapeutic relationship that results from the counselor's ability to convey total understanding, acceptance, and caring about the client and his problems.

support group. A group that provides people with a setting in which they can discuss their problems with other people who have similar concerns about a mutual problem such as illness.

supporting relationship. A relationship in which the helper approves of the actions of the client being helped. In *acceptance support* the listener validates the *person.* In *approval support* the listener validates the client's actions and experiences. In a counseling situation, acceptance support is the preferred patient approach.

suppression. A mature defense mechanism by which a conscious or semiconscious decision is made to delay paying attention to an unwanted conflict or impulse until a later time.

suspicious personality style. This personality style is characterized by the person who continually questions, complains, and finds fault in situations. The person's own internal anxieties and self-dislike are projected onto the environment, and he fears being put in a physically or mentally vulnerable position. When these traits are more pronounced, the person demonstrates traits of *paranoia.*

symbol. A single idea or object that represents another more complex thought or thing; there is a common association between them.

sympathy. The taking on of the feelings and circumstances of other people. The helper loses his own separate identity.

system. An assemblage or combination of parts (subsystems) forming a complex or unitary whole.

systems approach. A phrase describing an approach to patients that is consistent between all caregivers on all shifts. Ideally, a nursing care plan is executed using a systems approach.

tangentiality. A flow of spoken thoughts that results in many digressions, but the person never reaches a conclusion.

teaching relationship. A dominant–subordinate relationship in which the helper presents information about a subject that he believes the student needs to know.

termination. A psychological term for saying goodbye.

therapy group. A group in which all areas of a person's intrapsychic and interpersonal functioning are examined.

toxic brain syndrome. See *delirium.*

trait. See *personality trait.*

transaction. One part of a constantly changing relationship between man and his environment.

transference. An unconscious phenomenon in which the feelings, attitudes, and wishes originally linked with figures in one's early life are projected onto others.

"tree" approach to counseling. An open-ended questioning technique in which the helper takes his or her clues about the types of assessment questions to ask from the person needing help.

triad. A close relationship between three persons.

triangles. A three-person emotional configuration. It is the smallest stable relationship system.

trust. According to Erikson's developmental theory, trust is the first developmental challenge that occurs during the first year of life. If not fully attained, the child will develop with distrust of the environment, lack of hope, and lack of drive.

turnover. The departure of a nurse from his or her nursing position for any reason.

Type A personality style. A personality style frequently seen in patients with cardiac illness. It is characterized by aggressiveness, anxiety, repression of emotions, competitiveness, intense work involvement, and a high level of discipline.

unconditional positive regard. A genuine feeling of warmth for the person being helped. No judgments are made. The helper accepts the person as he is.

unconscious. A psychological process that a person is not aware of and cannot control. It consists of many repressed memories and experiences that surround a core of id drives.

undifferentiated ego mass. A commonly held feeling of two or more persons. As applied in family theory, when family members do not differentiate their own feelings and maintain their own separateness.

uninvolved personality style. The person with an uninvolved personality style appears distant, avoids encounters with others, and appears apathetic because of his bland emotional tone.

unitary man. A theoretical concept proposed by Martha Rogers in which man is described as an open system consisting of many elements or subsystems.

unresolved grief. A prolonged bereavement process in which the grieving person's quality of life is detrimentally affected beyond a 1-year period. (Also see *pathological bereavement.*)

waxy flexibility. The body maintains the position in which it is placed.

word salad. Disconnected mixture of unrelated words.

Bibliography

Abbey J: General systems theory: A framework for nursing. In Putt A (ed): General Systems Theory Applied to Nursing. Boston, Little, Brown & Co, 1978

Abse D, Wilkins M, van de Castle R et al: Personality and behavorial characteristics of lung cancer patients. J Psychosom Res 18:101, 1974

Ackerman N: Treating the Troubled Family. New York, Basic Books, 1966

Adam K: Interpersonal factors in suicide attempts: A pilot study in Christchurch. Aust NZ J Psychiatry 12:59, 1978

Agle D, Baum G: Psychological aspects of chronic obstructive pulmonary disease. Med Clin North Am 61:749, 1977

Aguilera D, Messick J: Crisis Intervention: Theory and Methodology, 3rd ed. St Louis, CV Mosby, 1978

Aldrich CK: Some dynamics of anticipatory grief. In Schoenberg B, Carr A, Kutscher A et al (eds): Anticipatory Grief. New York, Columbia University Press, 1974

Alexander F: Psychosomatic Medicine: Its Principles and Applications. New York, Norton, 1950

American Cancer Society: Cancer Facts and Figures, 1981. New York, American Cancer Society, 1980

American Cancer Society: Cancer Facts and Figures, 1979. New York, American Cancer Society, 1978

American College Dictionary. New York, Harper & Brothers Publishers, 1947

American Men and Women of Science: Social and Behavioral Sciences. New York, RR Bowker, 1973

Andreason N, Noyes R, Hartford C et al: Management of emotional reactions in seriously burned adults. N Engl J Med 286:65, 1972

Aponte H: Underorganization in the poor family. In Guerin P (ed): Family Therapy Theory and Practice. New York, Gardner Press, 1976

Appelbaum S: Exploring the relationship between personality and cancer. In Goldberg J (ed): Psychotherapeutic Treatment of the Cancer Patient. New York, The Free Press, 1981

Arieti S: The Intra-Psychic Self. New York, Basic Books, 1967

Arthur R: The response to life stress. In Usdin G, Lewis J (eds): Psychiatry in General Medical Practice. New York, McGraw-Hill, 1979

Ashley J: Hospitals, Paternalism, and the Role of the Nurse. New York, Columbia University Press, 1976

Babies: What do they know? When do they know it? The new Dr. Spock: A great dad. Time 122(7):57, August 15, 1983

Bahnson C: Stress and cancer. I. The state of the art. Psychosomatics 21:975, 1980

Bahnson C: Stress and cancer. II. The state of the art. Psychosomatics 22:207, 1981

Ballinger C: Psychiatric aspects of the menopause. In Campbell S (ed): The Management of the Menopause and Post-Menopausal Years. Baltimore, University Park Press, 1976

Ballou M: Crisis intervention and the hospital nurse. J Nurs Care 13:18, 1980

Barchha R, Stewart M, Guze S: The prevalence of alcoholism among general hospital ward patients. Am J Psychiatry 225:681, 1968

Barker M: Psychiatric illness after hysterectomy. Br Med J 268:91, 1968

Barry P: Grief in the general hospital. Unpublished paper, 1978

Barry P: Psychiatric consultation: A theoretical and clinical presentation of a patient with severe burns. Unpublished paper, 1978

Barry P: A comparison of the outcomes of primary and team nursing: Self-esteem, job satisfaction, involvement, and turnover rates. Master's thesis, Yale University, 1979

Barry P: Organic brain syndrome: An important etiological consideration in nursing diagnosis. In Kim M et al (eds): Classification of Nursing Diagnoses: Proceedings of the Fifth National Conference. St. Louis, CV Mosby (in press)

Bartrop RW, Luckhurst E, Lazarus L: Depressed lymphocyte function after bereavement. Lancet 1:834, 1977

Bateson G, Jackson D, Haley J et al: Toward a theory of schizophrenia. Behav Sci 1:251, 1956

Baxter R: Sex counseling and the SCI patient. Nursing '78 8:46, 1978

Bennis W, Benne K, Chin R (eds): The Planning of Change, 3rd ed. New York, Holt, Rinehart and Winston, 1976

Berger P: Management of depression and anxiety in primary care medicine. In Freeman A, Sack R, Berger P (eds): Psychiatry for the Primary Care Physician. Baltimore, Williams & Wilkins, 1979

Berger P, Tinklenberg J, Sack R: Management of the problem drinker. In Freeman A, Sack R, Berger P (eds): Psychiatry for the Primary Care Physician. Baltimore, Williams & Wilkins, 1979

Bertalanffy L von: General System Theory. New York, Braziller, 1968

Binger C, Ablin A, Feuerstein R et al: Childhood leukemia: Emotional impact on patient and family. N Engl J Med 280:414, 1969

Blanck G, Blanck R: Ego Psychology. II. Psychoanalytic Developmental Psychology. New York, Columbia University Press, 1979

Blockwood W, Corsellis JA (eds): Greenfield's Neuropathology, 3rd ed. Chicago, Year Book Medical Publishers, 1976

Boguslawski M: Therapeutic touch: A facilitator of pain relief. Top Clin Nurs 2:27, 1980

Bossert J, Freeman A: Emotional aspects of surgery. In Freeman A, Sack R, Berger P (eds): Psychiatry for the Primary Care Physician. Baltimore, Williams & Wilkins, 1979

Boszormenyi-Nagy I, Spark G: Invisible Loyalties: Reciprocity in Intergenerational Family Therapy. Hagerstown, MD, Harper & Row, 1973

Bowen M: Family therapy and family group therapy. In Kaplan H, Sadock B (eds): Comprehensive Group Psychotherapy. Baltimore, Williams & Wilkins, 1971

Bowen M: Toward the differentiation of a self in one's own family of origin. In Andres A, Lorio J (eds): Georgetown Family Symposia. Washington, DC, Georgetown University Medical Center, 1974

Bowen M: Family reaction to death. In Guerin P (ed): Family Therapy: Theory and Practice. New York, Gardner Press, 1976

Bowen M: Theory in the practice of psychotherapy. In Guerin P (ed): Family Therapy: Theory and Practice. New York, Gardner Press, 1976a

Bowen M: Principles and techniques of multiple family therapy. In Guerin P (ed): Family Therapy: Theory and Practice. New York, Gardner Press, 1976b

Bowen M: Family reaction to death. In Guerin P (ed): Family Therapy: Theory and Practice. New York, Gardner Press, 1976c

Bowen S, Miller B: Paternal attachment behavior as related to presence at delivery and parenthood classes: A pilot study. Nurs Res 29:307, 1980

Bowlby J: Processes of mourning. Int J Psychoanal 42:317, 1961

Bowlby J: Attachment and Loss, Vol 2, Separation. New York, Basic Books, 1973

Bowlby J: Attachment and Loss, Vol 3, Loss: Sadness and Depression. New York, Basic Books, 1980

Bozeman M, Orbach C, Sutherland A: Psychological impact of cancer and its treatment. III. The adaptation of mothers to the threatened loss of their children through leukemia. I. Cancer 8:1, 1955

Bracken M, Shepard M: Coping and adaptation following acute spinal cord injury: A theoretical analysis. Paraplegia 18:74, 1980

Brammer L: The Helping Relationship. Englewood Cliffs, NJ, Prentice-Hall, 1973

Brammer L, Shostrom E: Therapeutic Psychology: Fundamentals of Actualization Counseling and Psychotherapy, 2d ed. Englewood Cliffs, NJ, Prentice-Hall, 1968

Brand R, Rosenman R, Sholtz R, et al: Multivariate prediction of coronary heart disease in the Western Collaborative Study compared to the findings of the Framingham Study. Circulation 53:348, 1976

Brazelton R: Neonatal Behavioral Assessment Scale. Philadelphia, JB Lippincott, 1973

Brooke Army Medical Center: Interpersonal skills: Attending Behaviors (videocassette). Fort Sam Houston, TX, Academy of Health Sciences-TV, 1973

Brooke Army Medical Center: Interpersonal skills: Minimal Encourages to Talk (videocassette). Fort Sam Houston, TX, Academy of Health Sciences-TV, 1973

Brooke Army Medical Center: Interpersonal skills: Open-Ended Questions (videocassette). Fort Sam Houston, TX, Academy of Health Sciences-TV, 1973

Brooke Army Medical Center: Interpersonal skills: Reflection of Content (videocassette). Fort Sam Houston, TX, Academy of Health-Sciences-TV, 1973

Brooke Army Medical Center: Interpersonal skills: Reflection of Feeling (videocassette). Fort Sam Houston, TX, Academy of Health Sciences-TV, 1973

Brown M: Emotional response to the menopause. In Campbell S (ed): The Management of the Menopause and Post-Menopausal Years. Baltimore, University Park Press, 1976

Brown M: Distortions in Body Image in Illness and Disability. New York, John Wiley & Sons, 1977a

Brown M: Normal Development of Body Image. New York, John Wiley & Sons, 1977b

Brown R, Ramirez D, Taub J: The prescription of exercise for depression. Phys Sports Med 6:35, 1978

Brownell K: Differential diagnosis: Organic psychosis vs. functional psychosis. In Novello J (ed): A Practical Handbook of Psychiatry. Springfield, IL, Charles C Thomas, 1974

Bruhn J: Effects of chronic illness on the family. J Fam Pract 4:1057, 1977

Brunner L, Suddarth D: Textbook of Medical Surgical Nursing, 3rd ed. Philadelphia, JB Lippincott, 1975

Bungay G, Vessey M, McPherson C: Study of symptoms in middle life with special reference to the menopause. Br Med J 281:181, 1980

Cannon W: Bodily Changes in Pain, Hunger, Fear, and Rage, 2d ed. New York, Appleton, 1929

Caplan G: Principles of Preventive Psychiatry. New York, Basic Books, 1964

Carkhuff R, Truax C: Lay mental health counseling. The effects of lay group counseling. J Consult Psych 29:426, 1965

Carlson C: Loss. In Carlson C, Blackwell B (eds): Behavioral Concepts and Nursing Intervention, 2d ed. Philadelphia, JB Lippincott, 1978

Carnegie D: How to Win Friends and Influence People. New York, Simon and Schuster, 1936

Carney M: Serum folate values in 423 psychiatric patients. Br Med J 4:512, 1967

Carney M, Sheffield B: Associations of subnormal serum folate and vitamin B_{12} values and effects of replacement therapy. J Nerv Ment Dis 150:404, 1970

Carruthers M: Aggression and atheroma. Lancet 2:1170, 1969

Carson D: Personality development, conflict, and mechanisms of defense. In Usdin G, Lewis J (eds): Psychiatry in General Medical Practice. New York, McGraw-Hill, 1979

Cassel J: Studies of hypertension in migrants. In Oglesby P (ed): Epidemiology and Control of Hypertension. New York, Stratton Intercontinental Medical Book Corp, 1975

Cassem N: The dying patient. In Hackett T, Cassem N (eds): Massachusetts General Hospital Handbook of General Hospital Psychiatry. St. Louis, CV Mosby, 1978

Cassem N: Depression. In Hackett T, Cassem N (eds): Massachusetts General Hospital Handbook of General Hospital Psychiatry. St. Louis, CV Mosby, 1978a

Cassem N, Hackett R: Psychiatric consultation in a coronary care unit. Ann Intern Med 75:9, 1971

Castles M, Murray R: Dying in an Institution. New York, Appleton-Century-Crofts, 1979

Cay E: Psychological approach in patients after a myocardial infarction. Adv Cardiol 24:120, 1978

Chang F, Herzog B: A follow-up study of physical and psychological disability. Ann Surg 183:34, 1975

Charatan F, Fisk A: Mental and emotional results of strokes. NY State J Med 78:1403, 1978

Chenevert M: Special Techniques in Assertiveness Training for Women in the Health Professions. St. Louis, CV Mosby, 1978

Cherry L: An interview with Hans Selye: On the real benefits of eustress. Psychol Today 12:60, 1978

Chess T, Chess S: Temperament and Development. New York, Brunner/Mazel, 1977

Clark A, Affonso D: Mother child relationships. Matern Child Nurs J 1:93, 1976

Cleckley H: The Mask of Sanity, 4th ed. St. Louis, CV Mosby, 1964

Clemence Vaillot M: Existentialism: A philosophy of commitment. Am J Nurs 66:504, 1966

Cohen J, Cullen J, Martin L: Psychosocial Aspects of Cancer. New York, Raven Press, 1982

Cormier W, Cormier L: Interviewing Strategies for Helpers: A Guide to Assessment, Treatment, and Evaluation. Monterey, CA, Brooks/Cole Publishing Co., 1979

Coyne J, Lazarus R: Cognitive style, stress perception and coping. In Kutash I, Schlesinger L (eds): Handbook on Stress and Anxiety. San Francisco, Jossey-Bass, 1980

Crain A, Sussman M, Weil W: Effects of a diabetic child on marital integration and related measures of family functioning, J Health Hum Behav 7:122, 1966

Cropley C, Lester P, Pennington S: Assessment tool for measuring maternal attachment behaviors. Curr Pract Obstet Gynecol Nurs 1:16, 1976

Dartington T, Nurse G, Wilson M: Preparing nurses for counseling. Nurs Mirror 44:54, 1977

Davis J, Foreyt J: Mental Examiner's Handbook. Springfield, IL, Charles C Thomas, 1975

Dean A, Lin N: The stress-buffering role of social support: Problems and prospects for systematic investigation. J Nerv Ment Dis 165:403, 1977

Desiderata: St. Paul's Church, Baltimore, 1692

Detre T, Jarecki H: Modern Psychiatric Treatment. Philadelphia, JB Lippincott, 1971

Diagnostic and Statistical Manual of Mental Disorders, 3rd ed: Washington, DC, American Psychiatric Association, 1980

DiCaprio N: Personality Theories: Guides to Living. Philadelphia, WB Saunders, 1974

Donne J: Devotions upon emergent occasions. 1624 Folcroft, PA, Folcroft Library Editions, 1973

Donnelly J: The neuroses. In Usdin G, Lewis J (eds): Psychiatry in General Medical Practice. New York, McGraw-Hill, 1979

Donovan L: The shortage: Good jobs are going begging these days so why not be choosey. RN 43:20, 1980

Drotar D, Baskiewicz A, Irvin N et al: The adaptation of parents to the birth of an infant with a congenital malformation: A hypothetical model. Pediatrics 56:710, 1975

Dubin W, Stolberg R: Emergency Psychiatry for the House Officer. New York, SP Medical and Scientific Books, 1981

Dubois M, Keen D, Shuey B (eds): Larousse French-English Dictionary. New York, Washington Square Press, 1967

Dudley D, Glaser E, Jorgenson B et al: Psychosocial concomitants to rehabilitation in chronic obstructive pulmonary disease. Chest 77:413, 1980

Dudley D, Wermuth C, Hague W: Psychosocial aspects of care in the chronic obstructive pulmonary disease patient. Heart Lung 2:289, 1973

Duldt B: Anger: An alienating communication hazard for nurses. Nurs Outlook 29:640, 1981

Eaton J: Coping with staff grief. In Earle A, Argondizzo N, Kutscher A (eds): The Nurse as Caregiver For the Terminal Patient and His Family. New York, Columbia University Press, 1976

Eisendrath S, Dunkel J: Psychological issues in intensive care unit staff. Heart Lung 8:751, 1979

Elkind D: Egocentrism in adolescence. Child Dev 38:1025, 1967

Engel G: Is grief a disease? A challenge for medical research. Psychosom Med 23:18, 1961

Engel G: Psychological Development in Health and Disease. Philadelphia, WB Saunders, 1962

Engel G: Psychological Development in Health and Disease, 2d ed. Philadelphia, WB Saunders, 1968

Engel G: Sudden and rapid death during psychologic stress: Folk lore or folk wisdom? Ann Intern Med 74:771, 1971

Engel G: Memorial lecture: The psychosomatic approach to individual susceptibility to disease. Gastroenterology 67:1085, 1974

Engel G: Reactions to the Death of a Twin, pp. 4–12. Rochester Review, Fall 1975

Engel G: Psychologic stress, vasodepressor (vasovagal) syncope and sudden death. Ann Intern Med 89:403, 1978

Erikson E: Childhood and Society, 2d ed. New York, Norton, 1963

Estes N, Smith-Dijulio K, Heinemann M: Nursing Diagnosis of the Alcoholic Person. St. Louis, CV Mosby, 1980

Evans F: Psychosocial Nursing: Theory and Practice in Hospital and Community Mental Health. New York, Macmillan, 1971

Ezra J: Social and economic effects on families of patients with myocardial infarctions. Master's thesis, University of Denver, 1961

Farr K: Communication pitfalls in routine counseling. Pediatr Nurs 5:55, 1979

Fenichel O: The Psychoanalytic Theory of Neurosis. New York, Norton, 1945

Fields C: Despite problems, nursing research continues. Reflections 6:6, 1980

Finck K: The potential health care crisis of hysterectomy. In Kjervik D, Martinson I (eds): Women in Stress: A Nursing Perspective. New York, Appleton-Century-Crofts, 1979

Fink P: Psychiatric myths of menopause. In Eskin B (ed): Menopause: Comprehensive Management. New York, Masson, 1980

Flaherty J: Psychiatric complications of medical drugs. J Fam Pract 9:243, 1979

Flaskerud J, Halloran E, Janken J et al: Avoidance and distancing: A descriptive view of nursing. Nurs Forum 18:158, 1979

Fogarty T: Triangles. The Family 2:11, 1975

Fogarty T: Fusion. The Family 4:49, 1977

Framo J: Systematic research on family dynamics. In Boszormenyi-Nagy I, Framo J (eds): Intensive Family Therapy. New York, Harper & Row, 1965

Fredrickson P, Richelson E: Mayo seminars in psychiatry: Dopamine and schizophrenia—a review. J Clin Psychiatry 40:61, 1979

Freedman A, Kaplan H, Sadock B: Modern Synopsis of Comprehensive Textbook of Psychiatry II, 2d ed. Baltimore, Williams & Wilkins, 1976

Friedman M, Rosenman R: Type A Behavior and Your Heart. New York, Alfred A Knopf, 1974

Friedman M, Rosenman R: The key cause—type A behavior pattern. In Monat A, Lazarus R (eds): Stress and Coping. New York, Columbia University Press, 1977

Freud A: The Ego and the Mechanisms of Defense, rev. ed. New York, New International Universities Press, 1966

Freud S: Certain Neurotic Mechanisms in Jealousy, Paranoia and Homosexuality. In Collected Papers, Vol 22. London, Hogarth Press, 1924a

Freud S: Collected Papers: The Unconscious. London, London Institute of Psychoanalysis and Hogarth Press, 1924b

Freud S: The Ego and the Id. London, Hogarth Press, 1927

Freud S: New Introductory Lectures on Psychoanalysis. New York, Norton, 1933

Freud S: On the history of the psychoanalytic movement. In Collected Papers, Vol 1. New York, Basic Books, 1959

Frosch W: Psychoanalytic evaluation of addiction and habituation. J Am Psychoanal Assoc 18:209, 1970

Gates C: A Manual for Cancer. Boston, American Cancer Society, 1978

Gates E, Kernohan J: Metastatic brain abscess. Medicine 29:71, 1950

Geaga K, Amanth J: Responses of a psychiatric patient to vitamin B_{12} therapy. Dis Nerv Syst 36:343, 1975

Gillette R: Holistic medicine, wellness, and family medicine. J Fam Pract 10:1093, 1980

Gilroy J, Meyer J: Medical Neurology, 3rd ed. New York, Macmillan, 1975

Goldberg R: Strategies in Psychiatry for the Primary Care Physician. Darien, CT, Patient Care Books, 1980

Gomberg E: Prevalence of alcoholism among ward patients in a Veterans Administration hospital. J Stud Alcohol 36:1456, 1975

Goodstein R, Hurwitz R: The role of the psychiatric consultant in the treatment of burned patients. Int J Psychiatry Med 6:413, 1975

Gordon M: Historical perspective: The national conference group for classification of nursing diagnosis (1978, 1980). In Kim M, Moritz D (eds): Classification of Nursing Diagnoses: Proceedings of the Third and Fourth National Conferences. New York, McGraw-Hill, 1982

Gray S, Ramsey C, Villar-Real R et al: Adrenal influences upon the stomach and the gastric response to stress. In Fifth Annual Report on Stress: 1955-1956. New York, MD Publishing, 1955-1956

Greenbaum J, Lurie L: Encephalitis as a causative factor in behavior disorders of children. JAMA 136:923, 1948

Greenberg I: Studies of attitudes toward death. In Group for Advancement of Psychiatry, Death and Dying: Attitudes of Patient and Doctor. New York, Mental Health Materials Center, Vol 5, Symposium 11, 1965

Greene W: The psychosocial setting of the development of leukemia and lymphoma. Ann NY Acad Sci 125:794, 1966

Greenleaf N: The politics of self esteem. Nurs Digest 6:1, 1978

Greist J, Klein M, Eischens R et al: Running as a treatment for depression. Compr Psychiatry 20:44, 1979

Griffith E: Sexual dysfunctions associated with physical disabilities. Arch Phys Med Rehabil 56:8, 1975

Grissom J, Weiner B, Weiner E: Psychological correlates of cancer. J Consult Clin Psych 43:114, 1975

Grissum M, Spengler C: Womanpower and Health Care. Boston, Little, Brown & Co, 1976

Guerin P: Family Therapy: Theory and Practice. New York, Gardner Press, 1976

Guerin P, Guerin K: Theoretical aspects and clinical relevance of the multi-generational model of family therapy. In Guerin P (ed): Family Therapy: Theory and Practice. New York, Gardner Press, 1976

Gundle M, Reeves B, Tate S et al: Psychosocial outcome after coronary artery surgery. Am J Psychiatry 137:1591, 1980

Guttman L: Spinal cord injuries: Comprehensive management and research, 2d ed. Oxford, Blackwell Scientific Publications, 1976

Hackett T: Disruptive states. In Hackett R, Cassem N (eds): Massachusetts General Hospital Handbook of General Hospital Psychiatry. St Louis, CV Mosby, 1978

Hackett T: Beginnings: Liaison psychiatry in a general hospital. In Hackett T, Cassem N (eds): Massachusetts General Hospital Handbook of General Hospital Psychiatry. St Louis, CV Mosby, 1978a

Hackett T: The pain patient: Evaluation and treatment. In Hackett T, Cassem N (eds): Massachusetts General Hospital Handbook of General Hospital Psychiatry. St Louis, CV Mosby, 1978b

Hagnell O: The premorbid personality of persons who develop cancer in a total population investigated in 1947 and 1957. Ann NY Acad Sci 125:846, 1966

Hakel M, Hollman D, Dunnette M: Stability and change in occupational status of occupations in 21 and 42 year periods. Pers Guid J 46:762, 1968

Haley J: Changing Families. New York, Grune & Stratton, 1971

Hamburg D, Artz C, Reiss E et al: Clinical importance of emotional problems in the care of patients with burns. N Engl J Med 248:355, 1953

Hamburg D, Hamburg B, deGoza S: Adaptive problems and mechanisms in severely burned patients. Psychiatry 16:1, 1953

Hammond C: Menopause—an American view. In Campbell S (ed): The Management of the Menopause and Post-Menopausal Years. Baltimore, University Park Press, 1976

Hardy J, Wolff H, Goodell H: Studies on pain. A new method for measuring pain threshold: Observations on spatial summation of pain. J Clin Invest 19:649, 1940

Hatton D, Valente S, Rink A: Suicide Assessment and Intervention. New York, Appleton-Century-Crofts, 1977

Haug J, Kuntzman K, Seeger R: Socio-economic Fact Book for Surgery, 1981. Chicago, American College of Surgeons, 1981

Heidt P: Effects of therapeutic touch on anxiety level of hospitalized patients. Nurs Res 30:3207, 1981

Heller S, Frank K, Kornfeld D et al: Psychological outcome following open-heart surgery. Arch Intern Med 134:908, 1974

Hellerstein H, Friedman E: Sexual activity and the postcoronary patient. Arch Intern Med 125:987, 1970

Hicks C: Taking the Lid Off. Nurs Times 76:1681, 1980

Hinsie L, Campbell R (eds): Psychiatric Dictionary, 4th ed. New York, Oxford University Press, 1977

Hochberg S: The effect of running on depression in college students. Presented at Annual Research Day sponsored by Sigma Theta Tau, Yale University School of Nursing, 1980

Holmes R, Rahe R: The social readjustment rating scale. J Psychosom Res 11:213, 1967

Horne R, Picard R: Psychosocial risk factors for lung cancer. Psychosom Med 41:503, 1979

Horowitz M: Stress Response Syndromes. New York, Jason Aronson, 1976

Horvath T: Organic brain syndromes. In Freeman A, Sack R, Berger P (eds): Psychiatry for the Primary Care Physician. Baltimore, Williams & Wilkins, 1979

Houpt J: Death, dying, and the family. In Freeman A, Sack R, Berger P (eds): Psychiatry for the Primary Care Physician, Baltimore, Williams & Wilkins, 1979

Hurst M, Jenkins C, Rose R: The relation of psychological stress to onset of medical illness. In Garfield C (ed): Stress and Survival: The Emotional Realities of Life-Threatening Illness. St Louis, CV Mosby, 1979

Hysterectomy in women aged 15–44: 1970–78. Morbidity and Mortality Weekly Reports 30:173, 1981

Imara M: Dying as the last stage of growth. In Kübler-Ross E (ed): Death: The Final Stage of Growth. Englewood Cliffs, NJ, Prentice-Hall, 1975

International Health Foundation: The Mature Woman. A First Analysis of a Psychological Study of Chronological and Menstrual Aging. Geneva, International Health Foundation, 1973

International Health Foundation: La Ménopause/De Overgang-Sjaren. Etude Effectué En Belgique. Brussels, 1977

Iverson L: The chemistry of the brain. Sci Am 241:134, 1979

Jackson D: The eternal triangle: An interview with Don D. Jackson. In Haley J, Hoffman L (eds): Techniques of Family Therapy. New York, Basic Books, 1967

Jacobson E: Depression: Comparative Studies of Normal, Neurotic, and Psychotic Conditions. New York, International Universities Press, 1971

Jamison K, Wellisch D, Pasnau R: Psychosocial aspects of mastectomy. I. The women's perspective. Am J Psychiatry 35:432, 1978

Janov A: The Primal Scream. New York, Dell, 1971

Jasmin S, Trygstad L: Behavioral Concepts and the Nursing Process. St Louis, CV Mosby, 1979

Jeffers F, Verwoerdt A: How the old face death. In Busse E, Pfeiffer E (eds): Behavior and Adaptation in Late Life. Boston, Little, Brown & Co, 1969

Jenkins C: Psychosocial modifiers of response to stress. In Barrett J, Rose R, Klerman G (eds): Stress and Mental Disorder. New York, Raven Press, 1979

Jenney C, Scudder R, Baade E: Second Year Latin, 2d ed. Boston, Allyn and Bacon, 1979

Johnson J, Sarason I: Life, stress, depression, and anxiety internal-external control as a moderator variable. J Psychosom Res 22:205, 1978

Jones S: Family Therapy: A Comparison of Approaches. Bowie, MD, Robert J Brady, 1980

Jorgenson J, Brophy J: Psychiatric treatment modalities in burn patients. Curr Psychiatr Ther 15:85, 1975

Jouard S: The Transparent Self, rev ed. New York, Van Nostrand, 1971

Kahana R, Bibring G: Personality types in medical management. In Zinberg N (ed): Psychiatry and Medical Practice in a General Hospital. New York, International Universities Press, 1964

Kalisch B: What is empathy? In Sprodley B (ed): Contemporary Community Nursing. Boston, Little, Brown & Co, 1975

Kalish R: The onset of the dying process. Omega 1:57, 1970

Kalkman M, Davis A: New Dimensions in Mental Health. Psychiatric Nursing, 5th ed. New York, McGraw-Hill, 1980

Kanzer M: Object relations theory: An introduction. J Am Psychoanal Assoc 27:313, 1979

Kaplan D, Smith A, Grobstein R et al: Family mediation of stress. In Garfield C (ed): Psychosocial Care of the Dying Patient. New York, McGraw-Hill, 1978

Kaplan H, Sadock B: Modern Synopsis of Comprehensive Psychiatry/III, 3rd ed. Baltimore, Williams & Wilkins, 1981

Karmel M: Thank You Dr. LaMaze. Philadelphia, JB Lippincott, 1959

Kastenbaum R: The kingdom where nobody dies. Science 55:33, 1972

Kastenbaum R: In control. In Garfield C (ed): Psychosocial Care of the Dying Patient. New York, McGraw-Hill, 1978

Kearney T: Alcohol and general hospital patients. Am J Psychiatry 125:681, 1968

Keith C: Discussion group for posthysterectomy patients. Health Soc Work 5:59, 1980

Kellerman J, Rigler D, Siegel S: The psychological effects of isolation in protected environments. Am J Psychiatry 134:563, 1977

Kennell J: Birth of a malformed baby: Helping the family. Birth Family J 5:219, 1978

Kerr W, Thompson M: Acceptance of disability of sudden onset in paraplegia. Paraplegia 10:94, 1972

Kim M, McFarland G, McLane A: Classification of Nursing Diagnoses: Proceedings of the Fifth National Conference. St Louis, CV Mosby (in press)

Kim M, Moritz D: Classification of Nursing Diagnoses: Proceedings of the Third and Fourth National Conferences. New York, McGraw-Hill, 1982

Kimball C: Conceptual developments in psychosomatic medicine: 1939–1969. Ann Intern Med 73:307, 1970

Klaus M, Kennell J: Maternal-Infant Bonding. St Louis, CV Mosby, 1976

Klaus M, Kennell J: Parent-Infant Bonding. St Louis, CV Mosby, 1982

Kleegman S, Kaufman S: Infertility in Women. Philadelphia, FA Davis, 1966

Kornfeld D, Heller S, Frank K et al: Delirium after coronary artery bypass surgery. J Thorac Cardiovasc Surg 76:93, 1978

Kreigh H, Perko J: Psychiatric and Mental Health Nursing: A Commitment to Care and Concern. Reston, VA, Reston Pub Co, 1979

Krieger D: The Therapeutic Touch: How to Use Your Hands to Help or Heal. Englewood Cliffs, NJ, Prentice-Hall, 1979

Krieger D, Peper E, Ancoli S: Therapeutic touch: Searching for evidence of physiologic change. AJN 79:660, 1979

Kroger W: Hysterectomy: Psychosomatic factors of the pre-operative and post-operative aspects and management. In Kroger W (ed): Psychosomatic Obstetrics, Gynecology, and Endocrinology. Springfield, IL, Charles C Thomas, 1962

Krueger J, Hassell J, Goggins D et al: Relationship between nurse counseling and sexual adjustment after hysterectomy. Nurs Res 28:145, 1979

Krupp N: Adaptation to chronic illness. Postgrad Med 60:122, 1976

Kübler-Ross E: Death: The final stage of growth. Englewood Cliffs, NJ, Prentice-Hall, 1975

Kyes J, Hofling C: Basic Psychiatric Concepts in Nursing, 4th ed. Philadelphia, JB Lippincott, 1980

Labi M, Phillips R, Gresham G: Psychosocial disability in physically restored long-term stroke survivors. Arch Phys Med Rehabil 61:561, 1980

Landsman M: The patient with chronic renal failure: A marginal man. Ann Intern Med 82:268, 1975

Langsley D: The mental status examination. In Lewis J, Usdin G (eds): Psychiatry in General Medical Practice. New York, McGraw-Hill, 1979

LaViolette S: What does it take to stem turnover from the field? Mod Health Care 10:30, 1980

Lazarus R: Psychological Stress and the Coping Process. New York, McGraw-Hill, 1966

Lazarus R: Cognitive and personality factors underlying threat and coping. In Levine S, Scotch N (eds): Social Stress. Chicago, Aldine, 1970

Lazarus R: Cognitive and coping processes in emotion. In Monat A, Lazarus R (eds): Stress and Coping: An Anthology. New York, Columbia University Press, 1977

Lazarus R, Launier R: Stress-related transactions between person and environment. In Pervin L, Lewis M (eds): Perspectives in Interactional Psychology. New York, Plenum Press, 1978

LeBoyer F: Birth Without Violence. New York, Alfred A Knopf, 1975

Leigh H, Reiser M: Major trends in psychosomatic medicine: The psychiatrist's evolving role in medicine. Ann Intern Med 87:233, 1977

LeMasters E: Parenthood as crisis. In Parad H (ed): Crisis Intervention: Selected Readings. New York, Family Service Association of America, 1965

LeShan L: An emotional life history pattern associated with neoplastic disease. Ann NY Acad Sci 125:780, 1966

Levenson A: Basic Psychopharmacology. New York, Springer-Verlag, 1981

Levenson D: The Seasons of a Man's Life. New York, Ballantine Books, 1978

Levenstein S: The psychological management of the patient with chronic illness and his family. South Afr Med J 57:361, 1980

Levine J, Gordon N, Fields H: The mechanism of placebo analgesia. Lancet 2:654, 1978

Lewis A, Levy J: Psychiatric Liaison Nursing: The Theory and Clinical Practice. Reston, VA, Reston Publishing Co, 1982

Lewis M, Phillips T: The possible effects of emotional stress on cancer mediated through the immune system. In Tache J, Selye H, Say S (eds): Cancer, Stress, and Death. New York, Plenum Medical Book Co, 1979

Lidz T: The Person: His Development Throughout the Life Cycle. New York, Basic Books, 1968

Lindemann E: Symptomatology and management of acute grief. Am J Psychiatry 101:141, 1944

Lipkin G, Cohen R: Effective Approaches to Patients' Behavior, 2d ed. New York, Springer-Verlag, 1980

Lipowski Z: Review of consultation psychiatry and psychosomatic medicine. III. Theoretical issues. Psychosom Med 30:395, 1968

Lipowski Z: Consultation-liaison psychiatry: An overview. Am J Psychiatry 131:623, 1974

Lipowski Z: Organic brain syndromes: Overview and classification. In Benson D, Blumer D (eds): Psychiatric Aspects of Neurologic Disease. New York, Grune & Stratton, 1975

Lipowski Z: Delirium: Acute Brain Failure in Man. Springfield, IL, Charles C Thomas, 1979

Lipowski Z: A new look at organic brain syndrome. Am J Psychiatry 137:6, 1980

Lipton M, Jobson K: Psychopharmacology. In Usdin G, Lewis J (eds): Psychiatry in General Medical Practice. New York, McGraw-Hill, 1979

Lishman W: Organic psychiatry: The psychological consequences of cerebral disorder. Oxford, Blackwell Scientific Publications, 1978

Litwack L, Litwack J, Ballou M: Health Counseling. New York, Appleton-Century-Crofts, 1980

Locke S: Stress, adaptation, and immunity: Studies in humans. Gen Hosp Psychiatry 4:49, 1982

Loss and Grief, Part 2: The Grief Process (audiovisual slide series). Irvine, CA, Concept Media, 1977

Lustig F, Haas A, Castillo R: Clinical and rehabilitation regime in patients with COPD. Arch Phys Med Rehabil 53:315, 1972

Maas J: Clinical and biochemical heterogeneity of depressive disorders. Ann Intern Med 88:556, 1978

Mackinnon R, Michels R: The Psychiatric Interview in Clinical Practice. Philadelphia, WB Saunders, 1971

Maddi S: Personality Theories: A Comparative Analysis, 2d ed. Homewood, IL, Dorsey Press, 1972

Maddison D: The health of widows in the year following bereavement. J Pyschosom Res 12:297, 1968

Maddison D, Viola A, Walker W: Further studies in conjugal bereavement. Br J Psychiatry 113:1057, 1969

Mahler M: Symbiosis and individuation: The psychological birth of the human infant. Psychoanal Study Child 29:89, 1974

Mailick M: The impact of severe illness on the individual and family: An overview. Soc Work Health Care 5:117, 1979

Marks R, Sachar E: Undertreatment of medical inpatients with narcotic analgesics. Ann Intern Med 78:173, 1973

Marmot M, Syme S: Acculturation and coronary heart disease in Japanese Americans. Am J Epidemiol 104:224, 1976

Marriner H: The Nursing Process: A Scientific Approach to Nursing Care, 2d ed. St Louis, CV Mosby, 1978

Martin L: Overview of the psychosocial aspects of cancer. In Cohen J, Cullen J, Martin L (eds): Psychosocial Aspects of Cancer. New York, Raven Press, 1982

Martin M: Introduction: Psychiatric aspects of chronic illness. Postgrad Med 60:121, 1976

Martin M: Physical disease manifesting as psychiatric disorders. In Usdin G, Lewis J (eds): Psychiatry in General Medical Practice. New York, McGraw-Hill, 1979

Maslow A: Motivation and Personality, 2d ed. New York, Harper & Row, 1970

Mason J: A re-evaluation of the concept of non-specificity in stress theory. J Psychiatr Res 8:323, 1971

Mason J: The integrative approach in medicine—implications of neuroendocrine mechanisms. Perspect Biol Med 17:333, 1974

Masters W, Johnson V: Human Sexual Response. Boston, Little, Brown & Co, 1966

May R, Binswanger L, Ellen-Berger H: Existential psychotherapy and dasein analysis. In Sahakian W (ed): Psychotherapy and Counseling, 2d ed. Chicago, Rand McNally College Publishing Co, 1976

May W: The Metaphysical plight of the family. Hastings Cent Rep 2:19, 1974

Mayou R, Foster A, Williamson B: The psychological and social effects of myocardial infarcts on wives. Br Med J 1:699, 1978

McCaffery M: Nursing Management of the Patient With Pain, 2d ed. Philadelphia, JB Lippincott, 1979

McGeer P, Eccles J, McGeer E: Molecular Neurobiology of the Mammalian Brain. New York, Plenum Press, 1978

Medalie J, Snyder M, Groen J: Angina pectoris among 10,000 men: Five-year incidence and univariate analysis. Am J Med 55:583, 1973

Merriam-Webster Dictionary. New York, Pocket Books, 1974

Merskey H, Spear F: Pain: Psychological and Psychiatric Aspects. Baltimore, Williams & Wilkins, 1967

Meyer J: Sexual dysfunction. In Freeman A, Sack R, Berger P (eds): Psychiatry for the Primary Care Physician. Baltimore, Williams & Wilkins, 1979

Miller JB: Toward a New Psychology of Women. Boston, Beacon Press, 1976

Mims F, Swenson M: Sexuality: A Nursing Perspective. New York, McGraw-Hill, 1980

Minuchin S: Families and Family Therapy. Cambridge, Harvard University Press, 1974

Minuchin S, Montalvo B, Guerney B: Families of the Slums: An Exploration of their Structure and Treatment. New York, Basic Books, 1967

Minuchin S, Rosman B, Baker C: Psychosomatic Families, Anorexia Nervosa in Context. Cambridge, Harvard University Press, 1978

Moos R: Coping with the crisis of physical illness. In Freeman A, Sack R, Berger P (eds): Psychiatry for the Primary Care Physician. Baltimore, Williams & Wilkins, 1979

Moran S: Vaginal hysterectomy. RN 42:53, 1979

Morgan C, King R: Introduction to Psychology, 3rd ed. New York, McGraw-Hill, 1966

Morgan W, Roberts J, Brand F et al: Psychological effect of chronic physical activity. Med Sci Sports 2:213, 1970

Murray G: Confusion, delirium and dementia. In Hackett R, Cassem N (eds): Massachusetts General Hospital Handbook of General Hospital Psychiatry. St Louis, CV Mosby, 1978

Nagera H: Autoerotism, Autoerotic Activities, and Ego Development. Psychoanal Study Child 19:240, 1964

Nagy M: The child's view of death. In Feifel H (ed): The Meaning of Death. New York, McGraw-Hill, 1959

Nemiah J, Sifneos P: Affect and fantasy in patients with psychosomatic disorders. In Hill O (ed): Modern Trends in Psychosomatic Medicine. Scarborough, Ont, Butterworth & Co, 1970

Newsweek: Catecholamines: Depressive action. Newsweek Nov. 12, 1979

Norris C: Body image: Relevance to professional nursing. In Carlson C, Blackwell B (eds): Behavioral Concepts and Nursing Interventions, 2d ed. Philadelphia, JB Lippincott, 1978

Notman M: Midlife concerns of women: Implications of the menopause. Am J Psychiatry 136:1270, 1979

Nowycky M, Roth R: Presynaptic dopamine receptors. Arch Pharmacol 300:247, 1977

Nursing Shortage Linked to Hospital Environment: Hospitals 54:18, 1980

Pancheri R, Bellaterra M, Matteoli S et al: Infarct as a stress agent: Life history and personality characteristics in improved vs. not-improved patients after severe heart attacks. J Human Stress 4:16, 1978

Parad H, Caplan G: A framework for studying families in crisis. In Parad H (ed): Crisis Intervention: Selected Readings. New York, Family Service Association of America, 1965

Parkes C: Bereavement: Studies of Grief in Adult Life. New York, International Universities Press, 1972

Parkes C, Benjamin B, Fitzgerald R: Broken heart: A statistical study of increased mortality among widowers. Br Med J 1:740, 1969

Pattison E: The living-dying process. In Garfield C (ed): Psychosocial Care of the Dying Patient. New York, McGraw-Hill, 1978

Pattison E, Kaufman E: Alcohol and drug dependence. In Usdin G, Lewis J (eds): Psychiatry in General Medical Practice. New York, McGraw-Hill, 1979

Pearlin L, Schooler C: The structure of coping. J Health Soc Behav 19:2, 1978

Perley N: Problems of moral-ethical self: Guilt. In Roy C (ed): Introduction to Nursing: An Adaptation Model. Englewood Cliffs, NJ, Prentice-Hall, 1976

Physician's Desk Reference, 33rd ed: Oradell, NJ, Medical Economics Co, 1979

Piaget J, Inhelder B: Psychology of the Child. New York, Basic Books, 1969

Pierce C: Personality disorders. In Usdin G, Lewis J (eds): Psychiatry in General Medical Practice. New York, McGraw-Hill, 1979

Pincus J, Tucker G: Behavioral Neurology. New York, Oxford University Press, 1974

Powers R, Kutash I: Alcohol abuse and anxiety. In Kutash I, Schlesinger L (eds): Handbook on Stress and Anxiety. San Francisco, Jossey-Bass, 1980

A Psychiatric Glossary: The American Psychiatric Association, Washington, DC, 1975

Putt A: Introduction to general systems theory. In Putt A (ed): General Systems Theory Applied to Nursing. Boston, Little, Brown & Co, 1978

Rahe R, Lind E: Psychosocial factors and sudden cardiac death. A pilot study. J Psychosom Res 15:19, 1971

Rapaport R: Normal crises, family structure, and mental health. In Parad H (ed): Crisis Intervention: Selected Readings. New York, Family Service Association of America, 1965

Rawnsley M: Toward a conceptual base for affective nursing. Nurs Outlook 28:244, 1980

Rees W, Lutkins S: Mortality of bereavement. Br Med J 4:13, 1967

Reichel S: Severe Sustained Emotional Stress and Cancer. Unpublished paper, 1977

Reiser M: Changing theoretical concepts in psychosomatic medicine. In Arieti S (ed): American Handbook of Psychiatry, Vol 4, 2d ed. New York, Basic Books, 1974

Renneker R: Cancer and psychotherapy. In Goldberg J (ed): Psychotherapeutic Treatment of Cancer Patients. New York, The Free Press, 1981

Reres M: Editorial: coping with stress in nursing. Am Nurse 9:4, 1977

Reynolds E, Preece J, Bailey J et al: Folate deficiency in depressive illness. Br J Psychiatry 117:287, 1970

Rhodes E: Blood pressure and heart rate responses during sexual activity. Master's thesis, University of Washington, 1974

Richards F: Do you care for, or care about? AORN J 22:792, 1975

Richter C: On the phenomenon of sudden death in animals and man. Psychosom Med 19:191, 1957

Riehl J, Roy C (eds): Conceptual Models for Nursing Practice, 2d ed. New York, Appleton-Century-Crofts, 1980

Robertson D, Guttman L: The paraplegic patient in pregnancy and labour. Proc R Soc Med 56:381, 1963

Robinson L: Liaison Nursing: Psychological Approach to Patient Care. Philadelphia, FA Davis, 1974

Robinson L: Psychological Aspects of the Care of Hospitalized Patients, 3rd ed. Philadelphia, FA Davis, 1976

Roeske N: Hysterectomy and the quality of a woman's life after hysterectomy. Arch Intern Med 139:146, 1979

Rogers C: Non-directive counseling: Client-centered therapy. In Sahakian W (ed): Psychotherapy and Counseling, 2d ed. Chicago, Rand McNally College Pub Co, 1976

Rogers C: Carl Rogers on Personal Power. New York, Delacorte Press, 1977

Rogers M: The Theoretical Basis of Nursing. Philadelphia, FA Davis, 1970

Rosenbaum J: Widows and widowers and their medication use: Nursing implications. J Psychiatr Nurs 19:17, 1981

Rosenman R: Assessing the risk associated with behavior patterns. J Med Assoc Ga 60:31, 1971

Roy C: Adaptation as a model of nursing practice. In Roy C (ed): Introduction to Nursing: An Adaptation Model. Engelwood Cliffs, NJ, Prentice-Hall, 1976

Roy C: Historical perspective of the theoretical framework for the classification of nursing diagnosis. In Kim M, Moritz D (eds): Classification of Nursing Diagnoses: Proceedings of the Third and Fourth National Conferences. New York, McGraw-Hill, 1982

Rubin A, Babbott D: Impotence and diabetes mellitus. JAMA 168:498, 1958

Russell W, Schiller F: Crushing injuries to the skull. J Neurol Neurosurg 12:52, 1949

Sack R: Psychosomatic disorders. In Snyder S (ed): Biological Aspects of Mental Disorder. New York, Oxford University Press, 1980

Salk L, Hilgartner M, Granich B: The psychosocial impact of hemophilia on the patient and his family. Soc Sci Med 6:491, 1972

Sandroff R: A skeptic's guide to therapeutic touch. RN 43:25, 1980

Sarrel P: Psychosexual meanings of the climacteric. Presented at Symposium on The Menopause, Planned Parenthood League of Connecticut, 1981

Satir V, Stachowiak J, Taschman H: Helping Families to Change. New York, Jason Aronson, 1975

Schain W: Self-esteem, sexuality, and cancer management. In Goldberg J (ed): Psychotherapeutic Treatment of Cancer Patients. New York, The Free Press, 1981

Schmale A, Iker H: The psychological setting of uterine cervical cancer. Ann NY Acad Sci 125:807, 1966

Schneidman E: You and death. Psychol Today 5:43, 1971

Schoenberg B, Carr A, Kutscher A et al (eds): Anticipatory Grief. New York, Columbia University Press, 1974

Schowalter J: Pediatric nurses dream of death. In Earle A, Argondizzo N, Kutscher A (eds): The Nurse as Caregiver For the Terminal Patient and His Family. New York, Columbia University Press, 1976

Schwab J: Handbook of Psychiatric Consultation. New York, Appleton-Century-Crofts, 1968

Schwab J: Psychosomatic disturbances. In Usdin G, Lewis J (eds): Psychiatry in General Medical Practice. New York, McGraw-Hill, 1979

Selye H: The Stress of Life. New York, McGraw-Hill, 1956

Selye H: Stress Without Distress. Philadelphia, JB Lippincott, 1974

Selye H: Stress in Health and Disease. Scarborough, Ont, Butterworth & Co, 1976

Selye H: Stress without distress. In Garfield C (ed): Stress and Survival: The Emotional Realities of Life-Threatening Illness. St Louis, CV Mosby, 1979

Serban G: Psychopathology of Human Adaptation. New York, Plenum Press, 1976

Severne L: Psychosocial aspects of the menopause. In Haspels A, Musaph H (eds): Psychosomatics in Peri-Menopause. Baltimore, University Park Press, 1979

Shapiro D: Neurotic Styles. New York, Basic Books, 1965

Sheehan D: Extreme manifestations of anxiety in the general hospital: Phobic states, obsessive-compulsive neurosis, and anxiety neurosis. In Hackett T, Cassem N (eds): Massachusetts General Hospital Handbook of General Hospital Psychiatry. St Louis, CV Mosby, 1978

Sheehy G: Passages. New York, EP Dutton, 1974

Sheehy G: The happiness report. Redbook 153:29, 1978

Sheehy G: Pathfinders. New York, William Morrow, 1981

Shusterman R, Roseman L, Sechrest L: Attitudes of registered nurses toward death in a general hospital. Psychiatr Med 4:411, 1973

Siegel E: A critical examination of studies of parent-infant bonding. In Klaus M, Robertson M (eds): Birth, Interaction, and Attachment: The Proceedings of Pediatric Round Table 6. New Brunswick, NJ, Johnson & Johnson, 1982

Sifneos P: The Prevalence of alexithymic characteristics in psychosomatic patients. In Freyberger H (ed): Topics in Psychosomatic Research. Basel, S Karger, 1972

Siller J: Psychological situation of the disabled with spinal cord injuries. Rehabil Lit 30:290, 1969

Skinner B: Science and Human Behavior. New York, Macmillan, 1953

Skinner B: The Technology of Teaching. New York, Appleton-Century-Crofts, 1968

Skinner B: Beyond Freedom and Dignity. New York, Alfred A Knopf, 1971

Skynner R: The physician as family therapist. In Usdin G, Lewis J (eds): Psychiatry in General Medical Practice. New York, McGraw-Hill, 1979

Small L: The Briefer Psychotherapies. New York, Brunner/Mazel, 1979

Snyder S: Biological Aspects of Mental Disorders. New York, Oxford University Press, 1980

Soloff P: Denial and rehabilitation of the post-infarction patient. Int J Psychiatry Med 8:125, 1977

Solomon P, Patch V: Handbook of Psychiatry, 3rd ed. Los Altos, CA, Lange Medical Publications, 1974

Speeth K, Tosti D (eds): Introductory Psychology. San Rafael, CA, Individual Learning Systems, 1973

Spiegel D: Crisis points in family life. In Freeman A, Sack R, Berger P (eds): Psychiatry for the Primary Care Physician. Baltimore, Williams & Wilkins, 1979

Spinetta J: Anxiety in the dying child. Pediatrics 52:841, 1973

Spitz R: The First Year of Life. New York, International Universities Press, 1965

Stein R: Coital positions for coronary patients. Med Aspects Hum Sex 9:71, 1975

Stewart W: Nursing and counselling—a conflict of roles? Nurs Mirror 140:71, 1975

Storey P: Brain damage and personality change after subarachnoid hemorrhage. Br J Psychiatry 117:129, 1970

Strachey J: Collected Papers of Sigmund Freud. New York, Basic Books, 1959

Strub R, Black F: Organic Brain Syndromes: An Introduction to NeuroBehavioral Disorders. Philadelphia, FA Davis, 1981

Stuart G, Sundeen S: Principles and Practice of Psychiatric Nursing. St Louis, CV Mosby, 1979

Surman O: The surgical patient. In Hackett R, Cassem N (eds): Massachusetts General Hospital Handbook of General Hospital Psychiatry. St Louis, CV Mosby, 1978

Sweet E: Latin Workshop Experimental Materials. Ann Arbor, University of Michigan Press, 1964

Switzer D: The Dynamics of Grief. New York, Abingdon Press, 1970

Symington T, Currie A, Curran R et al: The reaction of the adrenal cortex in conditions of stress. In Ciba Foundations Colloquia on Endocrinology, Vol. 8. The Human Adrenal Cortex. Boston, Little, Brown & Co, 1955

Taves M, Corwin R, Haas J: Role Conception and Vocational Success and Satisfaction. Cleveland, Ohio University Press, 1963

Taymor M: Infertility. New York, Grune & Stratton, 1978

Taymor M, Bresnick E: Infertility counseling. In Taymor M (ed): Infertility. New York, Grune & Stratton, 1978

Telleen S: The church as a support to families under stress. In Lettermann H (ed): Health and Healing: Ministry of the Church. Chicago, Wheat Ridge Foundation, 1980

Thomas A, Chess S: The Dynamics of Psychological Development. New York, Brunner/Mazel, 1980

Thomas C (ed): Taber's Cyclopedic Medical Dictionary, 12th ed. Philadelphia, FA Davis, 1973

Thorn D, Von Salzen C, Fromme A: Psychologic aspects of the paraplegic patient. Med Clin North Am 30:473, 1946

Toffler A: Future Shock. New York, Bantam Books, 1970

Toman W: Family Constellation, 3rd ed. New York, Springer-Verlag, 1976

Topalis M, Aguilera D: Psychiatric Nursing, 7th ed. St Louis, CV Mosby, 1978

Treuting T: The role of emotional factors in the etiology and course of diabetes mellitus: A review of the recent literature. Am J Med Sci 244:93, 1962

Tully J: Breast cancer: Helping the mastectomy patient live life fully. Nursing '78 8:18, 1978

Udelman H, Udelman D: The family in chronic illness. Ariz Med 37:491, 1980

Ursin H: Activation, coping, and psychosomatics. In Ursin H, Baade E, Levine S (eds): Psychobiology of Stress: A Study of Coping Men. New York, Academic Press, 1978

Usdin G, Lewis J (eds): Psychiatry in General Medical Practice. New York, McGraw-Hill, 1979

Vaillant G: Adaptation to Life. Boston, Little, Brown & Co, 1977

Van Praag H: Central monoamine metabolism in depressions. II. Catecholamines and related compounds. Compr Psychiatry 21:44, 1980

Van Praag H: Central monoamine metabolism in depressions. I. Serotonin and related compounds. Compr Psychiatry 21:30, 1980

Van Vorst J, Root J: Hospital-affiliated wellness center stresses wholistic approach. Hosp Prog 61:59, 1980

Waechter E: Children's awareness of fatal illness. Am J Nurs 71:1168, 1971

Waechter E: Congenital anomalies. Nurs Forum 16:299, 1977

Watzlawick P, Coyne J: Depression following stroke: Brief problem-focused family treatment. Fam Process 19:13, 1980

Webb W, Gehi M: Electrolyte and fluid imbalance: Neuropsychiatric manifestations. Psychosomatics 22:199, 1981

Webster's New Collegiate Dictionary, 4th ed. Springfield, MA, G and C Merriam Co, 1977

Weisman A: Coping with illness. In Hackett T, Cassem N (eds): Massachusetts General Hospital, Handbook of General Hospital Psychiatry. St Louis, CV Mosby, 1978

Weisman A, Worden J: Risk-rescue rating. Arch Gen Psychiatry 26:555, 1972

Weisz A: Psychotherapeutic support of burned patients. Mod Treat 4:1291, 1967

Welch L: Planned change in nursing: The theory. Nurs Clin North Am 14:307, 1979

Welch M: Dysfunctional parenting of a profession. Nurs Outlook 28:724, 1980

Wellisch D, Jamison K, Pasnau R: Psychosocial aspects of mastectomy: II. The man's perspective. Am J Psychiatry 35:543, 1978

White R: Strategies of adaptation: An attempt at systematic description. In Coelho G, Hamburg D, Adams J (eds): Coping and Adaptation. New York, Basic Books, 1974

Wieder H, Kaplan E: Drug use in adolescents. Psychoanal Study Child 24:399, 1969

Wittkower E, Gingras G, Merglev L et al: A Combined psycho-study of spinal cord lesions. Can Med Assoc J 71:109, 1954

Woodell W: The Alcohol withdrawal syndrome. II. FCH/Alcoholism and Health 2:23, 1979

Woods J: Drug effects on human sexual behavior. In Woods N (ed): Human Sexuality in Health and Illness, 2d ed. St Louis, CV Mosby, 1979

Woods N: Human Sexuality in Health and Illness, 2d ed. St Louis, CV Mosby, 1979

Yalom I: The Theory and Practice of Psychotherapy. New York, Basic Books, 1975

Yearwood R, Yates S: Change in 28 days? Am J Nurs 79:1437, 1979

Zbilut J: Holistic nursing: The transcendental factor. Nurs Forum 19:45, 1980

Numbers followed by an *f* indicate a figure; *t* following a page number indicates tabular material.

Abstract thinking in mental status evaluation, 115, 167
Acceptance
  in bereavement process, 70
  dying patient and, 258
Acceptance support, 146
Achieving self, 63
Acting-out behavior, 38–39
Adaptation
  definition of, 7
  four modes of, 7
  physiological, 7, 8, 10
  psychosocial. *See* Psychosocial adaptation; Psychosocial maladaptation
Addiction. *See also* Alcohol abuse; Drug addiction
  dependent personality and, 50
  reinforcement techniques and, 27–28
Addison's disease, 124*t*
Advising relationship, 146
Affect, 16–17. *See also* Emotions
  definition of, 23
  in mental status evaluation, 112, 167
Aggression in mental status evaluation, 112
Aggressive drive, 15, 77
  affects and, 16
  Freud's psychosexual stages and, 28, 29
  id and, 17
  in Mahler's theory of development, 25
Aggressiveness vs. assertiveness in nurse, 286, 287*t*
Agitation in mental status evaluation, 12
Akathisia, 111
Akinesia, 111
Alarm reaction, definition of, 96
Alcohol abuse, 206–208
  conditions associated with, 206
  infantile roots of, 25
  nursing intervention in, 206–208
  and OBS, 132–133
  patient's history of, 164
  reinforcement and, 27–28
  withdrawal in, 206–207
Alexithymia, 45
Aloof personality. *See* Uninvolved personality
Altruism (defense mechanism), 45
Alzheimer's disease, 127, 218*t*
Ambivalence in mental status evaluation, 112
Amnesia, 114
Amputation, 228–229
  nursing approaches in, 229
  psychosocial issues in, 228–229
Anal stage, 28
Anger, 6, 12. *See also* Aggressive drive
  in bereavement process, 70
  after surgery, 10
Anniversary reaction, 262–263
Anomalies. *See* Congenital anomalies

Index

Anticipation (defense mechanism), 44
Anticipatory grief, 257–258
Antisocial personality, 56, 167, 184, 211
Anxiety, 6, 12, 198–201
  adaptive, 60
  in antisocial patient, 56
  in controlled patient, 51–53
  coping and, 95–106
  crisis and, 187–188
  defenses against. See Defense
    mechanisms
  definition of, 33
  in dementia, 122
  in dependent patient, 51
  in inadequate patient, 56
  infertility and, 220
  intervention and, 198–201
  medication management of, 200
  in mental status evaluation, 112
  patient's lack of control and, 68
  relaxation techniques for, 198, 199
  in suspicious patient, 53–54
  therapeutic touch for, 198–200
  too much support and, 184
  in uninvolved patient, 56
Anxiety neurosis, 41
Appearance in mental status
    evaluation, 111–112, 167
Approval support, 146
Assertiveness vs. aggressiveness in
    nurse, 286, 287t
Assessment. See Psychosocial nursing
    assessment
Attending behavior, 147–148
Autistic phase, 24
Autonomic nervous system, 8
  and mind–body bridge, 102–103
Aversive stimulus, 27
Avoidance, 39, 71, 145, 184
  in caregivers of dying patients, 277
Awareness level in mental status
    evaluation, 110, 111, 166–167

Bargaining in bereavement process, 70
Behavior in mental status evaluation,
    111–112, 167
Behavior modification, 28
  limit setting as, 212
Belle indifférence, la, 112
Belonging needs. See Love and
    belonging needs
Bereavement, 69, 202. See also Loss
  anniversary reaction to, 262–263
  Bowlby's stages of, 223, 229, 257–260
  conventional vs. anticipatory grief
    and, 257–258
  Kübler-Ross's stages of, 70, 223,
    229, 257, 258
  maladaptive response to, 263
  normal responses to, 260–262
  social attitudes toward, 260
  unresolved grief from, 69–70,
    263–264
Blocking, 113
Blunted affect, 112
Body image, 64–66, 169, 177
  amputation and, 228

burns and, 233–234
  isolation for infectious diseases or
    immunosuppressive conditions,
    235–236
  mastectomy and, 231–232
  ostomy and, 229–230
  feminine, and menopause and
    hysterectomy, 223–224
Body self, 63
Bonding, 19–21
Borderline states, 38
Boundaries in family system, 87
Bowlby, John, stages of bereavement
    of, 223, 229, 257–260
Burnout in nurses, 288–289
Burn patients, 6, 233–235
  nursing approaches to, 234–235
  psychosocial issues and, 233–234

Cancer, 241–244
  in etiology of OBS, 126–127
  nursing approaches in, 243–244
  psychosocial issues in, 241–243
  stress and, 104
Captivating personality. See
    Dramatizing personality
Cardiac disease. See also Coronary
    heart disease
  sexuality and, 246–247
  stress and, 104–105
  Type A personality in, 51–52
Castration anxiety, 29
Catastrophic reaction, 122
Catecholamine, 77, 102–103
Cerebral abscess, 131
Cerebral arteriosclerosis, 129
Cerebrovascular accident (CVA),
    127–129, 247–248
  nursing approaches in, 248
  psychosocial issues in, 247–248
Challenge, definition of, 97
Change, promotion of, 176–180,
    181t–182t
Childbirth as stressful event, 194
Chronic illness, 239–253. See also
    specific conditions
  family response to, 239, 241
  nurse's response to, 241
  patient's response to, 240–241
  stages of, 239–240
Circumstantiality, 113
Clarifying, 147, 148
Closed system, definition of, 76
Clouding of consciousness, 111
Cognitive appraisal, theory of, 96–98
Cognitive function(s). See also
    Thinking
  definition of, 23
  development of, Piaget's theory of,
    25–26
  evaluation of, for mental status,
    113–116, 167
  postoperative changes in, 137
Colostomy. See Ostomy
Coma, 110f, 111
Communicable diseases. See Isolation
    patients

Communication
  attending behavior, 147–148
  evaluation of, for mental status, 112,
    167
Compensation. See Reaction formation
Complaining personality. See
    Suspicious personality
Concrete operations, state of, 26
Concrete thinking in mental status
    evaluation, 115, 167
Conditioning, operant, 26–28
Confabulation, 114
Confusion, definition of, 111
Congenital anomalies, child with,
    221–223
  nursing approaches in, 223
  psychosocial issues and, 221–223
Conscious, 19
Consciousness
  clouding of, 111
  as ego function, 18
  level of, in mental status evaluation,
    110, 111
Constricted personality. See
    Controlled personality
"Content" in counseling, 144
Contracts, patient–nurse, 150–151
Control, 11, 13, 66–68
  personality style and, 169
  in specific conditions. See also
    Psychosocial issues, in specific
    physical conditions
Controlled/controlling personality,
    51–52, 68, 84, 112, 167–169, 184,
    190, 211, 265
Conversion, 45–46. See also
    Psychosomatic illness
Coping, 99–102. See also Defense
    mechanisms; Psychosocial
    adaptation
  anxiety and, 95–106
  cognitive–appraisal theory on, 97–99
  crisis and, 183–186
  definition of, 7
  inadequate. See also Psychosocial
    maladaptation; Stress
  and psychosomatic illness,
    102–105
  normal pattern of, as assessment
    factor, 10–12, 161, 165
  regression as, 26
  teaching of new skills for, 176
Coronary artery disease, 244–247
  nursing approaches in, 247
  psychosocial issues in, 244–247
  stress and, 105
Counseling, 139–154, 187
  appropriateness of, 140
  assessment approach in, 143–144
  attending behaviors in, 147–148
  "content" and "process" in, 144
  definition of, 147
  dynamics of relationship in, 144–146
  empathy vs. sympathy in, 140–141
  informal vs. formal, 141
  leading skills in, 148–150
  levels of relationship in, 144
  meaning of support in, 142–143

nurse-patient contracts in, 150-151
nurses's attitude toward, 142
patient's receptiveness to, 141
personal qualities needed in, 141-142
referral from, 151
referral vs., 140
Countertransference, 144-145
Creutzfeld-Jakob disease, 127, 128*t*
Crisis, 183-196
coping ability in, 184-186
factors in, 183-184
four stages of, 186
nursing process in, 187-191
assessment, 187-188
evaluation, 190
intervention, 190
limits of, 190-191
planning, 188-190
positive aspects of, 186-187
precipitating causes of, 191-196
developmental, 192, 193*t*
familial, 192
situational, 193-196
CVA. *See* Cerebrovascular accident

Death. *See also* Bereavement; Dying
patient
as critical event, 196
Decompensation, 38
Defense mechanisms, 33-47. *See also*
specific defenses
in caregivers of dying patients, 277
vs. coping, 35
development of, 35-36, 77
as ego function, 18, 271
immature, 36, 38-41
listed, 36, 262
mature, 36, 44-45
narcissistic, 36-38
neurotic, 36, 41-44
recognizing patient's use of, 34
resistance and, 145-146
stress and, 261, 282
Déjà vu, 114
Delirium, 120-121, 216*t*
definition of, 111
nursing intervention in, 217
Delusional projection, 38
Delusions, 38
types of, 113
Demanding personality. *See*
Dependent personality
Dementia, 121-122, 216*t*
nursing intervention in, 217
Denial, 37-38, 101, 145-146, 184
in alcoholic patient, 207
in bereavement process, 70, 257-258
in caregivers of dying patients, 277
in physician, 6
repression vs., 41
Dependent personality, 50-51,
167-169, 214
pain threshold in, 272
Depersonalization, 115
Depression, 6, 12, 67-68, 201-203. *See*
also Grief; Loss; Suicidal patient
adaptive, 60
in bereavement process, 70

body image changes and, 66
crisis and, 187-188
inadequate care of infant and, 24
medication for, 203
in mental status evaluation, 112
in newborn, 16
nursing intervention in, 202-203
psychotic, 37
rapprochement subphase and, 25
self-esteem and, 62
social judgment in, 116
after surgery, 10
Depressive neuroses, 41
Derealization, 115
Detoxification. *See* Withdrawal
Development, psychosocial. *See*
Personality, development of
Diagnosis(es), nursing, 155, 158,
169-172
categories of, 6, 13, 169-172,
295-323
of maladaptive coping in family,
264-265
professional language and, 6
Differentiation of self, 82-84
Differentiation subphase, 24
Disorganization stage of bereavement,
258-260
Displacement, 43, 184
"Distancing, professional," 142, 277
Distortion, 38, 145
Divorce as stressful event, 194
Documentation, psychosocial, 172
Dramatizing personality, 52-53, 168,
214
Dreamy state, definition of, 111
Drives, 15-16. *See also* Aggressive
drive; Libidinal drive
affect as sign of, 16
defenses against. *See* Defense
mechanisms
in Mahler's theory of development,
24-25
Drug addiction
hospital medication and, 214-215,
272
infantile roots of, 25
reinforcement and, 27-28
Drugs (medication)
for alcoholism, 207
for anxious patient, 200
dependency on, 214-215, 272
for depressed patient, 203
in etiology of OBS, 132-133,
134*t*-137*t*
and effects on sexual functioning,
209-210
Dying patient, 255-258
acceptance in, 258
age of, and conception of death, 256
alternatives to hospital for, 270-271
defenses in, 46
denial, 258, 268-269
family of. *See* Family, of dying patient
fears of, 256-257
nurse and. *See* Intervention,
nursing, with dying patient
religion and, 273

Dynamic(s), definition of, 76
Dyskinesia, 111
Dysphoria, 33, 112
Dystonic movement, 111

Echopraxia, 111
Ego, 17-18, 77
defenses of. *See* Defense
mechanisms
development of, 25, 30
functions of, listed, 18
in sensory disturbances, 217-218
weakening of, factors in, 177
Egocentricity
in adolescence, 29
Piaget's concept of, 26
Ego-syntonic vs. ego-dystonic
impulses, 34
Electra complex, 29, 52
Electrolyte imbalance in etiology of
OBS, 123, 125*t*-126*t*
Emotionally involved personality. *See*
Dramatizing personality
Emotional strength, 7
Emotions. *See also* Affect; *and*
specific emotions
control of, as ego function, 18
list of, 16-17
nursing vs. medical view of, 6-7, 13
patient's expression of, 12, 16
personality style and, 167
physiological adaptation and, 8-10
psychosocial assessment of, 167
Empathy vs. sympathy, 140-141
Encephalitis, 130-131
Encephalopathy. *See* Organic brain
syndrome
Endocrine system
in etiology of OBS, 123, 124*t*
and psychosomatic illness, 102-104
Enmeshment, 87
Epilepsy in etiology of OBS, 123-126
Erikson, Erik H., theory of psychosocial development of, 30-31, 60
Esteem needs, 32, 49, 63. *See also* Self-
esteem
Euphoria, 112
Evaluation in nursing process, 156,
182*t*
in crisis intervention, 190
Exaltation, 112
Exceptional children, 221-223
nursing approaches with, 223
psychosocial issues and, 221-223
Exhaustion stage, definition of, 96
Extended family, definition of, 82
Eye contact in counseling, 147

Failure to thrive syndrome, 20*f*, 21
Family
bonding and, 19-21
crises in, 192
of dying patient, 70, 255, 257-265.
See also Bereavement
anniversary reaction, 262-263
anticipatory grief, 257-258

Family, of dying patient *(continued)*
consequences of unresolved grief,
263–264
maladaptive grieving, 263
normal emotional responses,
260–262
nursing diagnosis of maladaptation
in, 264–265
social attitudes and, 260
guilt feelings of, 71
and inadequate patient, 57
promotion of change in, 179–180
responses to illness, 4, 12–13, 34,
241
right to information of, 63
separation from, 193–194
Family of origin, definition of, 82
Family relationships in psychosocial
assessment process, 163–164
Family rules, 86–87
Family secrets, 92
Family systems theory, 81–93
concepts of, 82–93
boundaries, 87
family rules, 86–87
family secrets, 92
feedback, 92–93
fusion, 87–89
homeostasis, 93
power, 91
scapegoating, 91–92
self-differentiation, 82–84
sibling position, 85–86
subsystem, 85
triangles, 89–91
terminology of, 82
Fear. *See also* Anxiety
in mental status evaluation, 112
Feedback, 92–93
Fixations, 30
Flat affect, 112
Flight of ideas, 113
Food addictions, 28
Formal thought, stage of, 26
Freud, Sigmund
developmental stages of, 28–30
structural theory of, 17–19
Fusion, 87–89. *See also* Self-
differentiation

General Adaptation Syndrome (GAS),
96
General paresis, 131
Genital stage, 29
Gestures in counseling, 147
Grief, 69. *See also* Bereavement; Loss
conventional vs. anticipatory,
257–258
maladaptive, in caregivers, 276–277
in mental status evaluation, 112
unresolved, 69–70, 263–264
Groups. *See* Support groups; Therapy
groups
Guarded personality. *See* Suspicious
personality
Guiding relationship, 146–147

Guilt
and ambivalence of grief, 258
personality style and, 55, 167, 169
as psychosocial issue, 11, 13, 70–72
in specific conditions. *See*
Psychosocial issues, in specific
physical conditions

Hallucinations, 38, 114–115
Hallucinogens, 133
Harm-loss, definition of, 97
Head-injury, OBS from, 129–130
Heavy metals, 133
Helping relationship. *See* Counseling
Hierarchy of human needs, Maslow's
theory of, 31–32, 49
Holistic approach, 8–9. *See also*
Systems theory
Holmes and Rahe Social Readjustment
Rating Scale, 99, 100*t*, 102
Homeostasis, 93
Hospices for dying patients, 271
Hospital policies
and mother–infant bonding, 19–21
and stress on nurses, 289–290
Humanistic psychology, 31
Humor (defense mechanism), 45
Huntington's chorea, 127, 128*t*
Hyperinsulinism, 124*t*
Hyperparathyroidism, 124*t*
Hypertension, stress and, 105
Hyperthyroidism, 124*t*
Hypoadrenalism, 124*t*
Hypochondriasis, 39–40
Hypomania, 111
Hypoparathyroidism, 124*t*
Hypothalamus, 8
Hypothyroidism, 124*t*
Hysterectomy, 223–227
nursing approaches and, 227
psychological consequences of,
224–225
Hysteria, 41

Id, 17, 77
defenses against. *See* Defense
mechanisms
Identification (defense mechanism), 42
with victim, 101
Identification self, 63
Illusions, 115
Immature defense mechanisms,
38–41. *See also specific defenses*
Immunosuppressive conditions. *See
also* Isolation patients
stress and, 104
Implementing phase in nursing
process, 156
Inadequate personality, 57
Infant. *See also* Personality,
development of
inadequate care of, 24
Infant, newborn, psyche of. *See*
Personality, foundations of

Infertility, 219–221
nursing approaches to, 221
psychosocial issues in, 220–221
Information
coping ability and, 184
dying patient and, 269
family's right to, 63
Instincts. *See* Drives
Intellectualization. *See* Isolation
Intelligence level of patient, 26
Interpersonal self, 63
Intervention, nursing, 181*t*. *See also*
nursing approaches *under*
specific conditions
with alcoholic patient, 206–208
with anxious patient, 198–201
in crisis. *See* Crisis, nursing
process in
with demanding or noncompliant
patients, 211–214
with depressed patient, 202–203
with dying patient, 267–278
communication issues, 273–275
control of dying process, 269–270
dealing with denial, 268–269
discussion of prognosis, 267–268
maintaining patient's choices, 270
nurse as patient advocate,
275–276
nurse's emotional involvement,
276–278
pain management, 271–273
religion, 273
withholding information, 269
with family of dying patient, 255–265
in medication dependency, 214–215
in OBS, 215–217
in sensory deprivation, 217–218
in sensory overload, 218
sexual acting out and, 210–211
and sexual functioning, 208–210
with suicidal patient, 204–205
with unmotivated patient, 206
Interviewing
in psychosocial nursing assessment,
158–159
relationship in, 146
Intimacy, 11, 13, 72–73
personality style and, 169
in specific conditions. *See* Psychosocial issues, in specific physical
conditions
"Intuition" in nurses, 4–5, 139
Isolation (rationalization; intellectualization), 42–43, 51, 145
in caregivers of dying patient, 277
as indication of personality style, 167
in relation to illness, 184
Isolation patients, 235–237
nursing approaches to, 236–237
psychosocial issues and, 235–236
Issues. *See* Psychosocial issues of
illness

Judgment
as ego function, 18

in mental status evaluation, 115–116, 167

Kübler-Ross, Elisabeth, stages of bereavement of, 70, 223, 229, 257

Lability, 112
Language, professional, 5–6
Latency stage, 29
Lazarus, Richard, theory of psychological stress of, 96–98
Le Chatelier principle, 95
Leading skills, 148–150
Liaison psychiatry, 3–4
Libidinal drive (drive for pleasure), 15–16, 77
  Freud's psychosexual stages and, 28–30
  id and, 17
  in Mahler's theory of development, 24–25
Life support systems, discontinuation of, 71
Limit setting, 56, 211–214
  and coping ability, 185–186
Locus of control, 66–67, 272
Long-suffering (self-sacrificing) personality, 54–55, 167–169
Loss, 101, 102. See also Bereavement; Depression
  of body function, 65–66
  and conversion, 45–46
  personality style and, 169
  physiological consequences of, 10
  as psychosocial issue of illness, 11, 13, 68–70
  in specific conditions. See Psychosocial issues, in specific physical conditions
Love and belonging needs, 32, 49
Lupus erythematosis, 127, 128t

Mahler, Margaret, theory of personality development of, 23–25
Maladaptation. See Psychosocial maladaptation
Mania, 110f
Manic-depressive illness, 37
Manipulative personality, 211
Marital status of patient, 163
Marriage as stressful event, 194
Maslow, Abraham, hierarchy of needs of, 31–32
Masochistic personality, 54, 71
Mastectomy, 12, 231–233
  nursing approaches to, 232–233
  psychosocial issues and, 231–232
Mature defense mechanisms, 44–45. See also specific defenses
Medication. See Drugs
Memory
  as ego function, 18
  evaluation of, for mental status, 114

impairment of, 114
  loss of, in OBS, 121t, 122
Meningitis, 131
Menopause, 223–227
  feminine body image and, 223–224
  psychosocial issues and, 225–227
Mental status examination, 107–117
  categories of, 110–116
    abstract thinking and judgment, 115–116, 167
    affect (mood), 112, 167
    appearance and behavior, 111–112, 167
    awareness and orientation, 110–111, 166–167
    memory, 114
    perception, 114–115, 167
    speech and communication, 112 167
    thinking process, 112–114, 167
  changes in status level, 108–109
  in psychosocial assessment process, 11, 162, 166–167
  suicide potential and, 116
Mind–body bridge. See Psychosomatic illness
Mobility as ego function, 18
Mood, 16. See also Affect
  in mental status evaluation, 112, 167
  postoperative changes in, 137
  swings in, 112
Mother–child interaction, 18
  in bonding theory, 19–21
  in Mahler's theory, 23–25
Motor skills, mastery of, as ego function, 18
Mourning. See Grief
Multiple infarct dementia, 129
Multiple sclerosis, 127, 128t
Myocardial infarct, stress and, 104–105

Narcissistic defense mechanisms, 37–38. See also specific defenses
Narcissistic personality, 55
Narcissistic supplies, 62
National Conferences on Nursing Diagnosis, categories of, 6, 13, 169–172, 295–323
Natural childbirth, 21
Needs, Maslow's hierarchy of, 31–32, 49
Negative reinforcement, 27–28
Neologisms, 113
Neuroendocrine system and psychosomatic illness, 102–104
Neurosis, 49
  definition of, 41
  phallic stage and, 29
Neurotic defense mechanisms, 41–44. See also specific defenses
Neurotransmitters, 77
  and mind–body bridge, 104
Neurovegetative function
  postoperative changes in, 137
  in psychosocial assessment process, 11, 161, 165–166
Newborn, psyche of. See Personality, foundations of

Noncompliant patient, 211–214
Normal-pressure hydrocephalus (NPH), 130
Nuclear family, definition of, 82
Nurses
  and bonding, 19
  as change agents, 176–177
  as counselors. See Counseling
  and detection of acute OBS, 119–120
  "intuition" of, 4–5, 139
  as monitors of psychosocial response, 4, 12–13, 60, 172
    documentation and, 172
    importance of, 108
    in stressed patient, 105–106
  as patient advocates, 7
  with dying patients, 275–276
  stress and, 281–292
    assertiveness vs. aggressiveness, 286–287
    basic rights of caregivers, 286
    burnout, 288–290
    caring for dying patient, 276–278
    changing hospital climate, 288–291
    defense mechanisms (coping style), 277, 282
    stress management, 281–282
    stress reduction, 285–286
    stress response, 283–285
    support groups, 277–278, 287–288
  use of professional language by, 5–6
  view of patient of, vs. physician's view, 6–7, 13
Nursing process, psychosocial. See also Evaluation; Intervention, nursing; Planning; Psychosocial nursing assessment
  in crisis. See Crisis, nursing process in
  four steps of, summarized, 155–156
  model for, 177–180, 181t–182t
  scope of, 175–177

Object constancy, 25, 26
Object relations, 17, 68–69
  as ego function, 18
OBS. See Organic brain syndrome
Obsessive–compulsive neurosis, 41
Obsessive thoughts, 113
Obstructive pulmonary disease, chronic, 249–250
  nursing approaches in, 249–250
  psychosocial issues in, 249
Occupation of patient, 163
Oedipus complex, 29, 52
Open system, definition of, 76
Operant conditioning, 26–28
Oral stage, 28, 30, 50
Orderly personality. See Controlled/controlling personality
Organic brain syndrome (OBS), 112, 119–138, 177, 190
  case examples of, 137–138
  causes of, 122–123

Organic brain syndrome (OBS)
    (continued)
  definition of, 119
  etiological categories of, 123–133
    arterial, 127–129
    degenerative, 127, 128*t*
    drug-related, 132–133, 134*t*–137*t*
    electrical, 123–126
    infectious, 130–132
    mechanical, 129–130
    metabolic, 123, 124*t*–126*t*
    neoplastic, 126–127
    nutritional, 132
  functional and organic, distinction
    between, 108, 120, 121*t*
  memory failure in, 114
  nursing intervention in, 215–217
  postoperative, 133–137
  social judgment in, 116
  types of, 120–122
    delirium, 111, 120–121, 216*t*, 217
    dementia, 121–122, 216*t*, 217
Organismic viewpoint, 77
Orientation in mental status
    evaluation, 110–111, 166–167
Osteoporosis, 226
Ostomy, 229–231
  nursing approaches to, 231
  psychosocial issues and, 230
  and sexual dysfunction, 208–209

Pain management with dying patient,
    271–273
Pain thresholds, 272
Paranoia, 110*f*
Paranoid personality, 53, 61
Paranoid psychosis, drug-induced,
    53, 54
Paraphrasing, 147–148
Paraplegia. *See* Spinal cord injury
Parasympathetic nervous system, 8
Parkinsonian movement, 111
Passive–aggressive behavior, 40
Penis envy, 29
Perception
  definition of, 23
  evaluation of, for mental status,
    114–115, 167
  as ego function, 18
Perception checking, 147, 148
Perseveration, 113
Personality
  definition of, 15
  development of, 23–32, 60
    crises in, 192, 193*t*
    Erikson's psychosocial stages,
      30–31, 60
    Freud's psychosexual stages,
      28–30
    Mahler's theory, 23–25, 61–62
    major issues in. *See* Psychosocial
      issues of illness
    Maslow's human needs, 31–32
    Piaget's theory, 25–26
    Skinner's operant-conditioning
      theory, 26–28
    systems theory applied to, 77

foundations of, 15–22
    affect, 16–17
    bonding, 19–21
    conscious, preconscious and
      unconscious, 19
    drive theory, 15–16
    id, ego, and superego, 17–19
    inborn characteristics, 21–22
    object relations, 17, 18, 68–69
Personality style(s), 3, 49–58, 177
  antisocial, 56, 167, 184, 211
  controlled/controlling, orderly, 68,
    84, 112, 184
    characteristics of, 51–52, 167–169
    crisis intervention and, 190
  dependent, demanding, 50–51,
    167–169, 211, 214, 272
  dramatizing, emotionally involved,
    captivating, 52–53, 168, 214
  immature defenses and, 38
  inadequate, 57
  listed, 50
  long-suffering, self-sacrificing,
    54–55, 167–169
  manipulative, 211
  masochistic, 54, 71
  narcissistic, 55
  paranoid, 53, 61
  pyschopathic, 56
  psychosexual stages and, 29, 30
  in psychosocial assessment process,
    162–163, 167–169
  psychosocial issues and, 168–169
  and response to organic change, 123
  schizoid, 56
  sociopathic, 56
  state vs. trait in, 50
  superior, 55, 167–169, 265
  suspicious, complaining, 53–54, 61,
    72, 167–169, 184, 265
  Type A, 51–52, 168, 184, 190
  uninvolved, aloof, 55–56, 72,
    167–169, 184, 265
Phallic stage, 29
Pheochromocytoma, 127
Phobias, 41
  types of, 113–114
Physical therapy, 12
Physicians
  professional language and, 4–5
  view of patient of, vs. nursing view,
    6–7, 13
Physiological needs, Maslow's concept
    of, 31, 49
Piagetian theory, 25–26
Pituitary disorders, 124*t*
Pituitary gland, 8
Placebos, 215
  antisocial patient and, 56
Planning phase in nursing process,
    155–156, 181*t*
  in crisis intervention, 188–190
Pleasure, drive for. *See* Libidinal drive
Positive reinforcement, 27–28
Posture in counseling, 147
Power, 91
Practicing subphase, 24–25
Preconscious, 19

Preoccupation of thought, 113
Preoperational thought, stage of,
    25–26
Problem-solving approach to stress,
    290–291
"Process" in counseling, 144
"Professional distancing," 142, 277
Professional language, 5–6
Projection, 40, 53, 184
  delusional, 38
Protest stage of bereavement, 258–259
Pseudo-self, 83
Psyche, definition of, 23
Psychiatric disorders. *See also*
    Neurosis; Organic brain
    syndrome; Psychosis; *and*
    specific disorders
  functional vs. organic, 37, 108, 117,
    120, 121*t*
  psychosocial maladaptation vs., 3
Psychiatric referral, 140, 151, 190–191,
    197, 202
Psychoanalytic theory
  Erikson's psychosocial stages,
    30–31
  on first two years of life, 23–25
  Freud's developmental stages,
    28–30
  on object relations, 17, 18, 68–69
  structural concepts (ego/id/
    superego) of, 17–19
  on women's intuition, 5
Psychopathic personality, 56
Psychosexual stages, Freud's theory
    of, 28–30
Psychosis, 49. *See also* Organic brain
    syndrome; Schizophrenia
  definition of, 37, 41
  functional vs. organic, 37, 108, 117,
    120, 121*t*
  paranoid, drug-induced, 53, 54
Psychosocial adaptation. *See also*
    Coping; Psychosocial mal-
    adaptation
  common themes in, listed, 99–101
  to critical events, 192–196
  definition of, 7
  major areas of conflict in. *See*
    Psychosocial issues of illness
  model for promotion of, 177–180,
    181*t*–182*t*
  patient's defenses and, 36–45
    immature mechanisms, 39
    mature mechanisms, 44–45
    narcissistic mechanisms, 37, 38
    neurotic mechanisms, 42–44
Psychosocial assessment. *See* Psycho-
    social nursing assessment
Psychosocial issues of illness, 59–73.
    See also Control; Guilt;
    Intimacy; Loss; Self-esteem;
    Trust
  in assessment process, 11, 163,
    168–169
  nurse's role and, 13
  personality style and, 168–169
  in specific physical conditions
    amputation, 228–229

burns, 233–234
cancer, 241–243
cerebrovascular accident
    (stroke), 247–248
chronic obstructive pulmonary
    disease, 249
coronary artery disease, 244–247
exceptional child/congenital
    anomalies, 221–223
hysterectomy/menopause,
    225–227
infertility, 220–221
isolation patients, 235–236
mastectomy, 231–232
ostomy, 230
spinal cord injury, 250–252
Psychosocial maladaptation, 59–60.
    See also Psychosocial issues
    of illness; Psychosocial nursing
    assessment
coping failures and, 101
definition of, 7
diagnosis of, 169–172. See also
    Diagnosis, nursing
in family of dying patient, 263–265
major types of, 197–217
    alcoholic patient, 206–208
    anxious patient, 198–201
    demanding or noncompliant
        patient, 211–214
    depressed patient, 201–203
    OBS patient, 215–217
    sensory disturbances, 217–219
    medication-dependent patient,
        214–215
    sexual dysfunction, 208–211
    suicidal patient, 203–205
    unmotivated patient, 205–206
nursing intervention vs. psychiatric
    referral in, 140
patient's defenses and, 34, 37–44
    immature mechanisms, 38–41
    narcissistic mechanisms, 37–38
    neurotic mechanisms, 42–44
professional language and, 5–6
psychiatric illness vs., 3
as response to crisis. See Crisis
Psychosocial nursing assessment,
    157–173, 181t
in crisis intervention, 187–188
definition of, 109, 155, 157
documentation of, 173
factors in. See also specific factors
    as basis of nursing process, 12–13
    listed, 10–11
importance of, 158
interview in, 158–159
process of, 159–172
    diagnosis, 169–172
    major issues of illness, 163,
        168–169
    mental status, 162, 166–167. See
        also Mental status examination
    neurovegetative functioning, 161,
        165–166
    normal coping ability, 161, 165
    patient's understanding of illness,
        161–162, 166

personality style, 162–163, 167–168
preadmission stress, 10, 11,
    160–161, 164–165, 191–196
rating scale, 160–163
social history, 159–164
structured vs. "free" approach to,
    143–144, 187
for suicide risk, 203–205
Psychosocial nursing process. See
    Nursing process, psychosocial
Psychosocial stages, Erikson's theory
    of, 30–31, 60
Psychosomatic illness, 46, 102–105
Psychotherapy, counseling vs., 147
Psychotic depression. 37

Quadriplegia. See Spinal cord injury
Querulous personality. See Suspicious
    personality

Rapprochement subphase, 25
Rationalization. See Isolation
Reaction formation, 43–44, 51
Reality, sense of, as ego function, 18
Referral. See Psychiatric referral
Reflection of content, 148
Regression, 40–41, 57, 84
    definition of, 26
Reinforcement, 27–28
Relaxation techniques for anxious
    patient, 198, 199
Religion of patient, 159–163
    and dying patient, 273
Reorganization stage of bereavement,
    258, 260
Repression, 29
    in caregivers of dying patients, 277
    as defense mechanism, 41–42, 84, 145
Resistance in counseling relationship,
    145–146
Resistance stage, definition of, 96
Respiratory disease, chronic, 28
Restraints, mechanical, 216–217

Safety needs, 31, 49
Scapegoating, 91–92
Schizoid personality, 56
Schizophrenia, 24, 37, 112
    concrete thinking in, 115
    social judgment in, 116
SCI. See Spinal cord injury
Secondary gain, 39
Sedation of anxious patient, 200
Seizures in etiology of OBS, 123–126
Self, definition of, 83
Self-actualization, need for, 32
Self-differentiation, 82–84
Self-esteem, 11, 13, 25, 61–66. See
    also Esteem needs
    body image and, 64–66
    four components of, 63
    in Maslow's hierarchy of needs, 32,
        49, 63
    narcissistic supplies and, 62
    personality style and, 168–169

in specific conditions. See Psycho-
    social issues, in specific physical
    conditions
Self-sacrificing (long-suffering)
    personality, 54–55, 167–169
Selye, Hans, theory of stress of, 96
Sensorimotor stage, 25
Sensory deprivation, 217–218
Sensory overload, 218
Separation–individuation phase, 24, 30
Sexuality, 72, 208–211
    of acting-out patient, 210–211
    amputation and, 229
    cancer and, 243
    cardiac patients and, 246–247
    drugs and, 209–210
    infantile, 28–30
    ostomy and, 229
    physical illness and, 208–209
    spinal cord injury and, 251, 252
    stroke patients and, 248
Sibling position, 85–86
Skinner, B. F., behavioral theories of,
    26–28
Sleep. See Neurovegetative functioning
Smoking, patient's history of, 164
Social history
    as assessment factor, 10, 11
    in psychosocial assessment process,
        159–164
Social judgment in mental status
    evaluation, 115–116, 167
Social Readjustment Rating Scale, 99,
    100t, 102
Sociopathic personality, 56
Solid self, 83
Somatization. See Conversion
Spinal cord injury (SCI), 250–252
    nursing approaches in, 252
    psychosocial issues in, 250–252
Splitting of hospital staff, 56
Stress, 3–4, 12, 95–106, 177. See also
    Crisis
    balancing factors and, 185f
    chronic illness and, 239–241
    comprehensive model for evaluation
        of, 105, 106t
    and coronary heart disease, 105
    defenses against. See Defense
        mechanisms
    definition of, 95
    emotional strength and, 7
    and inadequate patient, 57
    individual variation in response to,
        101–102
    Lazarus's cognitive-appraisal theory
        of, 96–98
    in model of psychosocial nursing
        process, 178, 179
    on nurses. See Nurses, stress and
    openness of system and, 77
    physiological responses to, 8
        in cognitive appraisal theory, 98
        Selye's theory of, 96
    preadmission, 10, 11, 160–161,
        164–165, 191–196
    psychosocial issues and, 11
    psychosocial mediation of, 99–102

Stress *(continued)*
and psychosomatic disorders, 46, 102–105
Social Readjustment Rating Scale for, 99, 100*t*, 102
systems approach to, 95–96, 102–106
Stressor, definition of, 95
Stroke. *See* Cerebrovascular accident
Structural theory, psychoanalytic, 17–19
Stupor, definition of, 111
Subdural hematoma, 130
Sublimation, 44
Subsystem, definition of, 76–77, 85
Suicidal patient, 203–205
Suicide potential, 116
Sun-downing, 121
Superego, 17–19, 30, 33, 77
of antisocial patient, 56
and level of guilt, 70–71
Superior personality style, 55, 167–169, 265
Support
coping ability and, 184
in counseling relationship, 142–143, 146
Support groups, 151–153
for infertile couples, 221
for nurses, 287–288
with dying patients, 277–278
Suppression (defense mechanism), 45, 145
Surgery, 10. *See also* Amputation; Hysterectomy; Ostomy; Mastectomy
as cause of OBS, 133–137
and sexual function, 208–209, 229

Suspicious personality, 53–54, 61, 72, 167–169
Symbolic phase, 24
Symbolic thought, 26
Sympathetic nervous system, 8
Sympathy vs. empathy, 140–141
Synapses, 104
Synergism, 133
Syphilis, 131–132
Systems theory, 8, 75–80
applied to family. *See* Family systems theory
applied to nursing practice, 78–80
history of, 77
and personality development, 77–78
and stress, 95–96, 102–105
"system" defined, 75–76
types of systems, 76

Tabes dorsalis, 131
Tangentiality, 113
Teaching relationship, 147
Terminal illness. *See* Dying patient
Termination of nurse–patient relationship, 151
Theapeutic touch treatment, 198–200
Therapy groups, 152
Thinking. *See also* Cognitive function(s)
as ego function, 18
evaluation of, for mental status, 113–116, 167
Threat, definition of, 97
Thyroid disease, 8
Toxic brain syndrome, 120, 121
Tranquilizers, 200
Transference, 144

"Tree" approach to assessment, 143–144, 187
Triangling, 89–91
Trust, 11, 13, 60–61, 150
in crisis intervention, 190
personality style and, 168
in specific conditions. *See* Psychosocial issues, in specific physical conditions
Tumors
benign, and OBS, 126
malignant. *See* Cancer
Type A personality, 51–52, 168, 184, 190

Unconscious, 19
Understanding of illness, patient's, 11, 161–162, 166
Undifferentiated ego mass, 82–83
Uninvolved (aloof) personality, 55–56, 72, 167–169, 184, 265
Unitary man, concept of, 8–9. *See also* Systems theory
Unmotivated patient, 205–206

Verbal attending behavior, 147–148
Vitamin deficiencies in OBS etiology, 132

Waxy flexibility, 111
Withdrawal, 54
alcoholic, 206–207
Word salad, 113